Abdominal Ultrasonography

Abdominal Ultrasonography
Second Edition

Edited by

Barry B. Goldberg, M.D.
Professor of Radiology
Director, Division of Ultrasound
  and Radiologic Imaging
Thomas Jefferson University Hospital
Philadelphia, Pennsylvania

A WILEY MEDICAL PUBLICATION
JOHN WILEY & SONS
New York · Chichester · Brisbane · Toronto · Singapore

The first edition of this book was published under
the title *Abdominal Gray Scale Ultrasonography.*

Library of Congress Cataloging in Publication Data

Main entry under title:

Abdominal ultrasonography.

  (A Wiley medical publication)
  Rev. ed. of: Abdominal ultrasonography.
  Includes bibliographical references and index.
  1. Abdomen—Radiography. 2. Diagnosis, Ultrasonic.
I. Goldberg, Barry B. II. Abdominal ultra-
sonography. III. Series. [DNLM: 1. Abdomen. 2. Ultra-
sonics—Diagnostics use. WI 900 A1339]
RC944.A194 1984   617'.5507'543   84-2257
ISBN 0-471-08569-3

Printed in the United States of America

10 9 8 7 6 5 4 3 2 1

To my wife, Phyllis, and our children, Marla and Mitchell. Their support and understanding have made this book possible.

Contributors

Peter L. Cooperberg, M.D., F.R.C.P.C.
Professor of Radiology
Director of Ultrasound
Vancouver General Hospital
Vancouver, British Columbia

Paul A. Dubbins, F.R.C.R.
Consultant-in-Charge
Department of Diagnostic Ultrasound
Plymouth General Hospital
Plymouth, England

Barry B. Goldberg, M.D.
Professor of Radiology
Director, Division of Ultrasound and Radiologic Imaging
Thomas Jefferson University Hospital
Philadelphia, Pennsylvania

Alfred B. Kurtz, M.D.
Professor of Radiology
Associate Director, Division of Ultrasound and Radiologic Imaging
Thomas Jefferson University Hospital
Philadelphia, Pennsylvania

George R. Leopold, M.D.
Professor of Radiology
Chief, Division of Diagnostic Ultrasound
University of California
San Diego, California

E. A. Lyons, M.D., F.R.C.P.C.
Director, Section of Ultrasound
Health Sciences Center
Winnipeg, Manitoba

Gordon S. Perlmutter, M.D.
Clinical Associate Professor of Radiology
Thomas Jefferson University Hospital
Philadelphia, Pennsylvania
Director of Diagnostic Ultrasound
The Reading Hospital and Medical Center
West Reading, Pennsylvania

M. Nathan Pinkney, B.S.
Physics Consultant
Thomas Jefferson University
Philadelphia, Pennsylvania

Howard M. Pollack, M.D.
Professor of Radiology
University of Pennsylvania Hospital and School of Medicine
Philadelphia, Pennsylvania

Matthew D. Rifkin, M.D.
Associate Professor of Radiology
Thomas Jefferson University Hospital
Philadelphia, Pennsylvania

Kenneth J. W. Taylor, M.D., Ph.D., F.A.C.P.
Professor of Diagnostic Radiology
Head, Ultrasound
Yale University School of Medicine
New Haven, Connecticut

Preface

In the seven years between the first and second editions of *Abdominal Ultrasonography*, ultrasound has continued to make rapid diagnostic and technological advances. As a diagnostic imaging modality, ultrasound's clinical usefulness has been proven in areas not even considered in the late 1970s. Pulsed Doppler duplex systems make it possible to sample blood flow and to identify and differentiate various structures within the body that might be vascular in origin. Flow direction and quantity of flow are also being investigated. Ultrasound tissue signature characterization (differentiating normal from abnormal tissue) is closer to becoming a reality. Now there is greater emphasis on the use of real-time gray scale ultrasound equipment. We are more aware of the need to select transducers properly in terms of their frequency and depth of focus. Endoscanning techniques (transesophageal, transrectal, and transurethral) make it possible to image structures within the body that are difficult or impossible to evaluate with a transducer applied to the skin's surface.

The new technology and increased clinical applications developed for ultrasound require the practitioner to keep abreast of these developments. The text of this second edition is based on the most recent advances in the field and is illustrated with new ultrasound images. These images are presented in a standardized format. Longitudinal images are shown as if one is looking at the patient from the right. Cephalad is to one's left. The letter H indicates the direction of the head; R and L indicate the right and left sides, respectively. When ultrasound images of the retroperitoneum and renal areas are obtained in the prone position, the left side of the patient will then be on the left side of the illustration. Coronal views are obtained by positioning the patient in the decubitus position and are labeled accordingly.

The result of our efforts is a comprehensive discussion of two-dimensional ultrasound imaging of the abdomen and pelvis. Radiologists specializing in ultrasound, physicians in other specialties, interns, residents, sonographers, and student technologists should find this to be a useful text. It will help the user to determine the appropriate ultrasound study to be performed and how to evaluate the information provided. As ultrasound becomes the primary imaging modality in more and more clinical examinations, this book should prove to be an important reference in planning diagnostic patient care.

Barry B. Goldberg

Acknowledgments

The authors wish to recognize the efforts of the following individuals whose help has made this book possible: Rosemarie Boccella and Teresa Dolan, as well as JoAnn Anderson and Joan Logan, for assistance in typing the manuscript; Thomas Aquilone, Steven Mervis, and Fred Ross for preparing the illustrations; and Steven Mervis and Robert Waxham for their editorial assistance.

Barry B. Goldberg

Contents

Abdominal Ultrasonography

1

Instrumentation

Gordon S. Perlmutter
M. Nathan Pinkney

INTRODUCTION

This chapter presents current concepts in ultrasound instrumentation. The discussion assumes the reader is conversant with the basic physical principles of ultrasound. These fundamentals have been covered in several excellent articles to which the reader is referred.[1-6]

All modern ultrasound instrumentation employs gray scale signal processing to display gradations of sound intensity. The signal response capacity or dynamic range of gray scale instrumentation is measured in decibels. A decibel is defined as $10 \times \log_{10}$ of the intensity of the ratio between two signals. Thus, the intensity difference between a given signal and another signal that is twice as intense is 3 decibels. A 10-decibel difference in signal strength signifies a 10-fold difference in intensity. The maximum intensity difference between ultrasound signals is given theoretically as approximately 100 decibels, that is a condition in which the strongest signal is approximately 10 billion times more intense than the weakest signal. From a practical standpoint, however, it is impossible to obtain an ultrasound imaging system capable of displaying more than 50 to 60 decibels in dynamic range.

An ultrasound imaging system can be thought of as a chain of components with the chain being only as strong as its weakest link. This analogy holds true for the dynamic range of an ultrasound scanning system as well, with the weakest link being the display components. The approximate dynamic range of the standard methods used to display ultrasound signals is as follows:

Scan converter	30 decibels
Cathode ray tube (CRT)	20 decibels
Television monitor	20–30 decibels
Bistable storage oscilloscope	0–5 decibels

Thus, it can be seen that the limiting factor in reproducing the sound intensity spectrum with older non-gray scale instruments was the restricted dynamic range of the bistable oscilloscope. For this reason, bistable technology has been abandoned except as an imaging option in gray scale units (Fig. 1-1).

Gray scale ultrasound equipment can be defined as an imaging system: (*1*) capable of producing images with a greater dynamic range than older bistable

1

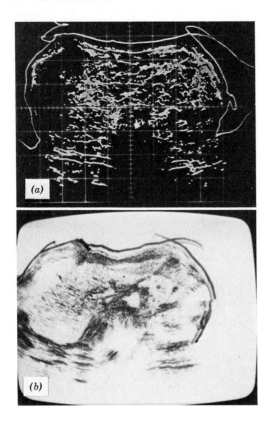

Figure 1-1 Examples of bistable (*a*) and gray scale (*b*) images demonstrating the relatively restricted dynamic range and resolution of the bistable display.

units, (*2*) having a dynamic range of 20 to 30 decibels, and (*3*) capable of yielding ultrasound images in several shades of gray.

NONSTORAGE GRAY SCALE IMAGING

Nonstorage gray scale imaging uses the broad dynamic range of the cathode ray tube (CRT). As noted previously, the CRT has an estimated dynamic range of 20 decibels. Stated differently, any one point on the surface of the CRT can be illuminated to any of approximately 10 degrees of brightness, or shades of gray, recognizable and distinguishable by the human eye. Although the dynamic range of the CRT display represents approximately a fivefold increase over the bistable oscilloscopes formerly used, it is still unable to display the full intensity range of echoes contained in a 60-decibel ultrasound signal. It is therefore necessary to compress or funnel the 60-decibel intensity spectrum of the ultrasound signal into a more restricted 20-decibel format. A simple method would be to divide the 60-decibel signal into three 20-decibel segments, displaying one-third of the potential signal range at any given time. This, of course, requires the simultaneous rejection of two-thirds of the information content of the signal, which is considered unacceptable. Another and more practical approach is to compress the 60-decibel signal spectrum electronically into a 20-decibel format using a device such as a logarithmic amplifier, or its equivalent, which amplifies signals as a function of intensity; the weaker signals being more highly amplified than the stronger signals. This is done in such a way that the ratio between the weakest and the strongest signal is brought within 20-decibels, thereby matching the dynamic range of the CRT display scope. Logarithmic amplification is used not only in nonstorage gray scale displays but also with analog and digital storage units to be discussed in the next section.

The CRT display is a real-time, nonstorage display such that, at any moment in time, a line of dots of varying brightness is displayed in the same spatial orientation as the transducer. There is no means of storing these signals once the transducer is moved. A time-exposure photograph, often referred to as the open-shutter technique, is the means most commonly employed for storing and integrating these instantaneous one-line displays to form a two-dimensional image. Since the brightness of any line or point on the photographic film is a function not only of the brightness of the dots on the CRT but also of the amount of time each dot is illuminated, it becomes necessary to employ a complex scanning method that ensures illumination of all points on the CRT for approximately the same period. This can be accomplished, although with considerable difficulty, with a rectilinear scanner by sweeping the transducer in a sectoring motion across the patient using a fixed velocity of sectoring motion and a fixed sectoring interval (Fig. 1-2). It is possible to produce excellent gray scale images with this technique; however, it is extremely difficult to fulfill these scanning requirements using a manually operated scanning arm. The problem has been solved in two ways: (1) by using scan converters for image integration and storage, and (2) by replacing manually operated scanning arms with automated scanning devices.

STORAGE GRAY SCALE IMAGING

At the heart of gray scale imaging is the scan converter. Similar in function to the photographic film used in nonstorage gray scale imaging, the scan converter acts as an image storage device for building up a two-dimensional scan. However, it has the added advantage of allowing real-time observation of the evolving two dimensional image and also permits a simple, convenient scanning technique not possible with the nonstorage photographic method. Nonstorage technology, therefore, has been largely replaced by scan conversion systems except in the lower cost automated units. Virtually all manual rectilinear scanners today have scan converter systems, which are available in two formats - analog and digital.

Analog Scan Converter

The analog scan converter functions by writing the scan image onto the surface of a scan converter tube which is accomplished by directing a stream of electrons across the tube from an electron gun at the back of the tube (Fig. 1-3). The imaging surface of the scan converter tube is composed of a matrix of approximately 1,000 × 1,000 elements, often composed of silicone dioxide, which are able to store electrical charges that vary in degree from element to

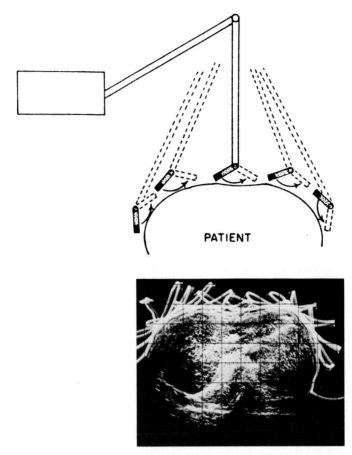

Figure 1-2 This is a schematic diagram of the sector scanning method using a rectilinear scanner with an open-shutter technique. An example of a typical scan is shown.

element. By operating the scan converter tube in such a way that any particular element does not accumulate electron charges additively but rather accepts only the most intense signal, it is possible to overwrite areas of the scan without creating serious image degradation. This mode of operation is called the *peak detection mode*. Since the surface of the tube is not composed of phosphors, it is not possible to see an illuminated image on the surface of the scan converter tube. To display the image, it is necessary to change the mode of operation of the tube from the "write" mode to the "read" mode. In the "read" mode, a stream of electrons is again directed toward the charged silicone-dioxide image surface, but at a different voltage than in the "write" mode. The beam of electrons is either attracted or repelled by the imaging surface depending on the charge accumulated by the silicone-dioxide elements. Repelled electrons are then captured by the collecting grid. The sweep of the electron beam in the "read" mode is synchronized with the raster of the standard 525-line commercial television monitor. It is thus possible to convert the data stored as a latent electronic image on the surface of a scan converter tube to a visible

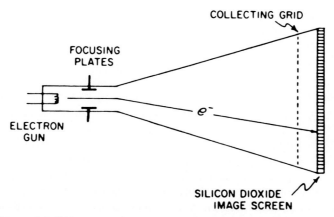

Figure 1-3 Diagrammatic representation of a scan converter tube.

image on a TV monitor. In practice, the analog converter tube is alternately switched between the "write" and "read" modes during image acquisition permitting real-time viewing of the scan process, but with a slight flicker. The typical analog scan converter tube can store images in 10 to 15 shades of gray.

Digital Scan Converter

Unlike the analog scan converters, digital scan converters store echo amplitude and position information in an electronic memory.[7-8] Because a vacuum tube storage target is not being used to record the received information, focus and gray scale drifting due to thermal aging and line voltage regulation problems, which are characteristics of analog scan converters, are virtually eliminated. The speed with which the digital circuitry can receive, store, and convert echo information permits flicker-free operation, a desirable feature usually not possible with analog systems.

The digital scan converter consists of an analog to digital (A to D) converter, a digital memory, a digital to analog (D to A) converter, and a microprocessor (Fig. 1-4). The purpose of the A to D converter is to accept the analog voltages that represent the varying amplitudes and positions of the received echoes, assign digital values to these variations, and write this information into the digital memory. Because the TV monitor operates as an analog display, the D to A converter reads the digital data that is recorded in the digital memory

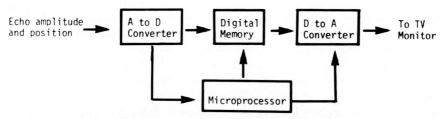

Figure 1-4 Block diagram of a digital scan converter.

and feeds this information in analog form to the TV monitor. The microprocessor controls the operation of the various components of the digital scan
converter. The microprocessor receives instructions from the operator of the
system. The digital scan converter not only stores the image, but can also
perform various operations on the image that might include preprocessing,
postprocessing, read and/or write magnification, alphanumeric character generation, video image polarity reversal, and other types of advanced signal
processing.

The typical digital memory consists of a matrix made up of a large number
of picture elements called pixels. A typical matrix might contain 512 pixels
horizontally by 512 pixels vertically. Each of the total of 262,144 pixels represents
a finite point within a scan plane. Each of these points contains anywhere from
four to eight bits of information. A four-bit system is capable of storing and
displaying up to 16 discrete gray scale levels. The number of gray scale levels
is determined by raising the number 2 to the power equal to the number of
bits. For example, $2^4 = 16$, $2^5 = 32$, and $2^6 = 64$.

Some systems are capable of magnifying an image that is already displayed
on the TV monitor. The scan converter performs this "read" magnification by
enlarging each of the displayed pixels, thus causing those pixels that are not
within the magnified region to be moved out of the display. The major
advantage of "read" magnification is the ability to obtain an enlarged image
that does not require an additional scan of the patient. Because "read"
magnification enlarges each pixel, the image may appear to have a coarse
texture. "Write" magnification, on the other hand, makes it possible to enlarge
the analog image before it is placed into digital memory. Some form of "write"
magnification is present in all commercial B scan systems either by choice of
scale factor or by magnification of a predetermined area of interest. In each
instance, an enlarged image can be obtained while still maintaining the total
number of normal-sized pixels on the display.

When the digital scan converter receives signals representing various echo
amplitudes, memory locations are assigned corresponding to discrete shades of
gray. The assignment of a range of gray scales to a given range of echo
amplitudes is a function of the preprocessing capability of the digital system.
Some systems offer the operator a choice of gray scale assignments for a given
range of echo amplitudes. Regardless of the operator's choice, the stronger
echoes are assigned to the higher gray scale levels and the weaker echoes are
assigned to the lower gray scale levels. Selectable preprocessing permits the
operator to alter the texture of the image by determining the gray scale
assignment before the scan is performed.

Once the gray scale assignment has been made and the information stored
in memory, it may be possible to alter the amount of emphasis that might be
given to a selected range of the gray scale. This emphasis is a function of the
postprocessing capability of the digital system. Selectable postprocessing permits
the operator to vary the amount of change in the intensity levels that would
normally be present between successive gray scale levels as displayed on the
TV monitor.

It is apparent that the digital scan converter is a definite improvement over
its analog predecessor in terms of reliability as well as in the ability to perform

manipulations of data obtained during the examination. Digital scan converters have completely replaced analog units on all storage gray scale ultrasound systems currently being manufactured.

Digital Freeze Frame

Digital freeze frame is a low-cost variation of the digital scan converter. It is similar to the digital scan converter in that it stores an ultrasound image in digital format. However, several features of the more expensive digital scan converter may be omitted, including selectable pre- and postprocessing, TV output, and magnification. The number of image matrix and memory bits is reduced in these units, resulting in images with larger pixels and fewer shades of gray. Digital freeze frame units are most commonly used as a stop-action image storage device in low-cost automated scanners.

GRAY SCALE INSTRUMENTATION

Several types of gray scale ultrasound machines are available. The various approaches different manufacturers have employed in developing gray scale imaging are described generically here, with no attempt made to judge the various claims and counterclaims made by the manufacturers regarding the performance characteristics of the machines.

Ultrasound instruments can be classified by several schemes: static versus real-time, contact versus water path, manual versus automated, portable versus fixed installation, mechanical versus electronic, etc. In this chapter, equipment is divided in the two major categories of static and real time with the other categories used as subgroupings.

The visual fusion rate of the human eye is 16 frames per second. Any instrument designed to present 16 or more images per second is therefore properly defined as real-time equipment. Instruments with slower frame rates are categorized as static scanners.

STATIC SCANNERS

The most prevalent static scanner is the standard rectilinear contact scanner. This instrument uses a 3-section mechanical arm with position sensors of various types that sense the direction of the sound beam by monitoring the angular orientation of the articulations of the arm (Fig. 1-5). This type of instrumentation is somewhat cumbersome to operate because of the mechanical restraints imposed by the arm. The quality of the scans obtained is highly dependent on the skill of the technologist operating it, which is considered to be an undesirable feature, particularly in regions where fully trained sonographers are scarce. Scans can be obtained in either the compound or sector mode or by using a combination of both techniques. Virtually all makes of this type of scanner come equipped with scan converters that integrate and store the image in the "store" mode or permit a nonintegrated image similar to a single frame of a real-time study in the "survey" mode.

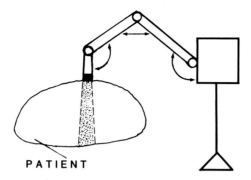

Figure 1-5 Rectilinear scanner.

STATIC AUTOMATED SCANNERS

Several approaches have been employed to automate the motion of the scanning arm in order to lessen operator dependency. One such unit, developed by George Kossoff and associates[9-11] at The Ultrasound Institute in Australia, uses eight transducers in a large water bath that are electromechanically swept in sector motion across an area of interest (Fig. 1-6). Sector scans can be obtained by activating only one transducer; compound scans are obtained when more than one transducer is activated. While earlier models of this unit used nonstorage photographic integration of the image, the newer models are equipped with a digital scan converter. Multiple angles and scan planes can be achieved by rotating and tilting the gantry to which the transducers are attached, but this must be done remotely from the scanner console since the transducers are submerged in the water bath. This can cause some consternation in terms of transducer orientation for the neophyte technologist accustomed to operating a static contact scanner, but this problem is quickly overcome with experience on the unit. The large water bath affords optimal focusing characteristics for the transducers, but the long pathway that the sound must travel limits the display rate to 1 to 2 frames per second.

REAL-TIME SCANNERS

Real-time scanners are units capable of generating images at a rapidity greater than the human visual fusion rate of 16 frames per second.[12] Some units mentioned fall slightly short of this mark but are also included in this section

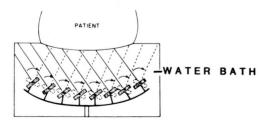

Figure 1-6 Automated scanner.

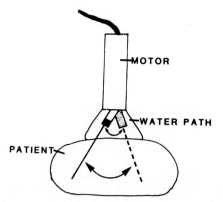

Figure 1-7 Oscillating sector scanner.

for simplicity. Real-time scanners can be divided into two major subcategories: mechanical and electronic scanners.

Mechanical Real-Time Scanners

Several varieties of mechanical scanners are available. Since there is mechanical motion of the transducer, almost all available mechanical units use a water-path standoff between the transducer and the patient. The less expensive units use direct photographic recording—"on the fly"—of the cathode ray tube, whereas the more expensive units incorporate digital freeze frame or scan converter units.

One of the least complex examples of this type of real-time unit is the mechanical sector unit developed by Bronson[13] and Turner (Fig. 1-7). This type of unit is available for ophthalmologic, cardiac, small parts, and general abdominal applications. It can be obtained as a stand alone unit or integrated into a static rectilinear scanning unit to provide added real-time capability. A variation of this is used by one manufacturer of breast scanners wherein a single transducer is incorporated into a water bath (Fig. 1-8).

Another approach to mechanical scanning was developed by Dr. Holm and his group at the Gentofte Hospital in Copenhagen, Denmark.[14] Current commercially available units have incorporated some modifications, but such units basically consist of multiple, usually three, transducers imbedded in a wheel that rotates within a water-filled housing (Fig. 1-9). In the Holm prototype unit, the wheel contained four transducers and was used in direct contact with

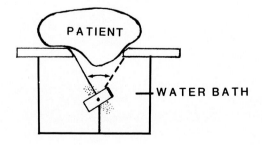

Figure 1-8 Automated breast scanner.

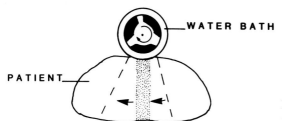

Figure 1-9 Multiple transducer rotating sector scanner.

the patient. By rotating a wheel with three transducers at greater than 5 cycles per second and consecutively firing the transducers as they become directed toward the patient, it is possible to develop frame repetition rates in excess of 15 frames per second for real-time viewing. In fact, very high frame rates in excess of 45 frames per second are achievable, making this type of unit ideal for cardiac as well as other applications. This technology has also been incorporated into a water bath breast scanner (Fig. 1-10).

A variation that affords a more rectangular field of view uses an acoustical mirror within a water housing. In this unit, multiple transducers rotate with the sound beam reflected from a parabolic mirror focusing system that converts the rotatory motion of the transducer to a linear sweeping motion within the patient (Fig. 1-11). Other units use a fixed transducer or transducers with an oscillating mirror system to accomplish the same purpose (Fig. 1-12). Alternatively, some units employ a fixed mirror or prism and an oscillating transducer (Fig. 1-13). Units of this design are available for abdominal imaging, but specialized units using this same concept have also been designed specifically for carotid artery imaging.

Another approach is to attach the transducer to a worm gear contained within a water housing. At this time, one manufacturer is using this technology in a small parts scanner (Fig. 1-14).

Electronic Real-Time Scanners

Electronic real-time scanners make use of a linear array of transducers that are electronically sequentially pulsed, in essence duplicating the effect of mechanically moving a single transducer across an area of interest. One of the first units of this type was developed by Dr. Bom of Holland[15] for use in cardiac evaluation. This unit consisted of a linear array of 20 transducers sequentially

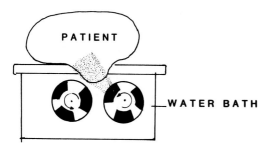

Figure 1-10 Automated breast scanner.

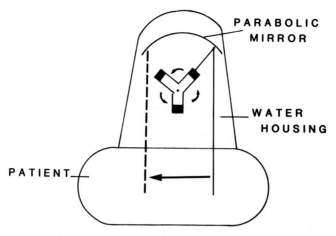

Figure 1-11 Multiple transducer rotational scanner with parabolic mirror.

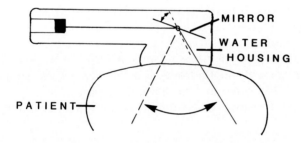

Figure 1-12 Sector scanner with oscillating mirror.

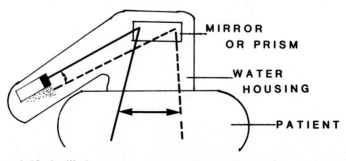

Figure 1-13 Oscillating sector scanner with stationary mirror or prism.

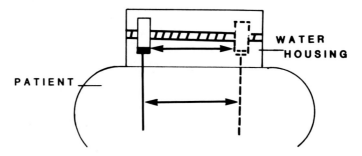

Figure 1-14 Translational small parts scanner.

pulsed to produce a frame repetition rate of 150 frames per second (Fig. 1-15). Images were rather coarse due to the fact that they consisted of only 20 lines of information corresponding to the 20 transducers in the array. Currently available units use a linear array of 64 or more elements in order to improve image resolution (Fig. 1-16). Since the transducer diameters are small, the sound beam tends to diverge unacceptably from the transducer surface. In order to improve beam geometry, transducers are commonly fired sequentially in groups of four or more, referred to as *multiplexed triggering* (Fig. 1-16). Further improvements in beam geometry have been effected by phase-firing transducers with the outer transducers of the group being fired slightly ahead of the central transducers. Additional transducers have been added to each side of the main transducer elements by some manufacturers in order to achieve phased focusing not only in the long axis but also in the short axis of the transducer (Fig. 1-17). Since no mechanical motion occurs with linear array units, they can be directly applied to the skin without an intervening water

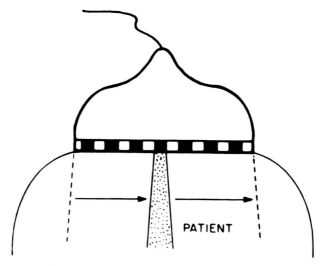

Figure 1-15 Electronic linear array scanner.

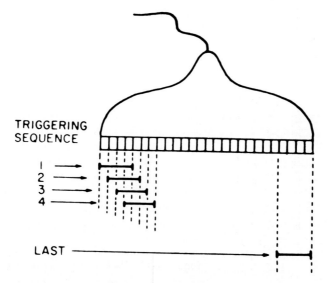

Figure 1-16 Multiplexed triggered electronic linear array scanner.

path. The length of the array determines the length of the field of view. The number of transducers determines the resolution. The frame repetition rate with linear array units of this type is 20 to 60 frames per second; however, the faster the frame repetition rate and the larger the number of transducers in the array, the smaller the possible depth of display.[10] Units for abdominal application use slower frame rates with resultant greater depth of penetration and line density than cardiac units that must use higher frame repetition rates in order to resolve fast-moving anatomic structures within the heart.

It is also possible to arrange the triggering sequence of a linear array of transducers in such a way that the sound beam sweeps through an arc of 45 to 90 degrees from the surface of the transducer array (Fig. 1-18). By phased

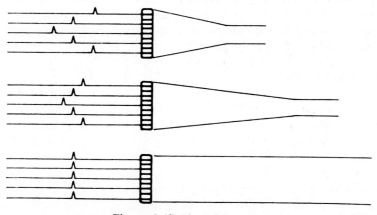

Figure 1-17 Phased focusing.

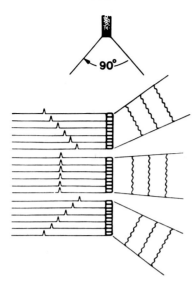

Figure 1-18 Phased sectoring or sweeping.

sweeping a beam in this fashion, it is possible to produce a sector image through a narrow acoustical window such as a rib interspace. This type of unit is particularly useful in cardiac imaging.

A prototype unit was developed by Dr. Thurstone at Duke University[16] called the *Thaumascan*, which used a computer not only to phase sweep the sound beam but also to phase focus the sound beam at varying depths, a technique referred to as *dynamic focusing*. Most linear array units currently available use some form of phased focusing. Some electronic array units also incorporate phased sweeping as well.

The Future

Newer forms of ultrasound instrumentation are actively being researched. Instruments that produce through transmission images rather than pulse-echo images are being developed. At least one laboratory is actively researching coupling through-transmission sound beams to a computer to produce ultrasound computed tomography, and units using this new technology may become commercially available in the not too distant future.

GRAY SCALE RECORDING

The most extensively used method of recording the gray scale image, whether it be from a CRT or TV monitor display, is by photographic film. Self-developing film provides almost immediate pictures without need for darkroom processing. Cameras compatible with self-developing film are inexpensive, and they are included as standard equipment on virtually all ultrasound units. Although considerable improvement has occurred in the resolution and latitude of self-developing film, single-emulsion photographic film is still somewhat better. Photographic film is less costly, but this saving is offset to some extent by the cost of maintaining a darkroom and purchasing a compatible roll film or multiimage camera. Roll film cameras are available in a variety of sizes including the popular 35-mm size, and hardware for mounting these cameras to the bezel of either a CRT or TV monitor is also available.

Multiimage cameras are photographic devices that are capable of placing more than one ultrasound image on a sheet of single-emulsion x-ray film. Although 8 × 10 inch film is commonly used, 11 × 14 inch systems are commercially available. The number of image positions that are available per sheet of film can range from 1 to 36, although 4, 6, or 9 images are normally preferred. A "single format" camera is provided with a fixed number of images. A "multiformat" camera offers the user more than one selection of the number of images per sheet of film. This is accomplished by using a front panel selector switch. The maximum size of each image is determined by the number of images selected.

The least expensive multiimage cameras operate by photographing the display directly from the face of a monitor that is part of the ultrasound unit. The camera may be designed to advance the image position on the film either manually or automatically.

Many multiimage cameras have a self-contained display monitor. This built-in monitor receives essentially the same electrical signal that is supplied to the display monitor on the ultrasound unit. Built-in monitors usually display a TV image. The ultrasound system must therefore be capable of providing a TV video signal at its output. While all gray scale B scan systems have this capability, some real-time scanners do not have TV video outputs. These scanners usually require some type of scan conversion system. The conversion process can be electronic, using digital methods, or it can be performed optically by mounting a TV camera on either the scanner's own viewing monitor or on an auxillary display monitor. The signal from the TV camera is then fed to the monitor built into the multiformat camera. Multiimage cameras, however, can also be purchased with built-in CRTs that function as slave monitors for use with scanners not equipped with scan converters.

In order to place each image in its proper positions on a sheet of film, a variety of mechanical, optical, and electronic methods are used. *Off-axis* is a term used to describe various photographic methods where the image and film planes are not always in complete optical alignment with the monitor. In some of these systems, a single motor-driven lens is moved across a stationary film cassette, stopping at the proper location before each exposure. Other systems perform sequential triggering of a series of mechanical shutters and lenses, each lens having been permanently positioned so that each exposure places an image at the proper location on the film (Fig. 1-19). The least amount of geometric distortion is present on the image at the center of the sheet of film. To reduce the geometric distortion of the images that are not near the center of the film, these off-axis cameras are manufactured with the film plane and lens at a substantial distance from the built-in TV monitor.

Multiimage cameras operate by photographing a static or frozen image. Real time "on the fly" photography can be accomplished only if the camera's exposure time does not exceed the frame rate of the real-time system and the photography is synchronized with the beginning of each TV frame. Because of the distance

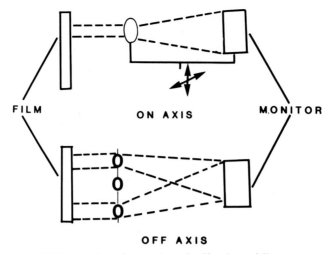

Figure 1-19 Examples of on-axis and off-axis multiimage cameras.

between the built-in TV monitor and the film plane, many multiimage cameras have light loss that does not permit exposures shorter than $\frac{1}{4}$ second.

An on-axis multiimage camera uses a shorter object-to-film distance. In some cases very short exposure times can be used. The term *on-axis* is used to describe a multiimage camera system where, during the duration of each exposure, all picture elements are parallel and positioned perpendicularly to a common axial line (Fig. 1-19). The result of this method is more uniform appearance of the images on the sheet of film and elimination of optical aberrations. An on-axis system might permanently couple a single lens to the TV display and index this complete assembly across the film to each image position. An equally effective method is to move the film about the lens-monitor axis to each image position. Another form of on-axis system uses the technique of mirror indexing and reflection from an axial lens-monitor axis. This system is subject to light absorption requiring higher monitor intensity levels and/or longer exposure time.

CONCLUSION

This chapter has outlined different approaches to gray scale imaging as used in various commercially available instruments. Great strides have been made in the past few years in improving the diagnostic quality of ultrasound images, and even greater improvements are anticipated in the foreseeable future.

REFERENCES

1. Ziskin MC: Basic physics, in Goldberg BB, et al: *Diagnostic Uses of Ultrasound.* New York, Grune & Statton, 1975, pp 1–30.

2. Ziskin MC: Basic physics of ultrasound, in Sanders RC, James AE: *The Principles and Practice of Ultrasonography in Obstetrics and Gynecology.* New York, Appleton Century Crofts, 1980, pp 1–14.

3. Sample WF, Erikson K: Basic principles of diagnostic ultrasound, in Sarti DA, Sample WF: *Diagnostic Ultrasound.* Boston, GK. Hall Co., 1980, pp 3–61.

4. Carlson EN: Ultrasonic physics for the physician: A brief review. *J Clin Ultrasound* 3:69, 1975.

5. Rose JL, Goldberg BB: *Basic Physics in Diagnostic Ultrasound.* New York, John Wiley & Sons, 1979.

6. Maginness MG: Signal processing, image storage, and display, in Wells PNT, Ziskin MC: *New Techniques and Instrumentation in Ultrasonography.* New York, Churchill Livingstone, 1980, pp 40–68.

7. Ophir J, Goldstein A: The principles of digital scan conversion and their application to diagnostic ultrasound. Presented at The World Federation for Ultrasound in Medicine and Biology (WFUMB), San Francisco, 1976.

8. Carlson EN, Slater JM, Nielsen IR, et al: An ultrasound/computer/video display and storage system. *J Clin Ultrasound* 1:236, 1973.

9. Kossoff G, Carpenter DA, Robinson DE, et al: Octoson: A new rapid general purpose echoscope, in White D, Barnes R (eds): *Ultrasound in Medicine.* New York, Plenum Press, 1976, vol 2, pp 330–340.

10. Carpenter D, Kossoff G, Garrett, WJ, et al: The UI Octoson: A new class of ultrasonic echoscope. *Aust Radiol* 21:85, 1977.

11. Garrett WJ, Kossoff G, Carpenter D: Clinical studies with the Octoson, in White DN, Brown RE (eds): *Ultrasound in Medicine.* New York, Plenum Press, 1977, vol. 3, pp 585–594.

12. Wells PNT: Realtime scanning systems, in Wells PNT, Ziskin MC (eds): *New Techniques and Instrumentation in Ultrasonography.* New York, Churchill Livingstone, 1980, pp 69–84.

13. Bronson NR: An ophthalmological ultrasonoscope. *Trans Am Acad Ophthalmol Otolaryngal* 71:360, 1967.

14. Holm HH, Kristensen JK, Pedersen JF, et al: A new mechanical real-time contact scanner. *Ultrasound Med Biol* 2:19, 1975.

15. Bom N, Lancee CT, Honkoop J: Ultrasonic viewer for cross-sectional analysis of moving cardiac structures. *Biomed Eng* 6:500, 1971.

16. Von Ramm OT, Thurstone FL: Thaumascan: Design considerations and performance characteristics. *J Clin Ultrasound* 2:251, 1974.

2

Abdominal Vasculature

Paul A. Dubbins
Barry B. Goldberg

INTRODUCTION

The ability of ultrasound to demonstrate the course and dimensions of major abdominal vessels accurately has long been known, having been accomplished even before the advent of gray scale signal processing.[1-3] However, it was such technologic advances as gray scale and real-time ultrasound that resulted in the regular identification of major branch vessels and their divisions[4-6] as well. These newer modalities led not only to the recognition of a variety of intrinsic pathologic changes in the aorta and inferior vena cava but also to the ability to appreciate displacement of these normal vascular structures by para-aortic and paracaval disease. In addition, the identification of the branch vessels of the aorta and inferior vena cava and the accurate anatomic delineation of the extrahepatic portal venous system facilitated recognition of the boundaries of such organs as the pancreas, thus permitting more reliable ultrasound demonstration of these organs.[4]

In the past, more attention was paid in the ultrasound literature to the evaluation of intraabdominal parenchymal organs than to the vessels. This was due in part to the fact that ultrasound added less information to the imaging of fluid-filled tubular structures than it did to the study of organs. The range of pathologic lesions that involve the vessels is limited, and in the past these lesions were not predicted by preoperative imaging procedures but rather were identified by their appearance at the time of operation. Now, however, several factors have contributed to a renewed interest in the investigation of intraabdominal vascular structures by ultrasound. The improved resolution of gray scale equipment achieved through advances in transducer design and computer technology, combined with advances in real-time imaging, has resulted in more reliable visualization of branch vessels and their course. The introduction of range-gated pulsed Doppler linked to either B-scan or real-time equipment affords the opportunity not only to image intraabdominal vessels but also to assess the velocity, direction and the nature of blood flow within these vessels.[7,8] Finally, improvements in surgical technique now allow the resection of extensive aortic aneurysms with subsequent reanastomosis of branch vessels. Careful planning of such extensive surgery is vital for a successful outcome; therefore,

19

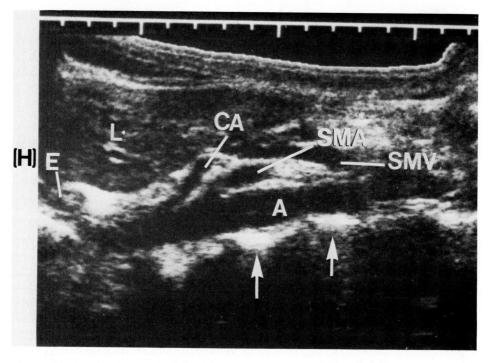

Figure 2-1 Normal aorta. Longitudinal scan 1 cm to the left of midline demonstrating the long tubular echo-free vessel with its anterior branches. The arrows point to the bright echoes of the second and third lumbar vertebral bodies. Note the apposition of the spine and aorta. A = aorta; E = gastroesophageal junction; L = liver; CA = celiac axis; SMA = superior mesenteric artery; SMV = superior mesenteric vein; H = toward patient's head.

accurate knowledge of the point of origin and course of aortic branch vessels is now mandatory.[9,10]

There is a current stimulus toward further enlarging the role of diagnostic ultrasound in the assessment of intraabdominal vessels and their pathology. Now that it is possible to detect branch vessels routinely and to analyze the nature and direction of flow within these vessels, it is not only feasible to identify their anatomic relationship to such pathology as aortic aneurysm but also to assess portal hypertension and perhaps, in the future, to detect aortic, peripheral, and branch occlusive disease as well.

TECHNIQUE

With its central position in the abdomen, the aorta is commonly visualized during routine imaging of intraabdominal structures.[4,6,11,12] The normal aorta is visualized in longitudinal plane by serial scans performed at 5-mm intervals, commencing approximately 4 cm to the left of midline and continuing to the midline (Figs. 2-1, and 2-2). If the scans are continued to the right of midline,

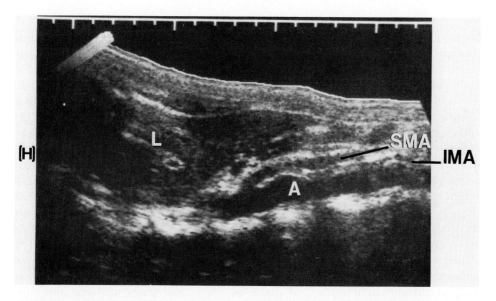

Figure 2-2 Longitudinal midline scan of a normal aorta (A) demonstrating two of its anterior branches, the superior mesenteric artery (SMA) and the inferior mesenteric artery (IMA). L = liver; H = toward patient's head.

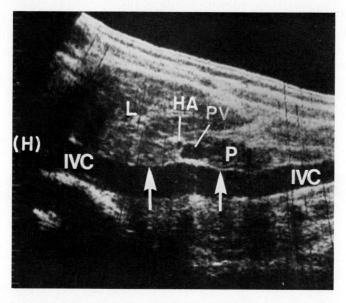

Figure 2-3 Normal inferior vena cava (IVC). Longitudinal scan 2 cm to the right of midline demonstrating the normal shape of the inferior vena cava in distended state. The structures anterior to the inferior vena cava are the liver (L), hepatic artery (HA), portal vein (PV), and the pancreas (P). Note the anterior impression on the surface of the IVC by the pancreas and liver demonstrated by arrows. H = toward patient's head.

21

the inferior vena cava will also be identified in longitudinal axis (Fig. 2-3).[13-16] Similarly, transverse scans can be obtained commencing at the xyphoid and continuing at 2-cm intervals caudad until the bifurcation is reached. This technique not only images the course and caliber of the major vessels of the abdomen, but also identifies the major anterior branches of the aorta: the celiac axis and superior mesenteric and inferior mesenteric arteries and the anterior tributaries of the inferior vena cava (i.e., the hepatic veins) (Figs. 2-4–2-9) Although transverse scans can identify lateral branches, these and the bifurcation are rather less well seen with the patient in the supine position than when the examination is performed with the patient in the lateral decubitus position (Fig. 2-10). Indeed, some workers report visualization of the renal arteries using this decubitus technique with a frequency as high as 75 percent (Fig. 2-11).[17] Similarly, the aortic bifurcation may be better demonstrated in the decubitus position, particularly when there is a prominent Riedel's lobe to act as an acoustic window.[18]

The extrahepatic portal venous system consists of the superior and inferior mesenteric veins, the splenic vein, and the extrahepatic portal vein. This system may be imaged in longitudinal plane by sequential scans at 1-cm intervals, commencing in the left anterior axillary line using an initial short subcostal sector scan with extension downward in a short sweep through the upper abdomen. Longitudinal scans should be continued to the porta hepatis, which although lying approximately 2 cm to the right of midline, varies with the size of the liver and its constituent lobes (Fig. 2-3 and 2-4a). Transverse scans may be performed at 5-mm intervals commencing at the xyphoid and continuing to the level of the transverse or third portion of the duodenum (Figs. 2-5, 2-7–2-9, and 2-12). Scanning in the oblique plane, such as one directed off transverse between 10 and 30 degrees from the right hip toward the left shoulder, may allow more complete visualization of the splenic vein as it courses posterior to the pancreatic body and tail (Fig. 2-13).[15,16,19]

Since vascular structures are fluid-containing tubes, they are eminently suitable for ultrasound assessment. The differences in acoustic impedance between the vessel wall, surrounding fat and connective tissue, and the fluid within the lumen produce a characteristic ultrasound appearance. In a plane sagittal to their long axis, vessels appear as echo-free tubes with brightly echogenic walls. The walls of the arteries and of the portal venous system are usually more brightly echogenic and thicker than those of the veins (Fig. 2-3, 2-6, 2-8, and 2-12). In the plane transverse to their axis, vessels appear as an echo-free ring.

Real time can be used to considerable advantage in the imaging of the intraabdominal vessels.[20] The course of a tortuous abdominal aorta or displacement of the inferior vena cava can be more rapidly and accurately identified. Branch vessels can be quickly identified and their course often assessed as far as the end organ. Further, the normal pulsations of the various intraabdominal vessels can be visualized and any abnormality in pulsations detected.

While continuous-wave Doppler has long been used for measurement of blood flow in peripheral vessels where the transducer can be directly applied to the skin surface over the superficial vessel, in the abdomen this type of Doppler suffers from an absence of range resolution. Thus, if two vessels are

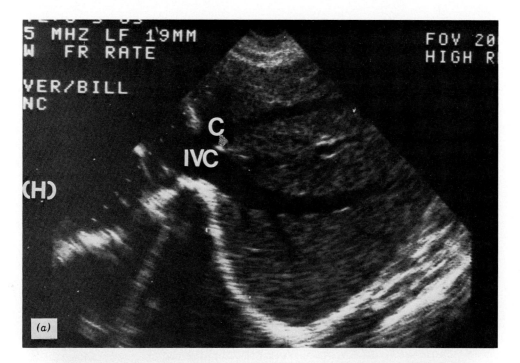

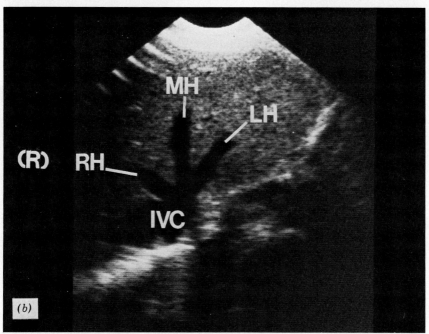

Figure 2-4 Normal inferior vena cava (IVC). Longitudinal (*a*) and transverse (*b*) scans of the inferior vena cava and its major hepatic venous tributaries. The venous confluence (C) of the hepatic veins is demonstrated on the longitudinal scan. On the transverse scan, the right hepatic (RH), the middle hepatic (MH) and the left hepatic (LH) veins join the IVC just below the right hemidiaphragm. R = toward patient's right side.

23

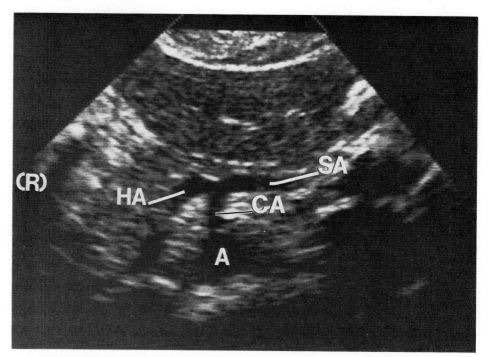

Figure 2-5 Transverse scan of the normal celiac axis (CA) arising from the anterior surface of the aorta (A) and branching in "T" fashion into the common hepatic artery (HA) and the splenic artery (SA) at the level of the T-12/L-1 vertebral bodies. R = toward patient's right side.

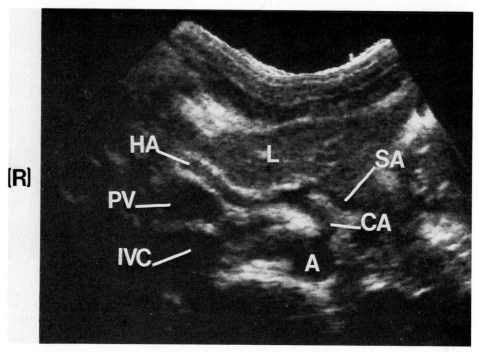

Figure 2-6 Normal transverse scan of the celiac axis (CA) demonstrating the hepatic artery (HA) and spenic artery (SA) at the level of the T-12/L-1 vertebral bodies. A long length of hepatic artery is identified. IVC = inferior vena cava; L = liver; A = aorta; PV = portal vein; R = toward patient's right side.

24

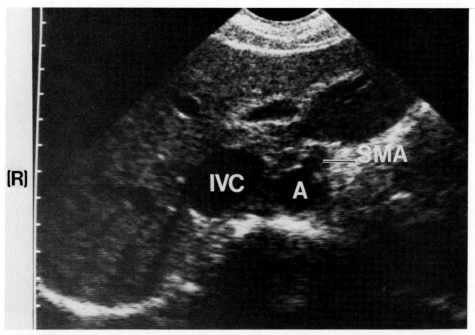

Figure 2-7 Transverse scan at approximately the level of the L-1 vertebral body showing the origin of the superior mesenteric artery (SMA) from the anterior surface of the aorta (A). IVC = inferior vena cava; R = toward patient's right side.

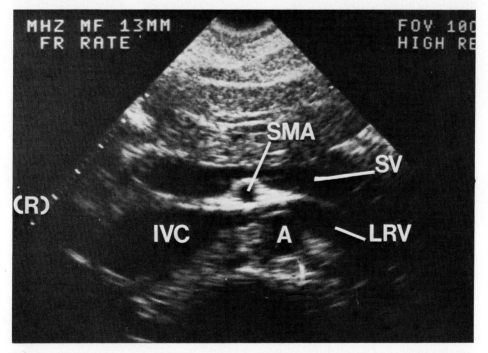

Figure 2-8 Transverse scan at approximately the level of the L-2 vertebral body demonstrating the course of the left renal vein (LRV) as it passes between the aorta (A) and the superior mesenteric artery (SMA) to reach the inferior vena cava (IVC). SV = splenic vein; R = toward patient's right side.

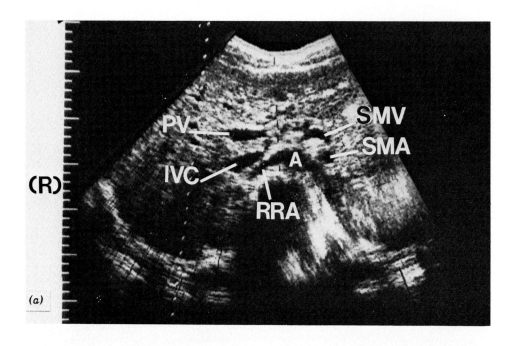

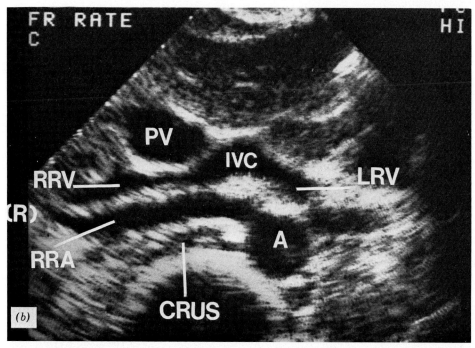

Figure 2-9 (*a*) Transverse scan of the upper abdomen at the level of the L-2 vertebral body showing the right renal artery (RRA) arising from the lateral surface of the aorta (A). Incidentally, a rather unusual, but normal left-sided location of the superior mesenteric artery (SMA) and superior mesenteric vein (ᴐMV) is seen. (*b*) In another case, the right renal artery (RRA) can be seen exiting the aorta (A) slightly more anterior in location. Its course lies behind the inferior vena cava (IVC) and the right renal artery (RRV). PV = portal vein; LRV = left renal vein; CRUS = crus of the diaphragm; R = toward patient's right side.

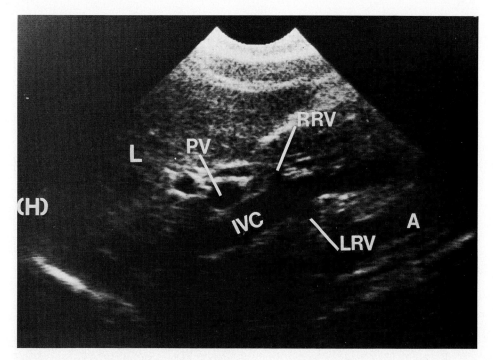

Figure 2-10 Longitudinal lateral decubitus scan of the inferior vena cava (IVC) demonstrating both the right renal vein (RRV) and left renal vein (LRV). L = liver; PV = portal vein; A = aorta; H = toward patient's head.

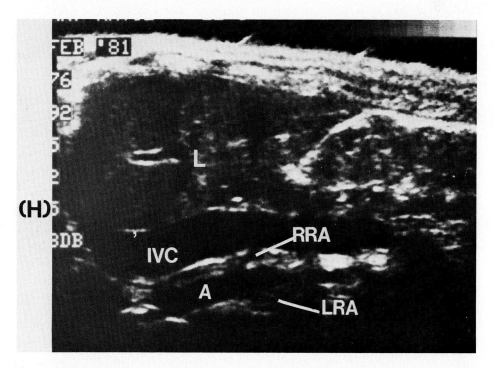

Figure 2-11 Longitudinal decubitus view of the normal major vessels demonstrating the origin of the right renal artery (RRA) and the left renal artery (LRA). A = aorta; IVC = inferior vena cava; L = liver; H = toward patient's head.

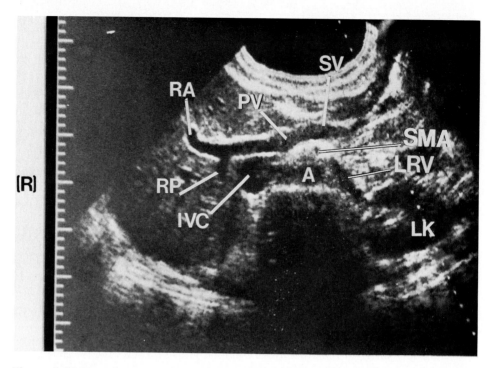

Figure 2-12 Transverse scan of the normal portal venous system demonstrating the splenic vein (SV) anterior to the superior mesenteric artery (SMA). The splenic vein courses transversely to the right and forms the main portal vein (PV) at the point it receives the superior mesenteric vein. The portal vein then continues to the right as the right main portal vein, which then branches into the right anterior (RA) and right posterior (RP) portal veins. A = aorta; LRV = left renal vein; IVC = inferior vena cava; LK = left kidney; R = toward patient's right side.

superimposed one on the other, the continuous-wave Doppler device will give an additive reading of flow that is proportional to the sum of average velocities within both vessels. Pulsed, range-gated Doppler, particularly when linked to a real-time imaging device, allows a previously imaged sample volume to be selected, with the Doppler assessing flow within that limited volume only.[21-25] Although, with most current equipment, quantitative assessment of rates of flow is subject to variations of up to 20 percent, relative velocity between different vessels can be compared, trends suggested when serial examinations are performed, and reversal of flow demonstrated. Furthermore, spectral analysis of the Doppler flow pattern from across the entire vessel lumen or from a selected volume within it may allow the detection of turbulence and eddy currents, thus predicting atheromatous and occlusive disease with greater accuracy. Therefore, even when used purely qualitatively, the simple detection of velocity within a vessel provides a considerable amount of useful information.

Real-time ultrasound is of use not only in rapidly identifying the course and position of the intraabdominal vessels but also in studying normal motion,

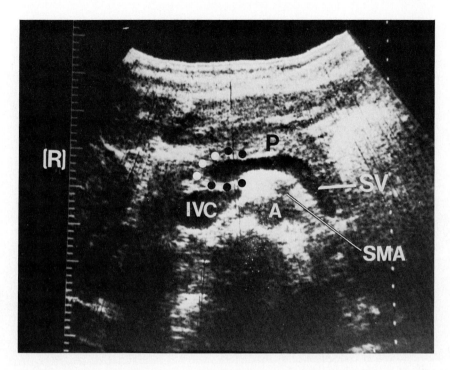

Figure 2-13 Transverse oblique scan from the right hip toward the left shoulder demonstrating the long axis of the splenic vein (SV) posterior to the body and tail of the pancreas (P). The splenic vein courses over the superior mesenteric artery (SMA) before joining with the superior mesenteric vein at the site of the local bulge (outlined by dots), the portal vein confluence. A = aorta; IVC = inferior vena cava; R = toward patient's right side.

distension, and intraluminal echoes. Vascular motion is transmitted from the heart; arteries show a sharp pulsation with each heartbeat so that the arterial walls may be observed to diverge slightly during each systole and can be recognized as distinct from the complex, bouncing, wavy pulsations seen in veins. These are sometimes recognized as corresponding to the *a*, *c*, and *v* waves of the jugular venous pulse. While the arteries tend to move as a unit with pulsation, veins show a definite opening and closing of their lumens.[26]

Occasionally, moving clusters of echoes may be identified within the lower-pressure venous and portal venous systems. These commonly appear to move more slowly at the periphery of the vessel than at center lumen; in the inferior vena cava, they may occasionally demonstrate a biphasic motion. The cause of these echoes has not been clearly established, although red cell rouleaux formation has been cited.[27] However, since many of the patients in whom this phenomenon is observed are asymptomatic and apparently normal, showing no evidence of rouleaux formation in peripheral blood smears, it may be instead that the appearances are due to turbulence.[28]

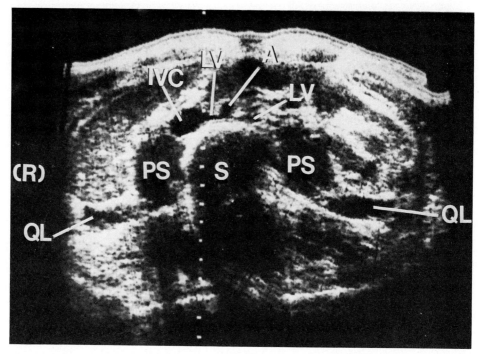

Figure 2-14 Transverse scan at the level of the L-3 vertebral body demonstrating an unusually prominent lumbar vein (LV) passing beneath the aorta (A) to join the inferior vena cava (IVC). L = liver; S = spine; A = aorta; PS = psoas muscle; QL = quadratus lumburum muscle; R = toward patient's right side.

NORMAL VENOUS ANATOMY[29]

The inferior vena cava (IVC) lies to the right of the aorta, just anterior and to the right side of the vertebral column. It is formed by the junction of the two common iliac veins posterior to the right common iliac artery. The inferior vena courses cephalad, lying anteriorly to the right lumbar arteries and right sympathetic trunk. It receives lumbar veins (the left ones passing behind the aorta), the right ovarian or testicular vein, right renal vein, right suprarenal veins, and the left renal vein. (The left suprarenal, inferior phrenic, and gonadal veins join the left renal vein before its adjunction with the IVC.) Just before the IVC disappears through the diaphragm to enter the heart, it receives the hepatic veins (right, left, and middle) from the liver and the right inferior phrenic vein (Fig. 2-4). Of these branches only the common iliac veins, the renal veins, and the hepatic veins are regularly visualized by ultrasound (Figs. 2-4, 2-8, and 2-12), although infrequently other branches such as a prominent lumbar vein can be identified (Fig. 2-14). On occasion, an oblique image of the inferior vena cava, scanned through the liver, offers more information than a supine scan (Fig. 2-15).

In the midabdomen, the inferior vena cava follows an almost horizontal course anterior to the lumbar spine. In the upper abdomen, it turns more

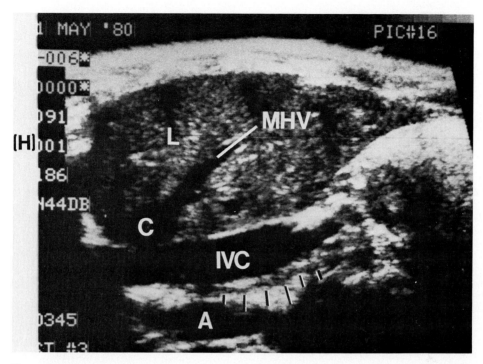

Figure 2-15 Longitudinal oblique scan of the major vessels demonstrating the middle hepatic vein (MHV) and the confluence of hepatic veins (C) as these drain into the inferior vena cava (IVC). The right crus is again identified by the lines between the IVC and the aorta (A). L = liver; H = toward patient's head.

anteriorly in a "hammock" configuration in intimate contact with the hepatic parenchyma until it passes through the caval hiatus of the diaphragm to enter the right atrium (Fig. 2-3, 2-4a, and 2-15). Normally, its smooth course is only interrupted by a small impression on the dorsal aspect caused by the right renal artery, periarterial fat, and fibrous tissue (Fig. 2-16).[6] The head of the pancreas may cause a small impression on the anterior surface of the IVC; although, if the impression is prominent, a pancreatic head mass should be suspected (Fig. 2-3).[35]

The caliber of the IVC usually increases as it courses cephalad, receiving blood from its various tributaries (Fig. 2-4). Changes in the dimensions of the IVC in response to the different phases of respiration are complex and can be observed either by sequential static scans during the different phases or by real time (Figs. 2-3 and 2-17). Most workers agree that at end inspiration the diameter of the IVC is decreased, while at end expiration Grant reports that the diameter is uniformly increased.[36] However, Grant also states that, in the majority of his patients, a Valsalva maneuver resulted in an overall decrease in the size of the IVC, in stark disagreement with all previous studies.[6,13,30–34,36] It is perhaps not surprising that there is disagreement in the observed response of the inferior vena cava to changes in respiration since the diameter of the IVC depends not only on intrathoracic pressure and right atrial pressure but

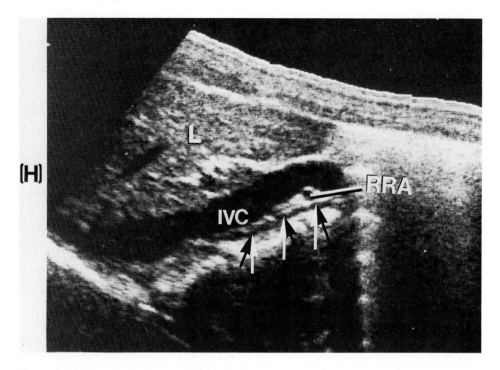

Figure 2-16 Longitudinal scan of the inferior vena cava (IVC) demonstrating the normal right renal artery (RRA) as it passes beneath the inferior vena cava (IVC) and anterior to the right crus (arrows) before turning dorsally to enter the renal hilum. L = liver; H = toward patient's head.

also on the intraabdominal pressure, and Cosgrove has reported that a Valsalva maneuver may produce either a markedly distended IVC or a completely collapsed state.[26]

It is therefore more appropriate to study the IVC in dynamic state during quiet respiration, using abnormalities in the opening and closing cycle, normally associated with cardiac pulsation, as suggestive evidence of disease.

TRIBUTARIES OF THE IVC

The Iliac Veins

The IVC is formed by the junction of the right and left common iliac veins, which in turn derive from the internal and external iliac veins that accompany arteries of the same name (Fig. 2-18).

The examination of the pelvis is, as usual, best performed with a filled urinary bladder. The course of the external iliac vein can usually be followed from the inguinal ligament cephalad and medially on the surface of the psoas muscle and medial to the corresponding artery, particularly if the transducer is angled laterally from the midline using the bladder as an acoustic window. The internal iliac vein may be infrequently imaged deep to the bladder and

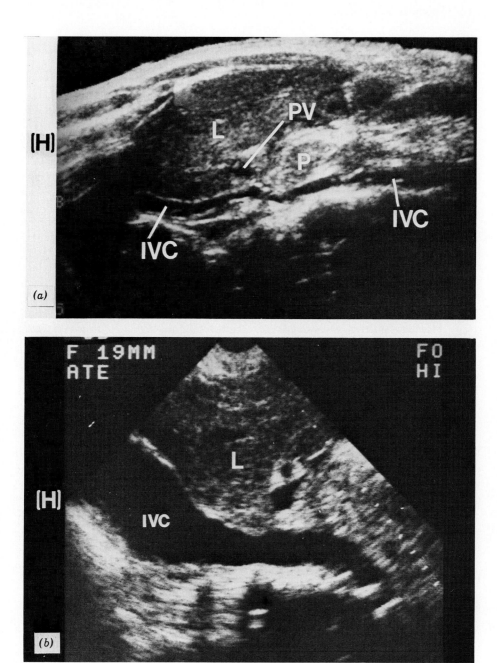

Figure 2-17 Longitudinal scan of the normal inferior vena cava (IVC) in collapsed state (*a*) and distended state (*b*). L = liver; PV = portal vein; P = pancreas; H = toward patient's head; R = toward patient's right side.

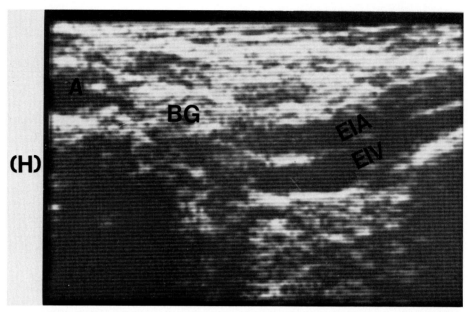

Figure 2-18 Longitudinal oblique scan of the iliac vessels with patient in semidecubitus position. The external iliac artery (EIA) and external iliac vein (EIV) are demonstrated as they course toward the inguinal ligament to become the femoral artery and veins. The common iliac artery and the internal iliac artery are obscured by bowel gas (BG). A = aorta; H = toward patient's head.

lateral to the ovary and broad ligament as it courses anteriorly, laterally, and cephalad to join with the external iliac vein and thus form the common iliac vein. Frequently, however, much of the common iliac vein is obscured by bowel gas, although the decubitus position may allow better visualization (Fig. 2-18).[18]

Visualization of the iliac veins depends on adequate distension. Occasionally their position can only be inferred from the position of the iliac arteries. The degree of distension of the iliac vein may be altered by changes in the phase of respiration, by changes in posture (e.g., standing the patient erect), and also by the presence of intraabdominal masses (e.g., pregnancy).

Renal Veins

Renal veins may be single or multiple. However, visualization of accessory renal veins are extremely difficult because of their small size, and it is not surprising that they have not been reported in the literature. The right renal vein is short (Fig. 2-10). It exits from the right renal sinus, coursing predominantly anteriorly and also slightly medially and cephalad to enter the posterolateral aspect of the IVC. The left renal vein is longer. It exits from the left renal sinus and courses at first anteriorly and medially to reach the anterolateral border of the aorta. It then continues more transversely, passing between the superior mesenteric artery and the aorta to enter the anterior and left medial aspect of the inferior vena cava (Figs. 2-8 and 2-12).[37] Occasionally, in patients of thin body habitus, the proximal portion of the left renal vein may become significantly distended,

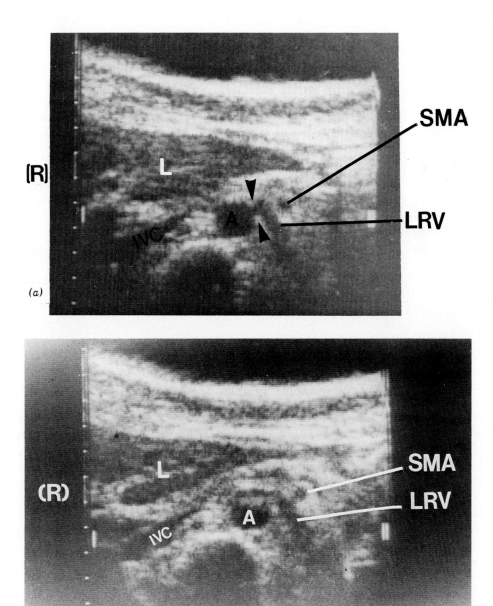

Figure 2-19 "Psuedoaneurysm effect" of the left renal vein. (*a*) Transverse scan at approximately the level of the second lumbar vertebral body in a patient of thin body habitus. There is focal dilatation of the left renal vein (LRV) and an apparent communication with the aorta (A), marked by arrowheads. That this is not a renal artery aneurysm can be confirmed by changing the plane of scan (*b*) or by applying compression to the abdomen during scanning. SMA = superior mesenteric artery; L = liver; IVC = inferior vena cava; R = toward patient's right side.

and that portion adjacent to the aorta may simulate a renal artery aneurysm in apparent continuity with the aorta (Fig. 2-19).[38,39] Such a false impression can usually be resolved by a change in scanning procedure, particularly through the use of anterior abdominal wall compression, which allows the renal vein to be imaged so that it can be seen to be clearly separate from the aorta. Also, pulsed Doppler examination will elicit normal venous sounds from within the sample volume rather than the turbulence characteristically found within an arterial aneurysm.[37]

The Hepatic Veins

The hepatic veins enter the inferior vena cava just before its passage through the caval hiatus into the right atrium (Fig. 2-4). The anatomy of the hepatic veins is extremely variable, but they are usually divisable into right, left, and middle veins.[15,16] The right hepatic vein normally enters the inferior vena cava on its right side, the middle vein anteriorly, and the left hepatic vein on the left side (Figs. 2-4b and 2-15). However, one or more of these hepatic veins may form a single trunk before draining into the IVC or, on occasion, may drain directly into the right atrium.

THE AORTA AND BRANCHES

The aorta enters the abdomen through the aortic hiatus and passes caudally, anterior to the vertebral column, and slightly to the left of midline to end by bifurcating in front of the lower part of the fourth lumbar vertebrae (Figs. 2-1 and 2-2). Because there is a normal lumbar lordosis in most people, the distal abdominal aorta is more anteriorly placed than the proximal aorta, and if the lordosis is marked, the aorta may be unusually close to the skin surface near its bifurcation (Fig. 2-2).

The aorta lies immediately anterior to the vertebral column except at its bifurcation where the left common iliac vein passes posterior to the aorta, interposing itself between the aorta and the vertebral column. The aorta bifurcates into the right and left common iliac arteries, which course slightly posteriorly, laterally, and caudally, lying anterior and lateral to their associated veins. Visualization of the common iliac arteries is usually incomplete and segmental due to bowel gas (Fig. 2-18) except when involved by aneurysm. With a full urinary bladder, segments of the internal and external iliac arteries can also be imaged in the pelvis.

It is not usually difficult to distinguish the aorta from the inferior vena cava because of its position, course, and branches. Similarly, the normal arterial pulsations characteristic of the aorta serve to distinguish it from the IVC. In cases of anomalous venous drainage with azygos continuation, a left-sided inferior vena cava can be diagnosed by the typical venous sounds detected with pulsed Doppler.[40,41]

The caliber of the aorta in spite of slight variations during systole and diastole remains fairly constant, tapering gradually from a maximum diameter at the level of the diaphragmatic hiatus to a minimum diameter at the bifurcation. Normal measurements for anteroposterior (AP) and transverse diameter based

Table 2-1 Comparison Between Aortography and Ultrasound in the Measurement of Aortic Diameter

Type of Procedure	Diameter (mm)			
	At 11th Rib	Above Renal Arteries	Below Renal Arteries	At Bifurcation
Aortography Transverse Diameter[a] Steinberg et al.[41]	24	21	19	17
Aortography AP diameter[a] Goldberg et al.[1]	25	22	19	15
Ultrasound Goldberg et al.,[1]	23	20	18	15

[a] Corrected for magnification.

on both contrast aortography and ultrasound are available (Table 2-1).[1,42] Comparison of true luminal diameter as assessed by caliper measurements of resected specimens demonstrates that ultrasound is at least as accurate as aortography.[1] For the most part, the AP diameter of the aorta is used for ultrasound measurements since the lateral resolution of the ultrasound beam causes indistinct lateral vessel margins when scanning is performed from the anterior abdominal wall. Similarly, if the aorta is tortuous, transverse ultrasound scans may exaggerate the true lateral dimensions, leading to an incorrect diagnosis of aneurysm.[12]

THE MAJOR VISCERAL ARTERIES

With modern gray scale signal processing, the major visceral arteries, that is, the celiac axis and its major branches, the common hepatic artery and the splenic artery, and the superior mesenteric artery and its proximal branches, are almost invariably seen. The right and left renal arteries may be seen in up to 75 percent of patients, particularly if the right lateral decubitus position is employed.[17] The inferior mesenteric artery is quite infrequently visualized and then only on longitudinal scans. While other visceral arteries are uncommonly seen, the advent of high resolution real-time equipment has allowed more frequent identification of the left gastric artery, the gastroduodenal artery, hepatic artery proper, the right gastric artery, and the pancreatic arcade.

The visceral arteries are often grouped anatomically into those arising from the anterior, lateral, and posterolateral surfaces of the abdominal aorta. These anatomic groupings are also convenient for ultrasound examination since different techniques are required to image the different groups. Those arising from the anterior surface, that is, the celiac, superior mesenteric, and inferior mesenteric arteries, are imaged by routine anterior abdominal wall scanning in both longitudinal and transverse axes (Figs. 2-1, 2-2, and 2-5–2-9). Conversely, those arising from the lateral or posterolateral aspect of the aorta, that is, the renal and the lumbar arteries, are usually visualized only on transverse scans or scans performed in the decubitus position (Figs. 2-9 and 2-11). The proximal right renal artery can frequently be visualized on longitudinal images posterior to the inferior vena cava as a rounded echo-free structure surrounded by the brightly echogenic vessel wall and retroperitoneal fat (Fig. 2-16).

When assessing the visceral branches of the abdominal aorta, a very flexible approach must be adopted, since it must be appreciated that variations in vascular anatomy are very common and that the appearance of aortic branches must therefore not be routinely expected to be classic.[42]

THE CELIAC ARTERY

The celiac artery arises from the ventral surface of the aorta, between the crura of the diaphragm and the aortic hiatus, usually opposite the disc space between the twelfth thoracic and first lumbar vertebrae (Fig. 2-1). It usually courses anteriorly for a variable distance above the upper margin of the pancreas before dividing into the common hepatic, left gastric, and splenic arteries (Fig. 2-1, 2-5, and 2-6). Occasionally, the length of the celiac trunk is so short that the common hepatic and the splenic artery appear to arise directly from the aorta.

The common hepatic artery follows an almost transverse course from its origin, running along the upper border of the head of the pancreas where it gives rise to the rarely visualized right gastric artery. At the upper margin of the duodenum, it courses anteriorly in the right hepatopancreatic fold, after having given off a major branch, the gastroduodenal artery. It then ascends to the liver in the free edge of the lesser omentum (hepatoduodenal ligament) where it is situated to the left and anterior to the main portal vein (Figs. 2-6 and 2-20). The gastroduodenal artery descends behind the first part of the duodenum anterior to the pancreas and may be used to identify the head of the pancreas during ultrasound examination. While the common hepatic artery usually arises from the celiac artery, approximately 40 percent of the normal population demonstrate variations; most commonly, an accessory hepatic artery still originates from the celiac axis or a replaced hepatic artery arises from the superior mesenteric artery (Figs. 2-21 and 2-22).[43]

The left gastric artery most commonly arises directly from the celiac axis but occasionally from the proximal portions of the common hepatic or splenic arteries (Fig. 2-23). It courses at first anteriorly, cephalad, and to the left toward the gastric cardia where it turns sharply downward and passes along the lesser curvature of the stomach toward the pylorus. Only the proximal portion of the left gastric artery is seen during routine ultrasound imaging.

The splenic artery, similar to the hepatic artery, follows a transverse course but toward the left, having a somewhat tortuous nature, particularly in older patients (Figs. 2-5 and 2-6). For this reason, the entire length of the splenic artery is rarely imaged on transverse or transverse-oblique scans, and only segments of the artery are visualized as it undulates in and out of the plane of scans. As it passes toward the left and somewhat cephalad to enter the splenic hilum, it lies posterior to the superior aspect of the body of the pancreas and is a reliable anatomic marker for this boundary.

The superior mesenteric artery arises from the ventral surface of the aorta, caudad to the celiac artery, at the level of the first lumbar vertebra, and dorsal

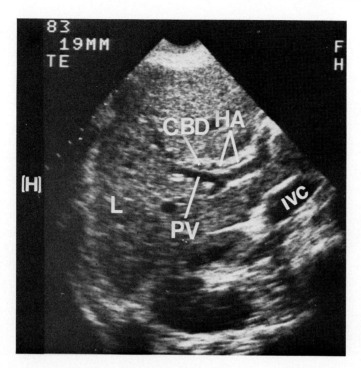

Figure 2-20 Transverse scan of the upper abdomen showing the normal relationship of the portal triad. The common bile duct (CBD) lies on the right anterior surface and the hepatic artery (HA), the left anterior surface of the portal vein (PV). L = liver; IVC = inferior vena cava; H = toward patient's head.

to the body of the pancreas and the splenic vein (Figs. 2-1, 2-2, and 2-7–2-9). It emerges from under the caudal border of the pancreas and passes anterior to the upper border of the third part of the duodenum. It descends caudad over the anterior surface of the uncinate process, usually giving rise to the middle colic artery just before it enters the small bowel mesentery. Occasionally, on real-time examination, branches of the superior mesenteric artery may be seen within the mesentery outlined by fat.

The inferior mesenteric artery may occasionally be imaged as it courses caudad toward the rectum from its origin from the central surface of the aorta at about the level of the third lumbar vertebra (Fig. 2-2).

The vessels arising from the lateral and posterior surface of the aorta include the renal and lumbar arteries. Of these, only the renal arteries are routinely imaged.

The right renal artery arises from the lateral or anterolateral surface of the aorta (Figs. 2-9 and 2-11). It passes dorsally, caudad, and to the right to pass between the right crux and the IVC where it may be imaged on longitudinal scans (Fig. 2-16). It then continues toward the renal hilum.

The left renal artery arises from the lateral or posterolateral surface of the aorta, coursing dorsally, caudally, and to the left to enter the renal hilum (Fig. 2-11).

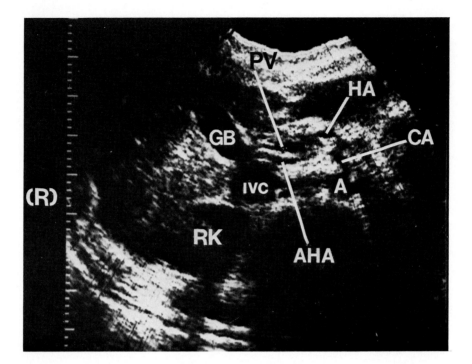

Figure 2-21 Transverse scan at the level of the T12/L1 vertebral bodies demonstrating a normal appearing celiac axis (CA) arising from the anterior surface of the aorta. The main hepatic artery (HA) is seen coursing to the right, anterior to the portal vein (PV). An accessory hepatic artery (AHA) also arising from the celiac axis (CA) is noted posterior to the portal vein (PV). This is an unusual anatomic variant. GB = gallbladder; A = aorta; RK = right kidney; IVC = inferior vena cava; L = liver; R = toward patient's right side.

Accessory renal arteries occur in about 20 percent of patients, usually below the main renal artery.[44] They have been detected by ultrasound although they are very small in caliber but, even if imaged, are often indistinguishable from prominent lumbar arteries (of Adamkiewitz).

Anatomic Relations of the Major Vessels

For the most part, the posterior relations of the major vessels are the vertebra and prevertebral fascia. The IVC as it courses anteriorly to the right atrium is also related posteriorly to the liver. The diaphragmatic crura are in close relationship to the upper part of the course of the major vessels (Figs. 2-4a, 2-10, 2-15, 2-16, 2-24). They originate as tendinous fibers from the upper three lumbar vertebrae on the right and from the first lumbar vertebra on the left. As the right crus passes cephalad, it may appear as a rounded structure on transverse scans in a posteromedial relationship to the inferior vena cava. It passes posterior to the right renal artery. and then the most medial fibers decussate with those of the left crus, forming an anterior sling over the surface of the aorta (Fig. 2-24).[45] From above down, the structures anterior to the

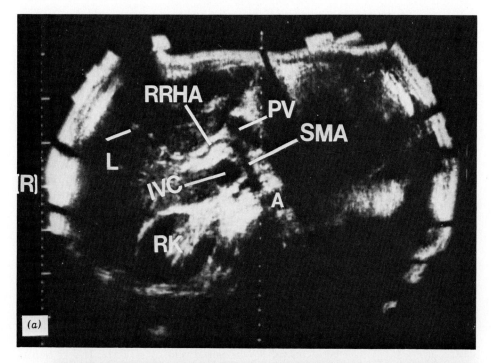

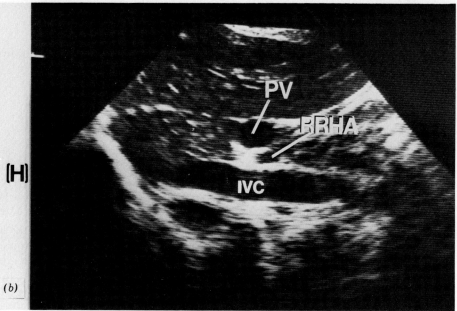

Figure 2-22 Replaced right hepatic artery. Transverse (*a*) and longitudinal (*b*) scans at approximately the level of the L2 vertebral body demonstrating a replaced right hepatic artery (RRHA) arising from the superior mesenteric artery (SMA) and passing between the inferior vena cava (IVC) and the portal vein (PV) on its way to the liver (L). RK = right kidney; A = aorta; R = toward patient's right side; H = toward patient's head.

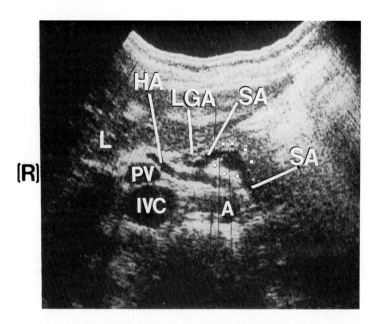

Figure 2-23 Transverse scan of the upper abdomen demonstrating the splenic artery (SA) with a branch aneurysm (outlined by dots). Incidentally, the origin of the left gastric artery (LGA) can be identified. PV = portal vein; A = aorta; HA = hepatic artery; IVC = inferior vena cava; R = toward patient's right side.

major vessels are the pancreas; the first, second, and third part of the duodenum; the root of the small bowel mesentery, and the small bowel.

THE PORTAL VENOUS SYSTEM[15,16,42]

The portal venous system conveys blood from the viscera to the liver and includes all the veins that drain the blood from the gastrointestinal tract, the spleen, pancreas, and gallbladder. The portal vein is about 8 cm long and arises from the junction of the superior mesenteric and splenic veins anterior to the inferior vena cava and posterior to the superior aspect of the duodenal bulb. At this point, it lies immediately cephalad to the junction between the head and neck of the pancreas. It ascends in the free edge of the lesser omentum at the aditus to the lesser sac to the porta hepatis where it divides into a right and left branch. In the lesser omentum, the main portal vein is related to the common bile duct on its right anterior aspect and the hepatic artery on its left anterior aspect.

The tributaries of the portal vein are

1. The splenic vein
2. The superior mesenteric vein
3. The coronary vein
4. The pyloric vein

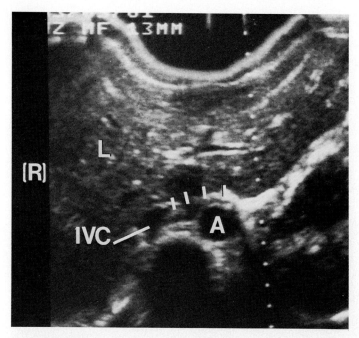

Figure 2-24 Normal transverse scan at the level of the T12/L1 vertebral bodies demonstrating the decussation of the right crus (small lines) over the surface of the aorta (A). IVC = inferior vena cava; L = liver; R = toward patient's right side.

5. The cystic vein
6. The paraumbilical veins

Of these, only the first two are regularly imaged by ultrasound in the normal patient. The splenic vein commences at the splenic hilum, passing from left toward the right, posterior to the superior part of the pancreas, and inferior to the splenic artery. Because of its position relative to the pancreas, it provides an accurate anatomic marker for this organ (Fig. 2-13). Of the tributaries of the splenic vein, only the inferior mesenteric vein draining the distal colon and rectum is imaged by ultrasound and then only occasionally at the variable point that it joins the splenic vein.

The superior mesenteric vein, which drains the small intestine and the proximal colon, can often be imaged to the right of the superior mesenteric artery as it courses from the right iliac fossa toward the neck of the pancreas where it unites with the splenic vein to form the portal vein (Figs. 2-1, 2-8, and 2-9)[15,16]

The coronary vein receives tributaries from both surfaces of the stomach, running from right to left along the lesser curvature of the stomach. At the esophageal opening of the stomach, it turns downward to enter the portal vein. This portion of the cornary vein may occasionally be imaged in normal patients, but may be more commonly imaged in portal hypertension when it is frequently enlarged.

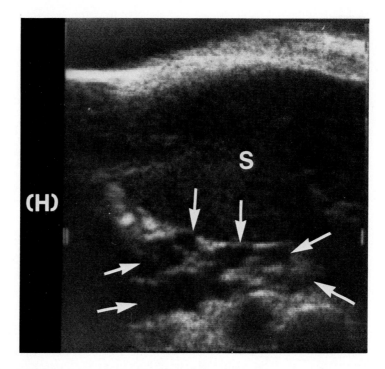

Figure 2-25 Longitudinal coronal image reveals an enlarged spleen (S) with multiple tortuous vessels (arrows) representing splenic retroperitoneal varices in the patient with proven portal hypertension. H = toward patient's head.

There are many portosystemic anastomoses that may become enlarged in the event of portal hypertension (Fig. 2-25).

1. Gastric-esophageal
2. Rectal-internal iliac
3. Veins of retzius in the small bowel mesentery
4. Gastric-adrenal and renal
5. Splenic-retroperitoneal
6. Recanalization of umbilical vein
7. Anastomosis via the liver capsule[42]

Any, or all, of these may be the site of an enlarged collateral vessel; therefore, while recanalization of the umbilical vein may be the most regularly demonstrated abnormality, recognition of an abnormally enlarged vessel in a known portal collateral pathway may assist in the diagnosis of portal hypertension.[46–48]

ABNORMAL VESSELS

Vessel pathology is significantly limited in its variety and is generally eminently suitable to examination by ultrasound. Generally, variations in blood vessel

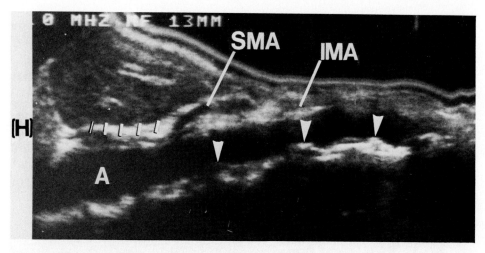

Figure 2-26 Atheromatous aorta. Longitudinal midline scan showing a slightly ectatic aorta (A) with evidence of significant irregularity of the contour (arrowheads). L = liver; SMA = superior mesenteric artery; IMA = inferior mesenteric artery; H = toward patient's head; Lines = crus of diaphragm.

caliber, presence of intraluminal echoes (either thrombus or tumor), and the presence of extra or unusual vessels may be investigated. In addition, knowledge of the normal position and relationship of intraabdominal vessels allows the assessment of displacement due to intraabdominal pathology such as lymph node enlargement. While variations in caliber, the presence and effects of intraluminal clot, etc., are discussed for each vessel system, vessel displacement is considered here as a separate topic.

THE AORTA

Atheromatous Disease

With advancing age, atheromatous disease becomes the rule rather than the exception, and the demonstration of aortic plaque in the elderly patient should not be considered abnormal.[49] The features of atheromatous disease that are demonstrable by ultrasound include the demonstration of luminal irregularities (which are representative of atheromatous plaque), tortuosity, and aortic wall calcification. Irregularity of the aortic and iliac vessel walls may be accompanied by intraluminal thrombus that is evidenced by low-level echoes within their lumens (Figs. 2-26 and 2-27). Calcification of the wall produces an area of very sharp reflectivity with distal acoustic shadowing due to sound reflection and absorption (Figs. 2-26 and 2-28). While demonstration of atheromatous plaques at the origin of branch vessels is possible, this is infrequently seen. In addition, the appearance may also be mimicked by beam-width artifact when there is an atheromatous plaque close to the ostium of a vessel. It is, therefore, an unreliable indicator of branch vessel disease unless accompanied by demonstrable stenosis,

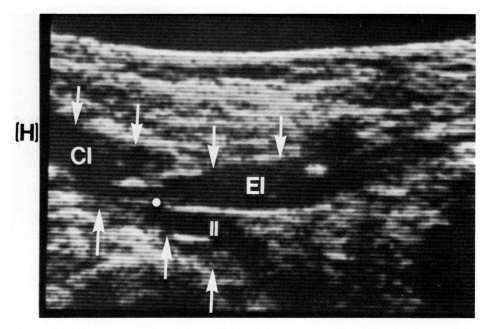

Figure 2-27 Atheroma and ectasia of iliac arteries. Longitudinal decubitus scan of the common iliac (CI), external iliac (EI) and internal iliac (IL) arteries. The course of the vessels is outlined by arrows with a dot at the bifurcation of the internal and external iliac arteries. There are numerous coarse bright echoes within the lumen of the vessels, particularly at the site of branching indicating severe atheromatous plaque formation. The low level echoes proximal to the bifurcation and in the internal iliac artery was thrombus. H = toward patient's head.

as evidenced by poststenotic dilatation or abnormalities of flow detectable by pulsed Doppler.

The aorta may be mildly or markedly tortuous. In such instances, demonstration of the course of the aorta is most easily performed with real-time ultrasound.[50] While deviating to the left in 80 percent of patients, aortic tortuosity may extend to the right across the midline, displacing the adjacent inferior vena cava.[51] On occasion, the aorta may even insinuate itself beneath the IVC at about the level of the right renal artery.[51] Because of tortuosity, there are times when it is very difficult to identify the aorta as a tubular structure, and the imaged rounded, fluid-filled structure may be confused with intraabdominal pathology (Fig. 2-29).

Dilatation and Aneurysm Formation

Perhaps the most frequent use of arteriosonography is in the demonstration of aortic aneurysm.[1,52–54] Before the advent of ultrasound and arteriography, detection of abdominal aortic aneurysm was dependent on careful examination of the AP and lateral plain abdominal x-ray film, which in turn depended to a large degree on the presence of calcification in the aneurysm wall. Detection rates were less than adequate, and underestimation of the size of aneurysm

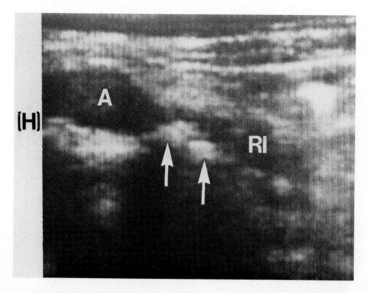

Figure 2-28 Oblique long-axis scan of the distal aorta (A) and right iliac artery (RI) demonstrating a stenosis secondary to calcified atheroma at the origin of the right iliac artery (RI). The atheroma (arrows) narrows the lumen, produces distal acoustic shadowing and causes poststenotic dilatation of the iliac artery H = toward patient's head.

was common. In one series, the preoperative diagnosis of aortic aneurysm was confirmed by lumbar spine films in only 72 percent and by ultrasound in all of the patients, while aneurysm size could be measured by a lumbar spine x-ray film in only 55 percent, whereas again ultrasound was able to measure the size in all cases.[55]

The diagnosis of aortic aneurysm by ultrasound depends on the accurate measurement of the AP diameter of the aorta. Leopold and Asher, using the figures achieved by Steinberg and Maloney citing unpublished data by Brown and Jeurgens, determined that a measurement of 3 cm should be considered the maximum AP diameter for the diagnosis of simple aortic ectasia, and that above this measurement the aorta should be considered aneurysmal.[42,55,56] In comparison with arteriography, ultrasound is able to image not only the true lumen but also the overall dimensions of the aneurysm (Fig. 2-30). In addition, ultrasound gives information comparable to computed tomography without the need for ionizing radiation or intravenous contrast techniques (Fig. 2-31).

Abdominal aortic aneurysms are usually arteriosclerotic in origin. They are most commonly fusiform in nature and commence below the origin of the renal arteries (Figs. 2-30 and 2-32). They usually project anteriorly and to the left of midline, the path of least resistance.[12] Aneurysms of the aorta may continue into the iliac vessels for a variable extent (Fig. 2-33). Saccular aneurysms of the abdominal aorta are rare (Fig. 2-34). Bowel gas frequently is displaced by large aneurysms; therefore, not uncommonly, the origin of the aneurysm and of the superior mesenteric and renal arteries becomes obscured (Fig. 2-30).

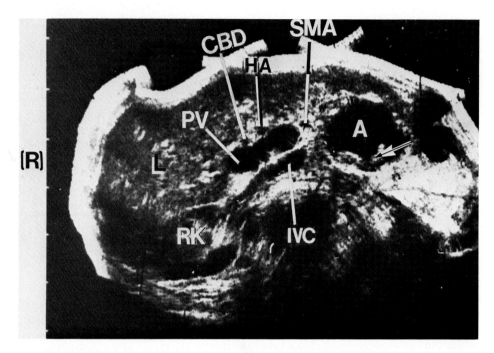

Figure 2-29 Transverse scan of the midabdomen. The aorta (A) is so tortuous that it is situated in the left upper quadrant. Note that it is located lateral to the superior mesenteric artery (SMA). The arrow denotes posteriorly located thrombus. PV = portal vein; L = liver; RK = right kidney; IVC = inferior vena cava; HA = hepatic artery; CBD = common bile duct; R = toward patient's right side.

Because of the abrupt change in aortic caliber at the site of an aneurysm, there is alteration of the laminar flow normally found within the aorta, giving rise to turbulence and eddy currents. This change in the character of flow can usually be detected by Doppler sampling across the vessel. Irregularities of flow significantly increase the likelihood of clot formation.

The amount of mural clot, which is variable, is demonstrable by ultrasound as the presence of low-level echoes within the aortic lumen; the true lumen remains as a echo-free space within the walls.[57] The mural clot may be circumferential or may predominate on the anterior wall (Figs. 2-30*b* and 2-31*a*). Calcification, evidenced by a brightly echogenic focus with distal shadowing, may be identified within the wall of the aneurysm. In addition, the calcification may be within the clot, at least partially explaining why plain abdominal radiography sometimes underestimates the size of the aneurysm.[57] Occasionally, anterior reverberation artifact may be confused for mural thrombus, and such artifact must be distinguished from true thrombus echoes on the basis of its characteristics and how the pattern responds to alterations in power and time-gain compensation curves.

Although aneurysms involving the renal arteries are rare (less than four percent in one series), an attempt should be made during the ultrasound examination to identify the renal arteries and assess their relationship to the

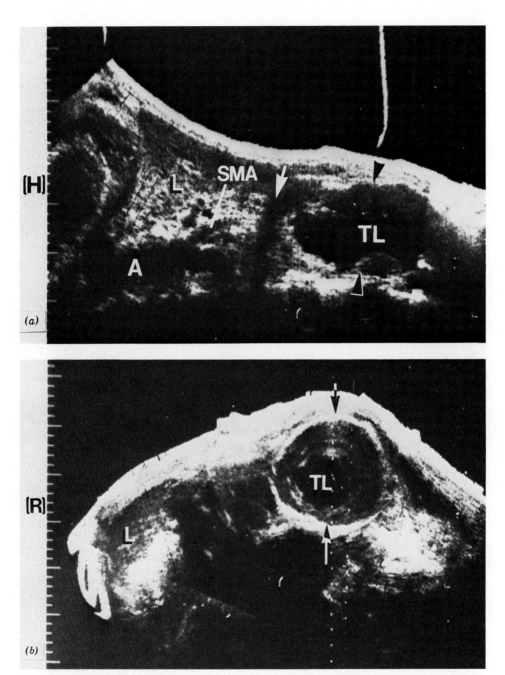

Figure 2-30 Fusiform abdominal aortic aneurysm with circumferential laminated clot. (*a*) Longitudinal midline scan demonstrates an aneurysm (arrowheads) of the distal abdominal aorta (A). Arrow denotes shadowing from bowel gas, obscuring the origin of the aneurysm. Note the overall dimensions and the true lumen (TL) of the aneurysm. (*b*) Transverse midabdominal scan shows the aneurysm (arrows) and the true lumen (TL). L = liver; SMA = superior mesenteric artery; H = toward patient's head; R = toward patient's right side.

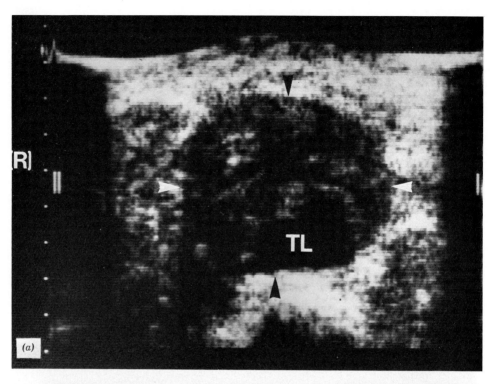

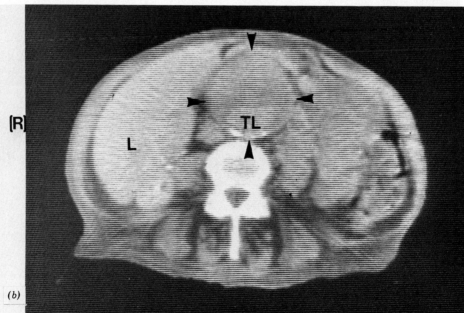

Figure 2-31 Abdominal aortic aneurysm. (a) represents the transverse ultrasound and (b) the postcontrast CT scan of the midabdomen in the same patient demonstrating the close correlation between the size of the aneurysm (arrowheads) and the size of the true lumen (TL). The clot is almost entirely anterior. L = liver; R = toward patient's right side.

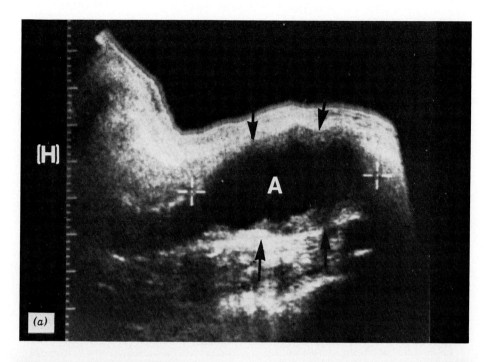

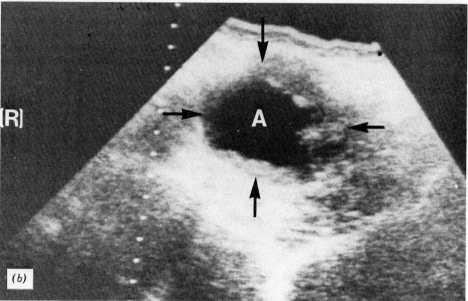

Figure 2-32 Fusiform aneurysm of the distal abdominal aorta. Midline longitudinal (*a*) and transverse midabdominal (*b*) are scans through a fusiform aneurysm (arrows) with considerably irregular intramural clot. A = aorta; H = toward patient's head; R = toward patient's right side.

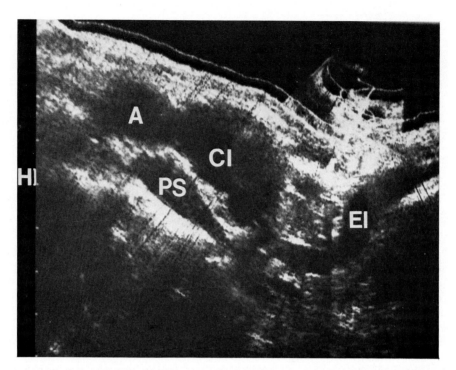

Figure 2-33 Oblique long-axis scan of the pelvis demonstrating an aneurysm of the right common iliac artery (CI) with ectasia of the external iliac artery (EI). The aneurysm of the iliac artery is an extension of an abdominal aortic aneurysm (A). PS = psoas muscle; H = toward patient's head.

level of takeoff of the aneurysm.[58,59] This is probably best performed on transverse supine scans and on longitudinal scans with the patient in the decubitus position. Although it is not always possible to demonstrate the exact relationship of the renal vessels to the aortic aneurysm, a high index of suspicion can be achieved, even if the renal arteries are not imaged, if the aneurysm approaches the origin of the superior mesenteric artery.

The morbidity and mortality rates of aortic aneurysm relate directly to the size of the aneurysm. However, although aneurysms less than 5 cm are said to rupture only rarely, in one study 10 percent of all ruptured aneurysms were 4 cm or less.[60] As aneurysms increase in size, the incidence of rupture did not rise significantly until a maximum diameter of 7 cm was reached, when rupture was reported in 60 to 80 percent of cases.[60] In addition, it has been shown that in small aneurysms, the likelihood of rupture becomes very much greater if significant enlargement is shown on sequential studies. It is, therefore, appropriate to reexamine even small aortic aneurysms 3 to 6 months after the initial diagnosis and at 12-month intervals thereafter to ensure that no significant increase in size has occurred.[61]

Not all aneurysms appear to grow in size during sequential examination. In one study, only one out of 12 showed significant enlargement over a period of 1 year, and these were subsequently resected.[62] Others, reviewing the growth

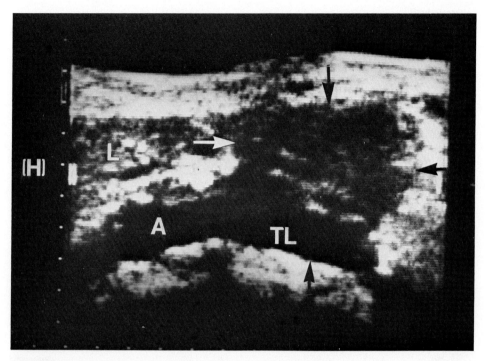

Figure 2-34 Longitudinal midline scan of saccular-type aneurysm (arrows) filled with clot. The true lumen (TL) of the aorta (A) is demonstrated. This type of aneurysm might be difficult to distinguish from an anterior tumor mass, and it is important in saccular aneurysms to identify the bright reflective aortic wall. L = liver; H = toward patient's head.

rate of small abdominal aortic aneurysms, concluded that there was a mean growth rate of approximately 0.4 cm per year.[61] Because of inherent inaccuracies in measurement and reproducibility, it is probably reasonable to consider only an increase in size of 5 mm or greater to be significant and, depending on the time course, a relative indication for surgical intervention.

Aortic Rupture

Symptoms and signs of aortic rupture are usually clinically obvious, there being severe central abdominal and back pain in association with a pulsating abdominal mass. Occasionally, there are signs of peritonism. Ultrasound can demonstrate aortic rupture with the identification of para-aortic hematoma, as evidenced by an echo-poor elliptical or rounded mass adjacent to the aortic wall. It is unusual to identify the site of the aortic rupture, although this may be inferred by the position of the hematoma.

The role of ultrasound, however, in the assessment of aortic rupture is dubious. Most surgeons would advocate emergency laparotomy in a patient suspected of aortic aneurysmal rupture, suggesting that delay for any diagnostic procedure produces a significant worsening of prognosis.[63] Thus, the technique

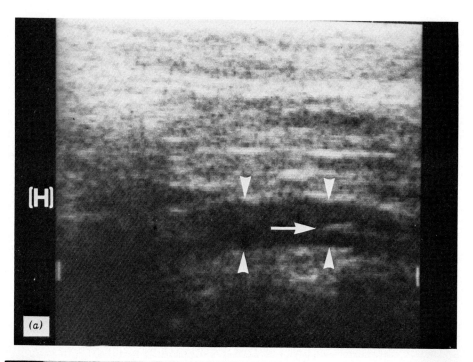

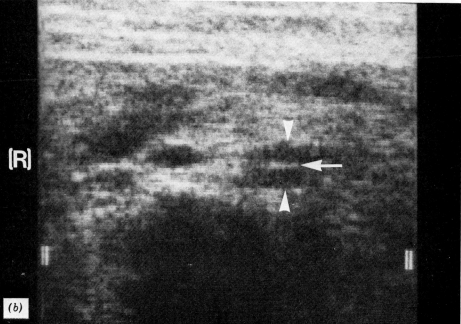

Figure 2-35 Longitudinal (*a*) and transverse (*b*) scans of an aortic dissection. The margins of the aorta are demonstrated by arrowheads. The intimal flap (arrows) was seen to move with each arterial pulsation on real time. H = toward patient's head; R = toward patient's right side.

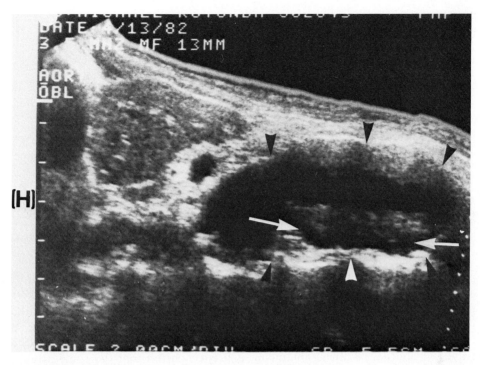

Figure 2-36 Longitudinal scan of a dissecting aortic aneurysm. The margins of the aneurysm are demonstrated by arrowheads. The area of the posterior dissection is indicated by arrows.

should be reserved for any case where there is reasonable doubt about the diagnosis.

Inflammatory aneurysms are an uncommon variant of atherosclerotic aneurysm, comprising between 5 and 10 percent of all abdominal aortic aneurysms. Patients have symptoms similar to acute aneurysmal rupture, and histology demonstrates prominent inflammatory cell infiltration of the aortic wall. Of importance is the fact that inflammatory aneurysms may be confused both clinically and by sectional imaging methods with either aortic rupture or dissection because of significant asymmetric thickening of the aortic wall.[64]

Aortic Dissection

Aortic dissection predominantly affects the thoracic aorta (types I and II), but may extend into the abdominal aorta (type III), where it may be demonstrated by ultrasound during routine abdominal examination (Figs. 2-35 and 2-36).[65] The intimal flap can be imaged as an echo-producing septum within the aortic lumen, and on real-time, motion of this intimal flap with aortic pulsation can be identified[66,67] It is not, however, possible to identify the true from the false lumen on the basis of this motion because, understandably, blood may be flowing through either channel in varying amounts.

SUMMARY OF INDICATIONS FOR ULTRASOUND OF THE AORTA[68]

1. Pulsatile palpable abdominal mass[69]
2. Questionable abdominal pulsation, particularly when the patient is difficult to examine and when the aorta may be unusually prominent in, for instance, a patient with kyphoscoliosis
3. Other clinical or radiologic findings suggestive of abdominal aortic aneurysm
4. Abdominal pain, particularly when referred to the back. In this instance, special attention should be paid to detection of leaking aneurysm or aortic dissection
5. Measurement and follow-up of known aortic aneurysm to assess interval growth
6. Following aneurysm repair to detect complications such as anastomotic aneurysm, hematoma, and infection

Although the use of ultrasound in the detection and assessment of abdominal aortic aneurysm is well established, with an accuracy of between 95 and 98 percent,[53,55] changes in surgical technique with improved morbidity and mortality rates, even for extensive aneurysms, may further enhance its role. At present, while ultrasound should be the modality of first choice in the investigation of abdominal aortic aneurysm, if it is suspected that the renal arteries are involved or that aneurysm is thoracoabdominal, then there should be no hesitation to perform contrast aortography. With improved resolution and the advent of pulsed Doppler linked to real-time gray scale equipment, it may be that intraabdominal aneurysms can be completely assessed by ultrasound. It is also possible that digital subtraction radiography will replace aortography in the assessment of thoracoabdominal aneurysms.

Aneurysms of Branch Vessels

Extension of aortic aneurysm into the iliac vessels can be frequently demonstrated, although if the aneurysm is small and localized then abdominal bowel gas may interfere with adequate imaging (Fig. 2-33).[70]

Aneurysms of the splenic artery are relatively common, but may be occasionally difficult to distinguish from adjacent bowel, especially if small (Fig. 2-23). Giant aneurysms of the superior mesenteric artery do occur, although they are rare, and have been demonstrated by ultrasound.[71] Similarly, renal artery aneurysms, most commonly due to fibromuscular dysplasia, may be demonstrated (Fig. 2-37).[51] It is important, however, to distinguish dilatation of the left renal vein and the associated aortic wall defect from a left renal artery aneurysm, and the distinction of this normal variant from an arterial aneurysm has been previously mentioned (Fig. 2-19)[37]

Vascular Stenosis and Occlusion

The presence of significant atheroma within the aortic lumen and within the branches of the aorta may produce aortic or branch stenosis. The addition of intraluminal clot may translate this stenosis into complete occlusion. Such

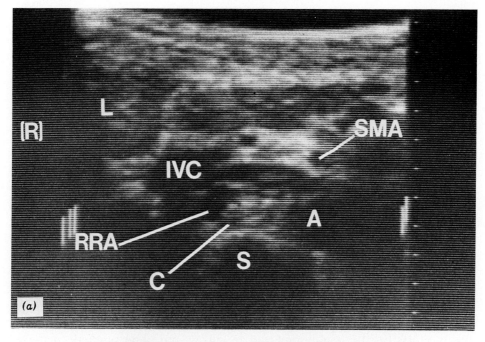

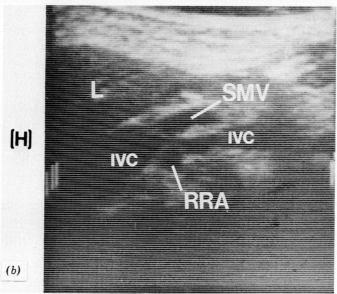

Figure 2-37 Branch aneurysm of the right renal artery (RRA) secondary to fibromuscular dysplasia. Transverse (*a*) and longitudinal (*b*) scans of the upper abdomen demonstrate an echo-free area beneath the inferior vena cava (IVC) representing the aneurysm. Note the rounded appearance of the distal right crus (C) on the transverse image. L = liver; S = spine; A = aorta; SMA = superior mesenteric artery; SMV = superior mesenteric vein; R = toward patient's right side; H = toward patient's head.

stenosis can usually be demonstrated in the aorta and within the iliac vessels if they are not obscured by abdominal bowel gas (Figs. 2-27 and 2-28).[49,52] Stenosis of other branch arteries is much less reliably demonstrated. Of particular interest, in this respect, are the renal vessels in the evaluation of systemic hypertension. There have been no reported cases of renal artery stenosis demonstrated by ultrasound, presumably due to the relative rarity of this entity and also due to the difficulty with which, by the standard approach, the renal artery is imaged. The use of the lateral decubitus position and duplex real-time/Doppler machinery will probably allow much more consistent identification in the future.

Occasionally, in the presence of fresh clot, complete occlusion of a vessel may not be detected by ultrasound.[72] Studies in the laboratory and in vivo have indicated that a fresh clot, for instance in hematomas, may be entirely echo free, thus mimicking the appearance of unclotted blood.[73] In one report, complete occlusion of the aorta was missed in three patients subsequently diagnosed by angiography and surgery.[72] It is to be expected that the use of pulsed, range-gated Doppler in the correct clinical situation would avoid this misdiagnosis.

Arterial Graft Surgery

Aortic grafts can be readily detected by ultrasound. The synthetic materials (usually Dacron) tend to generate high-amplitude echoes that are readily visible, and because the graft material is usually ribbed, it appears somewhat like an elongated concertina (Fig. 2-38). Postoperative complications can be identified, including anastomotic pseudoaneurysms, "aneurysms" in degenerated graft material, hematomas, seromas, and abscess formation (Fig. 2-38). The condition of the aorta proximal to the anastomosis may also be assessed.[74] Clinical findings may suggest a complication, but confirmation of the specific type and extent is essential for effective management. Pseudoaneurysms communicate with the lumen of the graft and usually are pulsatile masses. In most cases, ultrasound demonstrates abrupt termination of the graft wall in association with the fluid collection.[36] Pseudoaneurysms and hematomas frequently contain echoes attributable to clot aggregation. Abscesses and seromas are difficult to distinguish from hematomas except when the hematoma shows a considerable number of coarse echoes from clot aggregation. In this instance, a history of fever, leukocytosis, and local erythema suggests the diagnosis of abscess, while fine-needle aspiration confirms it.

Other Caliber Changes

Changes in caliber of the aorta and branch vessels are not always due to aneurysms or stenosis. Enlargement of branch vessels may be a result of enlargement of an organ (for instance, the spleen in hypersplenism), the presence of a large vascular tumor within an organ producing arteriovenous shunting (Fig. 2-39), or the presence of arteriovenous shunting from other causes (Fig. 2-40).[75] In these situations, both artery and vein are usually enlarged with the vein enlargement, due to its distensible walls, usually more marked.

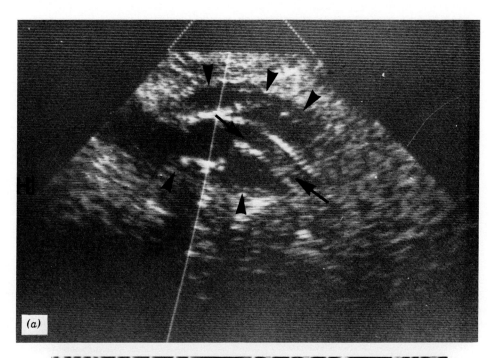

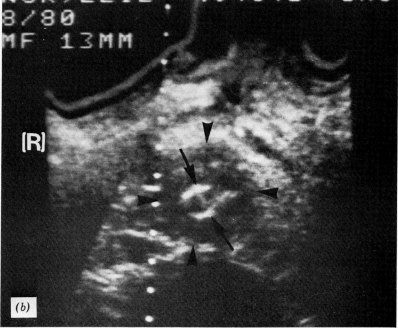

Figure 2-38 Longitudinal (*a*) and transverse (*b*) scans of the midabdomen demonstrate an aortic graft (arrows) surrounded by a complete area that proved to be a hematoma (arrowheads). H = toward patient's head; R = toward patient's right side.

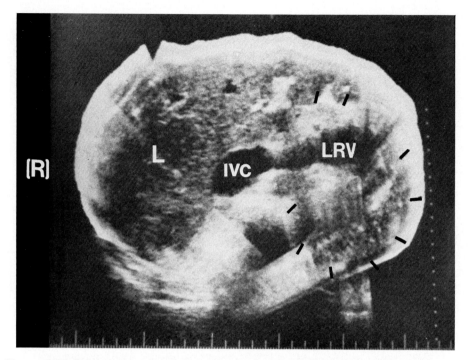

Figure 2-39 Transverse scan of the midabdomen demonstrating grossly enlarged left renal vein (LRV) as a result of arteriovenous shunting through a large vascular renal tumor (short lines). Note also the focal dilatation of the inferior vena cava (IVC). L = liver; R = toward patient's right side.

Reduction in caliber of the aorta or branch vessels is much less commonly seen, but in such disease entities as Takayasu's disease, neurofibromatosis, severe coarctation, or congenital infections, the aorta may be significantly narrowed throughout its length. The lumen is usually less than a centimeter in diameter. Comparison with branch vessels may reveal a similar diameter in such vessels as the superior mesenteric artery (Fig. 2-41).

ABNORMALITIES OF THE ABDOMINAL VENOUS SYSTEM

The Systemic Veins

The normal IVC can almost invariably be imaged in the upper abdomen, frequently throughout its entire length, and the normal changes in caliber of the inferior vena cava have already been discussed.[13,14,26,35] Reduction in caliber is difficult to assess, but there are few situations, such as IVC occlusion, capable of producing this effect. However, an increase in the caliber of the IVC occurs in two distinct situations: in increase in flow and in relative obstruction to flow. In congestive cardiac failure, venous return to the right heart is impaired, and the IVC is, therefore, significantly distended. In addition, there is reduction in

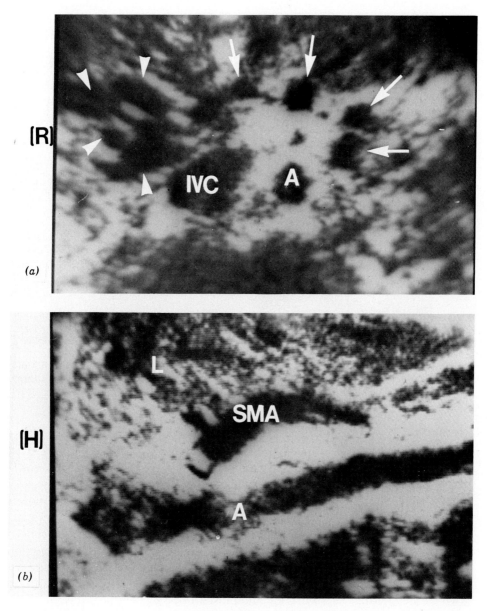

Figure 2-40 Spontaneous arteriovenous malformation of the abdomen. Transverse (*a*) and longitudinal (*b*) scans. The superior mesenteric artery (SMA) is demonstrated to be enlarged on the longitudinal scan. On the transverse scan, there are many large arteries (arrows) and veins (arrowheads). The patient was in high output cardiac failure with an audible bruit over the liver and upper abdomen. IVC = inferior vena cava; L = liver; A = aorta; R = toward patient's right side; H = toward patient's head.

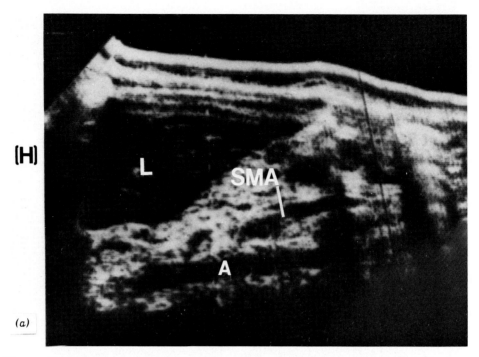

Figure 2-41 Takayasu's arteritis of the abdominal aorta. (*a*) Longitudinal midline ultrasonogram and (*b*) flush aortogram. Note the small aorta (A) and enlarged superior mesenteric artery (SMA). L = liver; H = toward patient's head.

the amount of variation in caliber that normally occurs with respiration and significant distension of the caval tributaries, particularly the hepatic veins.[34] When right heart failure is due to tricuspid insufficiency, there may be a significant increase in the transmitted venous pulse.[77] If the IVC distension is due to increased flow, this usually derives from abnormally high drainage through a tributary such as occurs in vascular tumors or arterial venous malformations (Fig. 2-39).[75] In these situations, there is significant dilatation of the venous tributary, for instance the renal vein in vascular renal tumors. There is often focal dilatation of the inferior vena cava at the site of junction between the IVC and its tributaries, and pulsed Doppler demonstrates torrential turbulent flow, which is only minimally affected by changes in respiration, through the affected vessel.

Demonstration of echoes within the inferior vena cava and its tributaries may represent evidence of either intraluminal clot or tumor thrombus (Figs. 2-42 and 2-43).[78,80,81,82] There is usually associated distension of the affected vessel with partial or complete occlusion (Fig. 2-43). It is not possible on ultrasound alone to differentiate between tumor and bland thrombus except in instances where the tumor invades the wall of the vessel and extends outside the vessel. When the diagnosis of venous occlusion is in doubt, Doppler has been used to demonstrate absence of flow.[80]

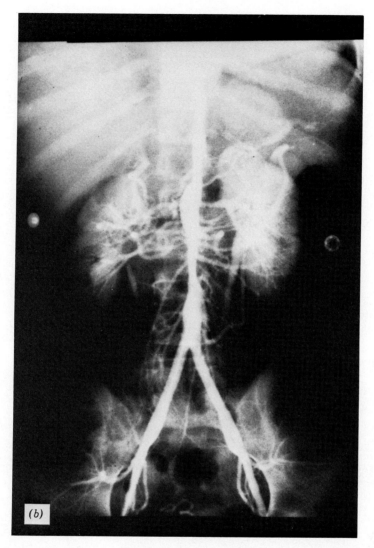

Figure 2-41 *(continued)*

Intraluminal echoes do not always derive from clot or tumor thrombus. The increase in use of caval umbrellas and similar devices produce bright intraluminal echoes, occasionally with distal acoustic shadowing.

Congenital abnormalities of the abdominal venous system are rare. Of these, the most common is absence of the normal right-sided IVC with hemiazigos continuation, appearing as an apparent left-sided IVC (Fig. 2-44). Similarly, a double IVC may occur, and while this must be distinguished from para-aortic adenopathy, it should not be too difficult to do so on longitudinal scan. There have been isolated cases reported of ultrasound demonstration of congenital vena caval abnormalities.[40,41]

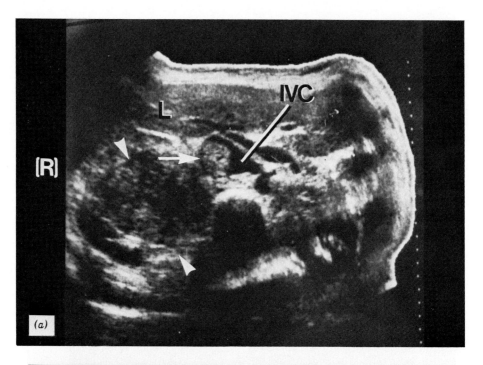

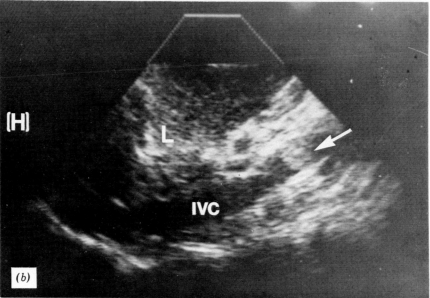

Figure 2-42 Supine transverse (*a*) and longitudinal (*b*) real-time sector scan 2 cm to right of midline demonstrate tumor thrombus (arrows) within the inferior vena cava (IVC) secondary to renal cell carcinoma (arrowheads). L = liver; H = toward patient's head; R = toward patient's right side.

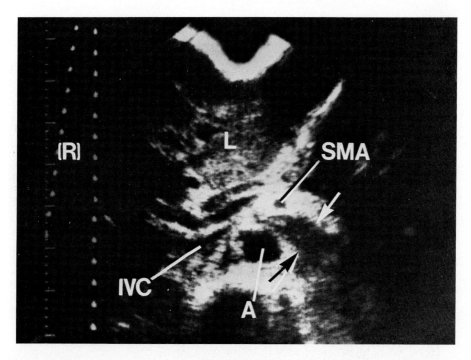

Figure 2-43 Transverse scan of the midabdomen demonstrating left renal vein thrombosis. The left renal vein is dilated (arrows) and contains low-level echoes in spite of the fact that the adjacent aorta (A) is completely echo-free. Variations in the phases of respiration did not alter the caliber of the left renal vein, and pulsed Doppler examination revealed no evidence of flow. Left renal vein thrombosis was confirmed by angiography. SMA = superior mesenteric artery; L = liver; IVC = inferior vena cava; R = toward patient's right side.

ABNORMALITIES OF THE PORTAL VENOUS SYSTEM

Although primary abnormalities of the portal venous system may occur, more commonly abnormalities of the portal vein and its tributaries are secondary to disease of the associated organs, specifically the liver and the spleen.

Portal Hypertension

Portal hypertension may be due to relative obstruction to venous flow in a posthepatic site (e.g., Budd-Chiari syndrome), hepatic site (e.g., cirrhosis), or prehepatic site (e.g., portal vein thrombosis). Of these, the hepatic causes for portal hypertension are the most common, but the vascular features of prehepatic, hepatic, and posthepatic portal hypertension are essentially similar.

In the past, diagnosis of portal hypertension by ultrasound has depended on the demonstration of an enlarged portal vein.[15] However, until recently there were no established normal values for the diameter of the portal vein as measured by ultrasound. Measurement of luminal diameter took origin from

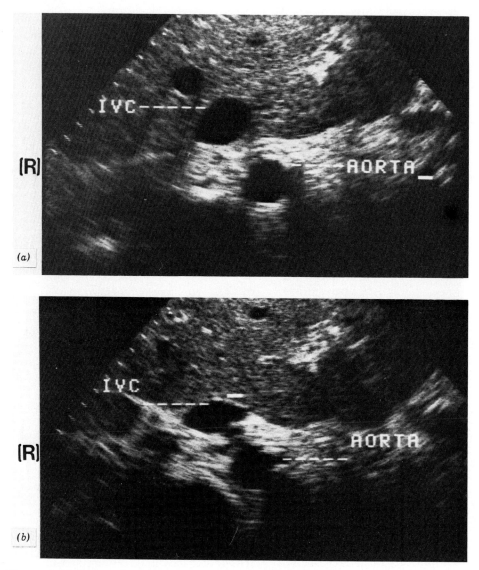

Figure 2-44 Series of transverse supine images demonstrating the proximal inferior vena cava in its normal position (*a* and *b*) then crossing to the left at the level of the left renal vein (*c*), finally becoming left sided (*d* and *e*). R = toward patient's right side.

comparison with morbid anatomic specimens and with portography, neither of which were strictly applicable to the ultrasound experience. However, in a recent series the normal cross-sectional diameter of the portal vein at its broadest point just distal to the union of the splenic superior mesenteric veins was established as 11 ± 2 mm.[85] It is suggested that a portal vein diameter outside this normal range is evidence of portal hypertension. Further corroborative evidence of portal hypertension includes the presence of splenomegaly and also the demonstration of portal venous collaterals. Thus far, the demon-

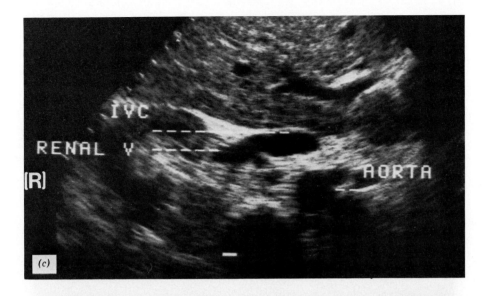

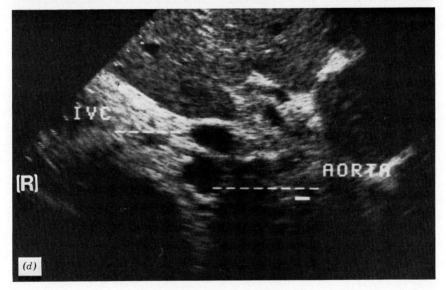

Figure 2-44 *(continued)*

stration of such collateral vessels has only been the subject of occasional reports.[47] However, recannalization of the umbilical vein has been shown to be reliable evidence of portal hypertension.[45,46] The frequency of umbilical vein recannalization in portal hypertension is unfortunately not documented, although Hale et al. noted that "in most examples of cirrhosis" the umbilical vein was patent.[86] Contrasted to this, however, a recent report noted the demonstration of a recanalized umbilical vein in only 11 percent of patients with cirrhosis secondary to alcohol abuse.[87] The visualization of the coronary vein, similarly, is more common in portal hypertension. However, it is also occasionally seen

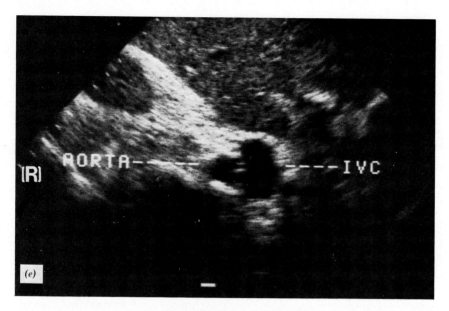

Figure 2-44 *(continued)*

in normal patients and, therefore, provides no absolute indicator of portal hypertension. Preliminary work on the use of duplex (real-time/Doppler) systems has shown that the assessment of portal venous flow is possible, and more specifically, the detection of reversal or hepatofugal flow is significant evidence of portal hypertension.[88] If Doppler findings are combined with recognition of the anatomic abnormality in portal hypertension, this may in the future be all that is needed for a diagnosis.[89]

Splenic enlargement is a usual concomitant of portal hypertension, but the spleen may be enlarged for reasons other than those associated with portal venous obstruction. In these cases, the portal vein may be similarly enlarged, simply due to increased flow as a result of the increased demands of the spleen.

Portal vein thrombosis usually occurs secondary to preexisting pathology. When it occurs in the newborn period, it is commonly the result of umbilical sepsis with propagation of infected clot along the umbilical vein into the left portal vein and thus into the main portal vein. While portal hypertension commonly ensues, there is generally only a finding of small intrahepatic portal veins within prominent fibrous portal tracts and evidence of portosystemic collateral communication. Not infrequently, however, there is cavernous transformation at the porta hepatis with collateral vessels providing direct communication between the patent portion of the extrahepatic portal venous system and the intrahepatic portal veins.[90]

In the older child and adult, portal vein thrombosis is usually caused by an acute abdominal infection or directly associated with hepatic pathology such as fulminant hepatitis. In these instances, liver swelling provides an acute relative obstruction to portal venous flow, and the subsequent stasis results in thrombosis. In this situation, intraluminal clot can be demonstrated within the portal

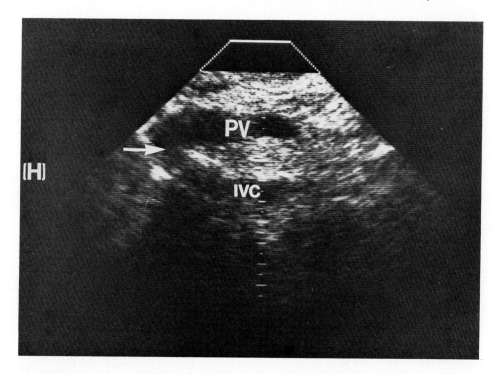

Figure 2-45 Supine longitudinal image demonstrates a portal-caval shunt (arrow). PV = portal vein; IVC = inferior vena cava; H = toward patient's head.

vein.[91,92] If the occlusion is complete, the outcome is fatal; if incomplete, then portal hypertension may ensue.

Portosystemic Shunts

Although the number of portosystemic shunt procedures performed has decreased in recent years, they are still used when the clinical situation requires diversion of portal venous flow. The demonstration of shunt patency is important to determine the efficacy of operations performed to decompress the portal venous system. Shunt procedures may involve the direct anatomosis of the portal vein or superior mesenteric vein with the inferior vena cava (Fig. 2-45). The status of these anastomoses is eminently suitable to evaluation by ultrasound.[93] Not only can the anastomosis be frequently identified directly, but also a focal dilatation of the inferior vena cava reflecting the increased blood flow at this level can be demonstrated. However, more recently, the procedure to divert blood from the proximal portion of the splenic vein into the left renal vein has been increasingly used. This anastomosis, occurring as it does in the "deep dark hole" of the left hypochondrium, is frequently very difficult to image by ultrasound. If ultrasound is to be used as an investigative procedure to evaluate the patency of such shunts, then pulsed Doppler techniques to assess the flow in the left renal vein would probably provide the most information. Indeed, this modality may be used to good effect in the

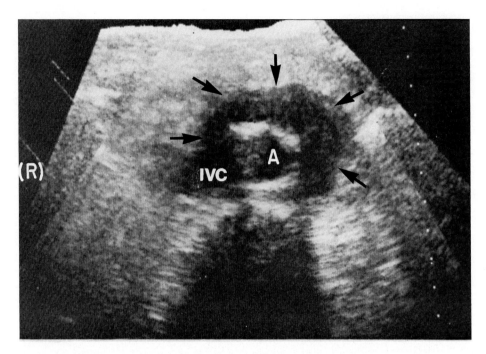

Figure 2-46 Transverse scan of the upper abdomen reveals a slightly nodular, poorly echogenic mass (arrows) draping over the aorta (A) and inferior vena cava (IVC) due to enlarged lymph nodes involved with lymphosarcoma.

assessment of all portosystemic shunts since alteration in flow may provide early warning of incipient shunt occlusion.

LESIONS DISPLACING THE MAJOR ABDOMINAL VESSELS

Since the major abdominal vessels course within the retroperitoneum, space-occupying lesions of the retroperitoneum may be expected to distort and displace the normal anatomy of these vessels. Although retroperitoneal inflammatory lesions, hematomas, and indeed spinal osteophytes may cause such displacement, the major causes are enlarged lymph nodes secondary to either metastatic disease or lymphoma and primary tumors of the retroperitoneum.

The Aorta

Para-aortic lymphadenopathy may occur in any of the lymph nodes that are present anterior, posterior, and to either side of the aorta (Figs. 2-46 and 2-47). The aorta may, therefore, be displaced anteriorly or laterally.[94] Because of the nature of the aortic wall and the fact that it is a high-pressure blood system, it is rarely, if ever, compressed. If there is extensive para-aortic lymphadenopathy, the aorta itself may be extremely difficult to visualize,[95] a

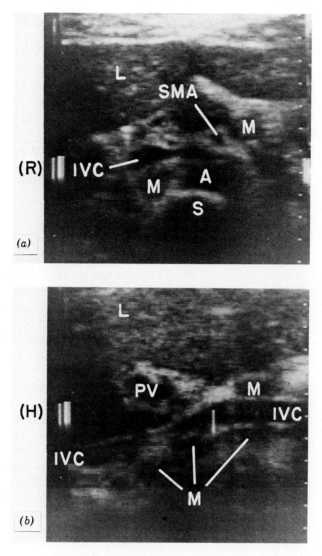

Figure 2-47 Transverse (*a*) and longitudinal (*b*) images demonstrate scattered enlarged lymph nodes involved with metastatic tumor (M). On the longitudinal scan, the enlarged lymph nodes are elevating the inferior vena cava (IVC). A = aorta; SMA = superior mesenteric artery; PV = portal vein, L = liver; S = spine.

feature that has been described as the "echo silhouette sign.[96]" This is probably the result of significant absorption of the ultrasound beam by the cellular tissue of the enlarged lymph nodes, except in those rare cases where the aortic wall itself is invaded by tumor. Displacement of the superior mesenteric artery and vein may provide valuable information as to the site of origin of a tumor in the region of the pancreas. Primary pancreatic tumors usually displace both vessels posteriorly, decreasing the angle between the superior mesenteric artery and the aorta, while adenopathy commonly displaces these vessels anteriorly.[97]

Rarely causing displacement of the aorta, but appearing ultrasonically as a relatively echo-free mantle anterior and lateral to the aorta, is the pathologic entity of retroperitoneal fibrosis. The appearances are of an anterolateral envelope of relatively echo-poor tissue without evidence of lobulation and without evidence of extension of disease posterior to the aorta, but occasionally with extension into the renal and paracolic fossae (Fig. 2-48).[98-100] Such an appearance is so characteristic of retroperitoneal fibrosis that it may provide a diagnosis without recourse to further investigation, particularly in the clinical setting of a patient having an ill-defined low back pain and medial deviation of the ureters on IVP. Not infrequently, retroperitoneal fibrosis is associated with other retroperitoneal pathology and occasionally with abdominal aortic aneurysm itself.[101]

The Inferior Vena Cava

The inferior vena cava may be displaced, compressed, and distorted by paracaval disease. The normal course of the IVC as a gentle sickle-shaped curve as it courses through the caval hiatus toward the right atrium has been described. Similarly, the normal impressions by the right renal artery, and occasionally by the head of the pancreas, have also been discussed. In cases of pancreatic carcinoma, involving the head of the pancreas, the impression on the anterior surface of the inferior vena cava becomes more marked and remains constant throughout all phases of respiration.[39]

Examination of the site of a posterior impression on the inferior vena cava may be of assistance in arriving at a differential diagnosis. In this context, Kurtz et al. have divided the inferior vena cava into three regions: (1) that lying cephalad to the portal vein representing the hepatic portion, (2) that between the portal vein and the inferior portion of the pancreas, the pancreatic region, and (3) below this, the intestinal region.[53] Lesions distorting the posterior aspect of the IVC in the hepatic portion can usually be ascribed to masses of adrenal or high retroperitoneal pathology; those in the pancreatic portion may result from a renal or vascular mass. Nodal masses and retroperitoneal tumors can occur in both of these areas, and these are the most common masses causing displacement in the intestinal part of the inferior vena cava (Fig. 2-49).[53]

Although many of the recent technological advances have resulted in greater improvement in the imaging of parenchymal organs than in the study of the tubular, echo-free structures that are vessels, certain recent developments have stimulated a recrudesence of interest in the further investigation of intraabdominal vascular structures. First, surgical techniques are being applied in a wider variety of intraabdominal vascular abnormalities. Second, improvement in resolution resulting from not only advances in digital processing but also in transducer design, including improved accuracy of transducer focus, half- and quarter-wave layered and matched transducers, and water-delay transducers, have allowed the smaller branch vessels to be identified with great frequency. The application of these technological advances to real-time equipment further enhances the applicability of this modality to intraabdominal vascular imaging. Third, the advent of duplex pulsed Doppler systems provides the facility for the assessment of blood flow within the abdominal vessels. In many instances

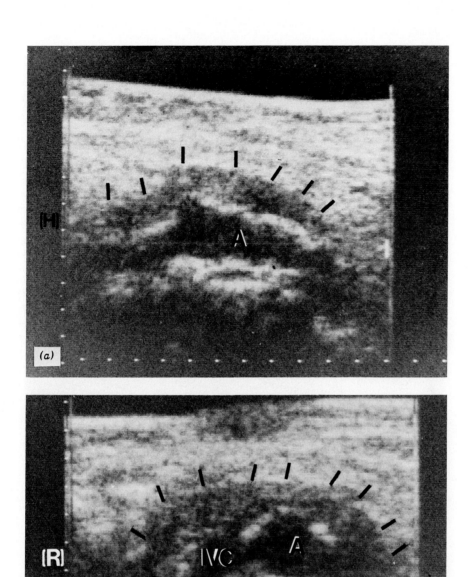

Figure 2-48 Retroperitoneal fibrosis. Longitudinal (*a*) and transverse (*b*) scans show an echo-poor mantle of proliferative fibrous tissue covering the anterior and lateral surfaces of the aorta (lines). The masses do not insinuate posterior to the aorta (A) whose posterior relationship to the spine remains constant. IVC = inferior vena cava; R = toward patient's right side; H = toward patient's head.

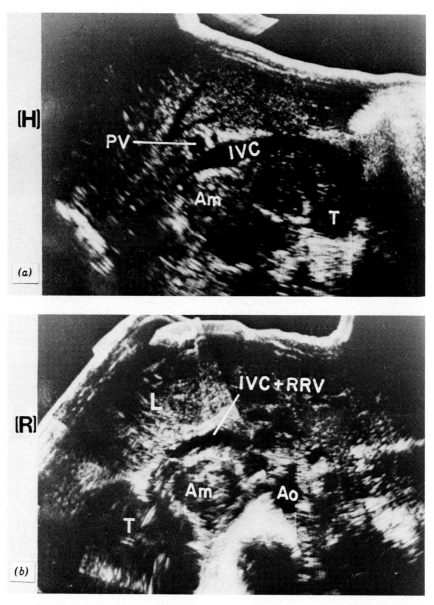

Figure 2-49 Renal cell carcinoma with adrenal metastasis. Longitudinal (*a*) and transverse (*b*) scans demonstrate anterior displacement and compression of the inferior vena cava (IVC) in both hepatic and renal portions by a primary renal carcinoma (T) that had extended posterior to the inferior vena cava. Just superior an enlarged right adrenal mass (Am) can be seen, due to metastic involvement, which is also elevating the inferior vena cava. RRV = right renal vein; A = aorta; L = liver; R = toward patient's right side; H = toward patient's head.

Doppler examination is largely qualitative, but this in itself is of value in the demonstration of patency or occlusion of vessels and in alteration of the nature or direction of flow. With the anticipated further improvement in ultrasonic image resolution and with the development of techniques for quantitative measurement of blood flow, ultrasound should remain a viable alternative to more invasive methods for the accurate delineation of vascular structures.

REFERENCES

1. Goldberg BB, Ostrum BJ, Isard HJ: Ultrasonic aortography. *JAMA* 198:353–358, 1966.
2. Segal BL, et al: Ultrasound diagnosis of an abdominal aortic aneurysm. *Am J Cardiol* 17:101–103, 1966.
3. Leopold GR: Ultrasonic abdominal aortography. *Radiology* 96:9–14, 1970.
4. Filly RA, Carlsen EN: Newer ultrasonography in the upper abdomen II. The major systemic veins and arteries with a special note on localization of the pancreas. *J Clin Ultrasound* 4:91–96, 1976.
5. Filly RA, Goldberg BB: Normal vessels, in: Goldberg BB (ed): *Abdominal Gray Scale Ultrasonography.* New York: John Wiley & Sons, 1977, pp 19–56.
6. Leopold GR: Gray scale ultrasonic angiography of the upper abdomen. *Radiology* 117:665–671, 1975.
7. Taylor KJW, Atkinson T, deGraff CS, et al: Clinical evaluation of Pulsed Doppler device linked to gray scale B-scan equipment. *Radiology* 129:745–749, 1978.
8. Barber FE, Baker DW, Strandness JR, et al: Duplex Scanner II: For simultaneous imaging of artery, tissues, and flow. *IEEE Ultrasonics Symposium Proceedings*, pp 744–748, 1974.
9. Crawford ES, Schuessler JS: Thoraco-abdominal and abdominal aortic aneurysm involving celiac, superior mesenteric, and renal arteries. *World J Surg* 4:643–652, 1980.
10. Darling RC, Brewster DC: Elective treatment of abdominal aortic aneurysms. *World J Surg* 4:661–667, 1980.
11. Sample WF: Techniques for the improved delineation of normal anatomy of the upper abdomen and high retroperitoneum with gray scale ultrasound. *Radiology* 124:197–202, 1977.
12. Raskin MM: Ultrasonography of the abdominal aorta, in Sarti DA, Sample WF (eds): *Diagnostic Ultrasound.* New York, G.K. Hall & Co., 1980, pp 226–243.
13. Taylor KJW: Ultrasonic investigation of inferior vena caval obstruction. *Br J Radiol* 48:1024–1026, 1975.
14. Gosink BB: The inferior vena cava: Mass effects. *AJR* 130:533–536, 1978.
15. Sanders RC, Conrad MR, White RI: Normal and abnormal upper abdominal venous structure as seen by ultrasound. *AJR* 128:657–662, 1977.
16. Carlsen EN, Filly RA: Newer ultrasonographic anatomy in the upper abdomen I. The portal and hepatic venous anatomy. *J Clin Ultrasound* 4:85–90, 1976.
17. Isikoff MB, Hill MC: Sonography of the renal arteries: Left lateral decubitus position. *AJR* 134:1,177–1,179, 1980.
18. Athey PA, Tamez L: Lateral decubitus position for demonstration of the aortic bifurcation. *J Clin Ultrasound* 7:154–155, 1979.

19. Marks WM, Filly RA, Callen TW: Ultrasonic anatomy of the liver: A review with new applications. *J Clin Ultrasound* 7:137–146, 1979.

20. Bartrum RJ Jr, Crow WHC: Real-time ultrasound: Its role in abdominal examinations. *Radiology* 133:823–824, 1979.

21. Atkinson T, Wells PNT: Pulsed Doppler ultrasound and its clinical application. *Y J Biol Med* 50:367–373, 1977.

22. McDicken WN, Anderson T, McHugh R, et al: An ultrasonic real-time scanner with pulsed Doppler and T-M facilities for fetal breathing and other obstetrical studies. *Ultrasound Med Biol* 5:333–339, 1979.

23. Loh C, Atkinson T, Halliwell M: The differentiation of bile ducts and blood vessels using a pulsed Doppler system. *Ultrasound Med Biol* 4:37–49, 1978.

24. Gill RW: Pulsed Doppler with B-mode imaging for quantitative blood flow measurement. *Ultrasound Med Biol* 5:223–235, 1979.

25. Kossoff G: Doppler. Its use in the abdomen and pelvis. The leading edge in diagnostic ultrasound. Atlantic City, NJ, 1981.

26. Cosgrove DO: Real-time: Its use in identifying abdominal tissues based on their motion. The leading edge in diagnostic ultrasound. Atlantic City, NJ, 1981.

27. Finberg H: Ultrasonic visualization of in vivo flow phenomena without introducing contrast material. Presented at the AIUM 1981.

28. Dubbins PA, Kurtz AK, Darby J, Goldberg BB: Ureteric jet effect: The echographic appearance of urine entering the bladder: A means of identifying the trigone and assessing ureteral function. *Radiology* 140:513–515, 1981.

29. Hollinshead WH: The abdomen and the pelvis, in Hollinshead WH (ed): *Textbook of Anatomy, ed. 3.* Hagerstown, Md, Harper & Row, 1974, pp. 655–666, 677–699.

30. Bartrum RJ Jr, Crow HC: *Gray Scale Ultrasound: A Manual for Physicians and Technical Personnel.* Philadelphia, WB Saunders, 1977.

31. Goldberg BB: Abdominal ultrasonography: Retroperitoneal structures, in Goldberg BB, Kotler MN, Ziskin MC, Waxham RD (eds): *Diagnostic Uses of Ultrasound.* New York, Grune & Stratton, 1975, pp 243–339.

32. Hassani N: *Ultrasonography of the Abdomen.* New York, Springer, 1976, pp 72–85.

33. Holm HH, Kirstensen JK, Rasmussen SN, et al: *Abdominal Ultrasound.* Copenhagen, Munksgaard, 1976, pp 75–87.

34. Weill S, Maurat P: The sign of the vena cava: Echosonographic illustration of right cardiac insufficiency. *J Clin Ultrasound* 2:27–32, 1974.

35. Walls WJ, Templeton AW: The ultrasonic demonstration of inferior vena caval compression: A guide to pancreatic head enlargement with emphasis on neoplasm. *Radiology* 123:165–167, 1977.

36. Grant E, Rendano F, Sevinc E, et al: Normal inferior vena cava: Caliber changes observed by dynamic ultrasound. *AJR* 135:335–338, 1980.

37. Sample WF: Renal, adrenal, retroperitoneal, and scrotal ultrasonography, in Sarti DA, Sample WF (eds): *Diagnostic Ultrasound Text and Cases.* Boston, G.K. Hall & Co., 1980, pp 268–279.

38. Kurtz AB, Dubbins PA, Zegel HG, et al: Normal left renal vein mimicking left renal artery aneurysm. *J Clin Ultrasound* 9:105–108, 1981.

39. Buschi AJ, Harrison RB, Brenbridge AN, et al: Distended left renal vein. CT/Sonographic Normal Variant. *AJR* 135:339–342, 1980.

40. Garris, JB, Kangarloo H, Sample WF: Ultrasonic diagnosis of infra-hepatic interruption of the inferior vena cava with azygos (hemi-azygos) continuation. *Radiology* 134:179–183, 1980.

41. Steinberg CR, Archer M, Steinberg L: Measurement of the abdominal aorta after intravenous aortography in health and artero-sclerotic peripheral vascular disease. *AJR* 95:703, 1965.

42. McNulty JG: *Radiology of the Liver.* New York, W.B. Saunders, 1977, pp 9–23.

43. Michels NA: *Blood Supply and Anatomy of the Upper Abdominal Organs.* Philadelphia, Lippincott, 1955.

44. Marchal G, Kint E, Nijssens M, Baert AL: Variability of the hepatic arterial anatomy: A sonographic demonstration. *J Clin Ultrasound* 9:377–381, 1981.

45. Ralls PW, Quinn MF, Rogers W, et al: Sonographic anatomy of the hepatic artery. *AJR* 136:1,059–1,063, 1981.

46. Rogoff SM, Lipchik EO: The normal lumbar aortogram, in Abrams HL (ed): *Angiography.* Boston, Little, Brown & Company, 1971, pp 732–733.

47. Callen TW, Filly RA, Sarti DA, Sample WS: Ultrasonography of the diaphragmatic crura. *Radiology* 130:71–74, 1979.

48. Glazer GM, Laing SC, Brown TW, Gooding GA: Sonographic demonstration of portal hypertension; The patent umbilical vein. *Radiology* 136:161–163, 1980.

49. Funston MR, Goudi E, Richter IA, et al: Ultrasound diagnosis of the re-canalized umbilical vein in portal hypertension. *J Clin Ultrasound* 8:244–246, 1980.

50. Kim YC, Handler SJ, Conroy RM, Glen WV: Multiplanar demonstration of spontaneous portal systemic shunt by ultrasound and computerized tomography. *CT, J Comput Tomogr* 4:10–18, 1980.

51. Fasani S, Bard R, Vonmieski LI: Ultrasonic investigation of the geriatric aorta. *Geriatrics* 30:154–155, 1975.

52. Winsberg F, Cole-Beuglet C, Mulder DS: Continuous ultrasound B-scanning of abdominal aortic aneurysms. *AJR* 121:626–633, 1974.

53. Kurtz AB, Rubin C, Goldberg BB: Ultrasound diagnosis of masses elevating the inferior vena cava. *AJR* 132:401–406, 1979.

54. Gordon DH, Martin EC, Schneider M, et al: The complementary role of sonography and arteriography in the evaluation of the atheromatous abdominal aorta. *Cardiovasc Radiol* 1:165–171, 1978.

55. Nusbaum JW, Freimanis AK, Thomsord NR: Echography in the diagnosis of abdominal aortic aneurysms. *Arch Surg* 102:385–388, 1971.

56. Wheeler WE, Beachley MC, Ranniger K: Angiography and ultrasonography: a comparative study of abdominal aortic aneurysms. *AJR* 126:95–100, 1976.

57. Maloney JD, Pairolero TC, Smith BE, et al: Ultrasound evaluation of abdominal aortic aneurysms. *Circulation* 56(II)80–85, 1977.

58. Leopold GR, Asher WM: Aorta, in Leopold GR, Asher, WM (eds): *Fundamentals of Abdominal and Pelvic Ultrasonography.* Philadelphia, W.B. Saunders, 1975, pp 146–163.

59. Raskin MM, Cunningham JB, Vining P, et al: Abdominal aortic aneurysms: Ultrasound versus computed tomography, in White D, Brown RE (eds): *Ultrasound in Medicine.* New York, Plenum Publishing Corporation, 1977, pp 531–532.

60. Lee RK, Wall WJ, Martin NI, Templeton AW: A practical approach to the diagnosis of abdominal aortic aneurysm. *Surgery* 78:195–201, 1975.

61. Sutton D, Gasner R: Ultrasound in the diagnosis and measurement of aneurysms of the abdominal aorta. *Postgrad Med J,* 53:741–744, 1977.

62. Darling RC, Messina CR, Brewster DC, Pottinger LW: Autopsy study of unoperated abdominal aortic aneurysm: The case for early resection. *Circulation* 56(II)161–164, 1977.

63. Berstein ES, Dilley RB, Goldberger LE, et al: Growth rates of small abdominal aortic aneurysm. *Surgery* 80:765, 1976.

64. Goldberg BB, Lehman JS: Aortosonography: Ultrasound measurement of the abdominal and thoracic aorta. *Arch Surg* 100:652–655, 1970.

65. Laurie GM, Crawford ES, Morris GC Jr, Howell JS: Progress in the treatment of ruptured abdominal aortic aneurysm. *World J Surg* 4:653–660, 1980.

66. Aiello MR, Cohen WN: Inflammatory aneurysm of the abdominal aorta. *J Comput-Assist Tomogr* 4(II)265–267, 1980.

67. Debakey ME, Henly WS, Cooley DA, et al: Surgical management of dissecting aneurysm of aorta. *J Thorac Cardiovasc Surg* 49:130–149, 1965.

68. Bresnihan ER, Keats PG: Ultrasound and dissection of the abdominal aorta. *Clin Radiol* 31:105–108, 1980.

69. Kumari SS, Pillari G, Mandon V, Bank S: Occult aortic dissection: Diagnosis by ultrasound. *Br J Radiol,* 53:1,093–1,095, 1980.

70. Hattery RR, Williamson B Jr, Wallace RB: Ultrasonic and computed tomographic imaging of the abdominal aorta. *World J Surg,* 4:511–519, 1980.

71. Shawker TH, Steinfeld AD: Ultrasonic evaluation of pulsatile abdominal masses. *JAMA* 239(V):419–422, 1978.

72. Gooding GA: Ultrasonography of the iliac arteries. *Radiology* 135:161–163, 1980.

73. Passariello R, Simonetti G, Rovighi L, Ciolina A: Characteristic CT pattern of giant superior mesenteric artery aneurysms. *J Comput Assist Tomogr* 4(V):621–626, 1980.

74. Anderson JC, Baltax E, Wolfe GL: Inability to show clot: One limitation of ultrasonography of the abdominal aorta. *Radiology* 132:693–696, 1979.

75. Wicks JD, Silver TM, Bree RL: Gray scale features of hematoma: An ultrasonic spectrum. *AJR* 131:977–980, 1978.

76. Wolson AH, Kaupp HA, McDonald K: Ultrasound of arterial graft surgery complications. *AJR* 133:869–875, 1979.

77. Thomas JL, Bernadino ME: Neoplastic-induced renal vein enlargement: Sonographic detection. *AJR* 136:75–79, 1981.

78. Thomas JL, Lymberis MEB, Hunt TH: Ultrasonic features of acquired renal arterovenous fistula. *AJR* 132:653–655, 1979.

79. Weill S, Eisencher A: Echo-angio structure hepatique: Etude echo-anatomique des structures canalaires intra parenchymateuses. *J Radiol Electrol* 57:311–319, 1976.

80. Sonnenfeld M, Finberg HJ: Ultrasonographic diagnosis of incomplete inferior vena caval thrombosis secondary to periphlebitis: The importance of a complete survey examination. *Radiology* 137:743–744, 1980.

81. Braun B, Weilemann LS, Weigand W: Ultrasonographic demonstration of renal vein thrombosis. *Radiology* 138:157–158, 1981.

82. Weinreb J, Kumari S, Phillips G, Pochaczgvsky R: Portal vein measurements by real time sonography. *AJR* 139:497–499, 1980.

83. Rosenfield AT, Zeman RK, Cronan JJ, Taylor KJW: Ultrasound in experimental and clinical renal vein thrombosis. *Radiology* 137:735–741, 1980.

84. Greene D, Steinbach HL: Ultrasonic diagnosis of hypernephroma extending into the inferior vena cava. *Radiology* 115:679–680, 1975.

85. Goldstein HM, Green D, Weaver RM: Ultrasonic detection of renal tumor extension into the inferior vena cava. *AJR* 130:1,083–1,085, 1978.

86. Hales MR, Allan JS, Hall EM: Injection-corrosion studies of normal and cirrhotic livers. *Am J Pathol* 35:909–941, 1959.

87. Schabel SI, Rittenberg TM, Javid LH, et al: The "bullseye" falciform ligament: A sonographic findings of portal hypertension. *Radiology* 136:157–159, 1980.

88. Foster DN, Herlinger H, Miloszewski KJA, Losowsky MS: Hepatofugal portal flow in hepatic cirrhosis. *Ann Surg* 187:179–182, 1978.

89. Tallett P, Wilson K: The investigation of portal vein haemodynamics in man using a duplex scanner. CV 114 Presented at International Congress of Radiology, Brussels, 1981.

90. Sassoon C, Douillet P, Cranfalt AM, et al: Ultrasonographic diagnosis of portal cavernoma in children: A study of twelve cases. *Br J Radiol* 53:1,047–1,051, 1980.

91. Babcock DS: Ultrasound diagnosis of portal vein thrombosis as a complication of appendicitis. *AJR* 133:317–319, 1979.

92. Merrit CRB: Ultrasonographic demonstration of portal vein thrombosis. *Radiology* 133:425–427, 1979.

93. Goldberg BB, Patel J: Ultrasonic evaluation of porta caval shunt. *J Clin Ultrasound* 5:304–306, 1977.

94. Spirt B, Skholnick I, Carsky E, et al: Anterior displacement of the abdominal aorta: A radiographic and sonographic study. *Radiology* 111:399–403, 1974.

95. Freimanis AK: Echographic diagnosis of lesions of the abdominal aorta and lymph nodes. *Radiol Clin North Am* 13:557–572, 1975.

96. Asher W, Freimanis A: Echographic diagnosis of retroperitoneal lymph node enlargement. *AJR Rad Ther Nucl Med* 105:438–445, 1969.

97. Weill S, Rohmer T, Zeltner S, Bihr E: Diagnostic ultrasonore des adenopathies lymphomateuses retroperitoneales: le Signe de la veine mesenterique. *Ann Radiol* 21:531–537, 1978.

98. Sanders RC, Duffy T, McLaughlin MG, Walsh TC: Sonography in the diagnosis of retroperitoneal fibrosis. *J Urol* 118:944–946, 1977.

99. Fagan, CJ, Larrieu AJ, Amparo EG: Retroperitoneal fibrosis: Ultrasound and CT features. *AJR* 133:239–243, 1979.

100. Bowie JD, Bernstein JR: Retroperitoneal fibrosis: Ultrasound findings and case report. *J Clin Ultrasound* 4:435–437, 1976.

101. Henry LG, Daust B, Korns ME, Bernhard VM: Abdominal aortic aneurysm and retroperitoneal fibrosis: Ultrasonographic diagnosis and treatment. *Arch Surg* 113:1,456–1,460, 1978.

Color Plates

SECTIONAL ABDOMINAL ANATOMY
E. A. Lyons

This section of the book is a small tribute to that which is consistent and perfect—the human body. The entire book is a large collection of the best gray scale images that can be produced by today's level of ultrasonic instrumentation. As has been witnessed since the 1970s, the prize pictures of the present rapidly become hopelessly unacceptable studies in the future.

The following pages display selected anatomical sections and labelled line diagrams. No representative ultrasound scans were used due to a space restriction as well as a strong feeling that even the best examples would only be a compromise on what we eventually will be capable of producing given the proposed, rapid advances in instrumentation. Anything short of an exact duplication of the anatomical specimen would be a compromise. Post mortem scans were attempted and were found to be unsatisfactory, due to an abundance of very strong interfaces, probably associated with changes in the fat planes. We were fortunate in that each post mortem specimen was received in the anatomy department within 24 hours of death. The criteria for our selection included the restrictions that no prior surgery had been performed and that the individuals should have died from causes that would not irrevocably distort their abdominal anatomy, although each one does, however, exhibit some deviations from the norm. To prepare the body, a special declotting solution was used to flush out the system and pulmonic vessels, followed by the introduction of red or blue latex solutions into the arteries or veins respectively.

In diagnostic ultrasound and, to a lesser extent, in computed tomography, recognition of the position of upper abdominal vessels is a great aid in delineating pathologic features.

A major advantage of this over other texts is that the user has greater ability to recognize readily arteries and veins by their artificial coloring and all other organs by their natural coloring.

The large number of structures labelled required the use of abbreviations. Because no standard nomenclature of anatomical abbreviations exists, one was created.

All of the individuals used in the following pages donated their bodies to the Anatomy Department at the Health Sciences Center in Winnipeg. This program was successfully initiated and promoted by Professor I. M. Thompson, Professor Emeritus and head of the Department of Anatomy, University of Manitoba, Winnipeg. We are indebted to him for his efforts and to the many individuals who have recognized the value of this program and have contributed to its success.

Finally, we would like to express our appreciation to the Medical Photography Department for its superb work, to Mr. Syd Bradbury for preparing the specimens, and to the Department of Anatomy for their continuing support and cooperation. Color photographs have been reproduced with the permission of E. A. Lyons. From Lyons, EA: *Color Atlas of Sectional Anatomy*, St. Louis: C. V. Mosby Co., 1977. Copyright 1982 by E. A. Lyons.

ABBREVIATIONS

access. spl. accessory spleen
acet. acetabulum
add. brev. m. adductor brevis muscle
add. gp. m. adductor group muscles
add. mag. m. adductor magnus muscle
ant. ext. ven. plexus anterior external venous plexus
ant.-lat. abd. m. anterolateral abdominal muscles
ant. long. lig. anterior longitudinal ligament
ant. rect. sh. anterior rectus sheath
ao. aorta
ao. aneur./thromb. aortic aneurysm (mural thrombus)
apon. ext. obl. aponeurosis of external oblique muscle
apoph. jt. apophyseal joint
asc. colon ascending colon
az. v. azygos vein
b. duct bile duct
cath. catheter
cath. bulb catheter bulb
caud. eq. cauda equina
c. b. d. common bile duct
cec. cecum
cel. a. celiac artery
c. i. a. & v. common iliac artery and vein
c. med. conus medullaris
corp. cav. (clit.) corpus cavernosum (clitoris)
corp. cav. pen. corpus cavernosum penis
corp. cav. (uret.) corpus cavernosum (urethral portion)
cost. cart. costal cartilage
costo-diaph. rec. costo-diaphragmatic recess
crus. diaph. crus of diaphragm
c. v. jt. costovertebral joint
d. d. p. v. deep dorsal penile vein
desc. colon descending colon
diaph. diaphragm
d. r. gang. dorsal root ganglion
duod. duodenum
doud. bulb duodenal bulb
e. i. a. external iliac artery
e. i. v. external iliac vein
emph. bulla emphysematous bulla
epicard. fat epicardial fat
erect. sp. m. erector spinae muscles
es. a. esophageal artery
esoph. esophagus
ext. obl. m. external oblique muscle
falc. lig. falciform ligament
fiss. lig. teres. fissure for ligamentum teres
f. p. a. first perforating artery
f. term. filum terminale
f. v. femoral vein
gastrolien. lig. gastrolienal ligament
g. blad. gall bladder

g. d. a. gastroduodenal artery
gem. m. gemelli muscles
g. e. vessels gastroepiploic vessels
gl. max. m. gluteus maximus muscle
g. med. m. gluteus medius muscle
gl. min. m. gluteus minimus muscle
gr. oment. greater omentum
h. a. hepatic artery
h. a. (br.) branch of hepatic artery
h. duct hepatic duct
hemiaz. v. hemiazygos vein
h. flex. (asc. colon) hepatic flexure (ascending colon
h. v. heptic vein
i. i. v. (br.) branch of internal iliac vein
i. l. a. & v. iliolumbar artery & vein
iliac. m. iliacus muscle
ilium ilium
i. m. a. inferior mesenteric artery
i. m. v. inferior mesenteric vein
inf. art. proc. inferior articular process
inf. pub. ram. inferior pubic ramus
intercost. a. & v. intercostal artery & vein
intercost. m. intercostal muscles
interv. disc. intervertebral disc
interv. for. intervertebral foramen
int. obl. m. internal oblique muscle
i. v. c. inferior vena cava
jej. jejunum
L1 lumbar vertebra (1st)
lab. maj. labium majorum
lam. lamina
lat. dorsi. m. latissimus dorsi muscle
l. c. i. a. left common iliac artery
l. c. i. v. left common iliac vein
lev. ani. m. levator ani muscle
l. g. a. (br.) branch of left gastric artery
lin. alba linea alba
l. oment. lesser omentum
l. o. v. left ovarian vein
l. r. a. left renal artery
l. r. v. left renal vein
lt. suprar. gl. left suprarenal gland
lt. suprar. v. left suprarenal vein
lumbar n. lumbar nerve
lum. pl. nerve of lumbar plexus
lym. n. lymph node
nuc. pulp. nucleus pulposus
obt. ext. m. obturator externus muscle
obt. for. obturator foramen
obt. int. m. obturator internus muscle
oment. bur. omental bursa
pamp. plex. pampiniform plexus
panc. pancreas
panc. (body) pancreas (body)

panc. (head)   pancreas (head)
par. perit.   parietal peritoneum
par. pl.   parietal pleura
pect. m.   pectineus muscle
pericard. eff.   pericardial effusion
pericard. fat   pericardial fat
periren. fat   perirenal fat
perit. cav.   peritoneal cavity
phrenic v.   phrenic vein
pir. m.   piriformis muscle
pl. cav.   pleural cavity
pl. rec.   pleural recess
prost.   prostate
ps. maj. m.   psoas major muscle
pubis   pubis
p. v.   portal vien
pyl.   pylorus
quad. lumb. m.   quadratus lumborum muscle
r. a.   rènal artery
r. c. i. a.   right common iliac artery
r. c. i. v.   right common iliac vein
rect. abd. m.   rectus abdominus muscle
rect. sh.   rectus sheath
ren. pyr.   renal pyramid
retrop. fat   retropubic fat
r. o. a. & v.   right ovarian artery & vein
r. r. a.   right renal artery
r. r. v.   right renal vein
rt. cor. lig.   right coronary ligament
rt. gast. a. & v.   right gastric artery & vein
rt. suprar. gl.   right suprarenal gland
rt. triang. lig.   right triangular ligament
r. v. sept.   rectovaginal septum
sac. canal   sacral canal
sem. ves.   seminal vesicles
ser. ant. m.   serratus anterior muscle
ser. post. inf. m.   serratus posterior inferior muscle
s. g. a. & v.   superior gluteal artery & vein

sig. colon   sigmoid colon (feces)
s. m. a.   superior mesenteric artery
s. m. v.   superior mesenteric vein
sp. cord   spinal cord
sperm. cord   spermatic cord
sph. ani ext.   sphincter ani externus
sph. ani int.   sphincter ani internus
spl. a.   splenic artery
spl. a. (br.)   branch of splenic artery
spl. flex. (desc. colon)   splenic flexure (descending colon)
spl. v.   splenic vein
sp. proc.   spinous process
st. gast. a. & v.   short gastric artery & vein
sup. art. proc.   superior articular process
sup. epig. a. & v.   superior epigastric artery & vein
sup. pub. ram.   superior pubic ramus
symph.   symphysis
symp. tr.   sympathetic trunk
T12   thoracic verterbra (12th)
test.   testes
thor. duct   thoracic duct
t. ileum   terminal ileum
trans. abd. m.   transversus abdominus muscle
trans. colon   transvcrse colon
trap. m.   trapezius muscle
urin. blad.   urinary bladder
u. r. pouch   uterorectal pouch
ut. cx.   uterine cervix
ut. fund.   uterine fundus
u. v.   uterovesical pouch
vag.   vagina
vag. n.   vagus nerve
vert. can.   vertebral canal
visc. perit.   visceral peritoneum
visc. pl.   visceral pleura
xiphoid proc.   xiphoid process

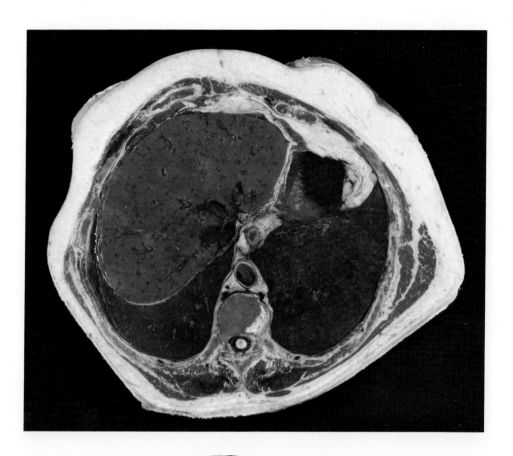

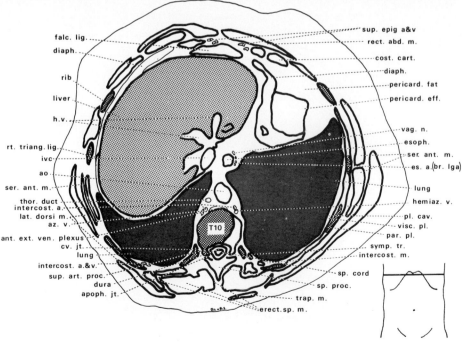

falc. lig.
diaph.
rib
liver
h.v.
rt. triang. lig.
ivc
ao
ser. ant. m.
thor. duct
intercost. a.
lat. dorsi m.
az. v.
ant. ext. ven. plexus
cv. jt.
lung
intercost. a.&v.
sup. art. proc.
dura
apoph. jt.

T10

sup. epig a&v
rect. abd. m.
cost. cart.
diaph.
pericard. fat
pericard. eff.
vag. n.
esoph.
ser. ant. m.
es. a.(br. lga)
lung
hemiaz. v.
pl. cav.
visc. pl.
par. pl.
symp. tr.
intercost. m.
sp. cord
sp. proc.
trap. m.
erect.sp. m.

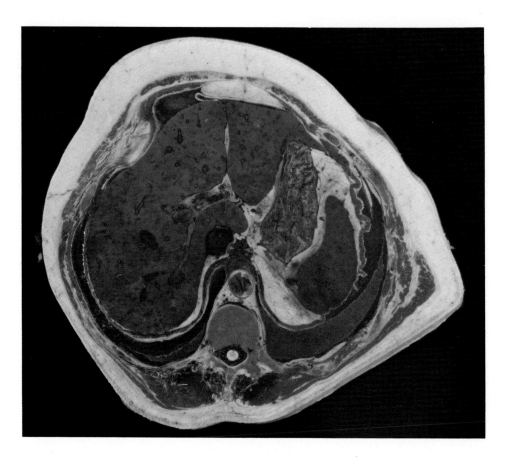

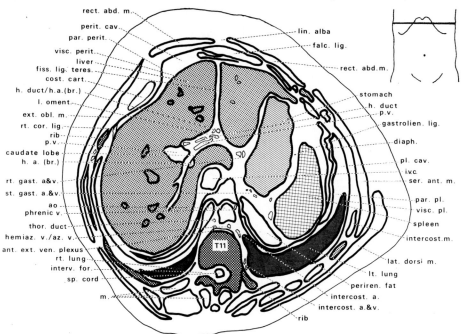

rect. abd. m.
perit. cav.
par. perit.
visc. perit.
liver
fiss. lig. teres.
cost. cart.
h. duct/h.a.(br.)
l. oment.
ext. obl. m.
rt. cor. lig.
rib
p.v.
caudate lobe
h. a. (br.)
rt. gast. a&v.
st. gast. a.&v.
ao
phrenic v.
thor. duct
hemiaz. v./az. v.
ant. ext. ven. plexus
rt. lung
interv. for.
sp. cord
m.

lin. alba
falc. lig.
rect. abd.m.
stomach
h. duct
p.v.
gastrolien. lig.
diaph.
pl. cav.
i.v.c.
ser. ant. m.
par. pl.
visc. pl.
spleen
intercost.m.
lat. dorsi m.
lt. lung
periren. fat
intercost. a.
intercost. a.&v.
rib

T11

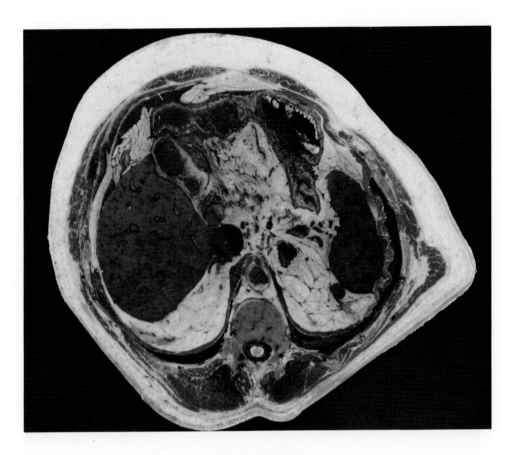

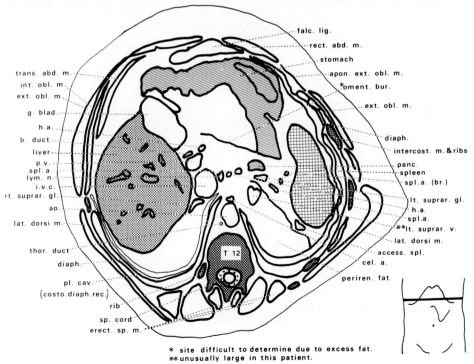

falc. lig.

rect. abd. m.

stomach

apon. ext. obl. m.

*oment. bur.

ext. obl. m.

diaph.

intercost. m.&ribs

panc.

spleen

spl.a. (br.)

lt. suprar. gl.

h.a.

spl.a.

**lt. suprar. v.

lat. dorsi m.

access. spl.

cel. a.

periren. fat

trans. abd. m.

int. obl. m.

ext. obl. m.

g. blad.

h.a.

b. duct

liver

p.v.

spl. a.

lym. n.

i.v.c.

rt. suprar. gl.

ao.

lat. dorsi m.

thor. duct

diaph.

pl. cav.

(costo.diaph.rec.)

rib

sp. cord

erect. sp. m.

T 12

* site difficult to determine due to excess fat.
** unusually large in this patient.

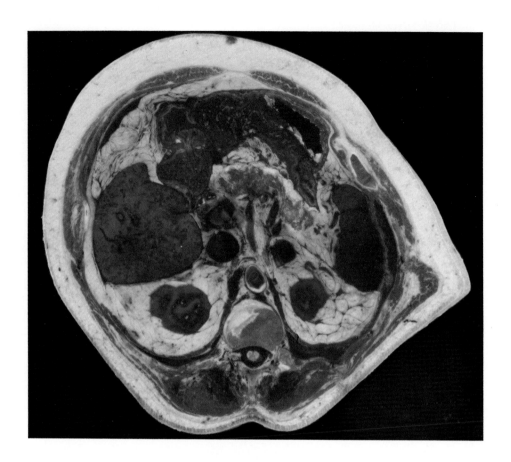

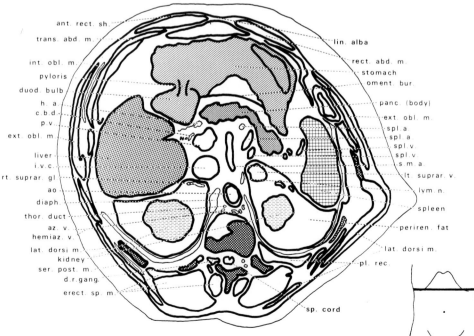

ant. rect. sh
trans. abd. m.
int. obl. m
pyloris
duod. bulb
h. a.
c.b.d.
p.v.
ext. obl. m
liver
i.v.c.
rt. suprar. gl
ao
diaph.
thor. duct
az. v.
hemiaz. v.
lat. dorsi m.
kidney
ser. post. m.
d.r.gang.
erect. sp. m.

lin. alba
rect. abd. m.
stomach
oment. bur.
panc. (body)
ext. obl. m.
spl. a
spl. a
spl. v
spl. v
s.m.a
lt. suprar. v.
lym. n.
spleen
periren. fat
lat. dorsi m.
pl. rec.

sp. cord

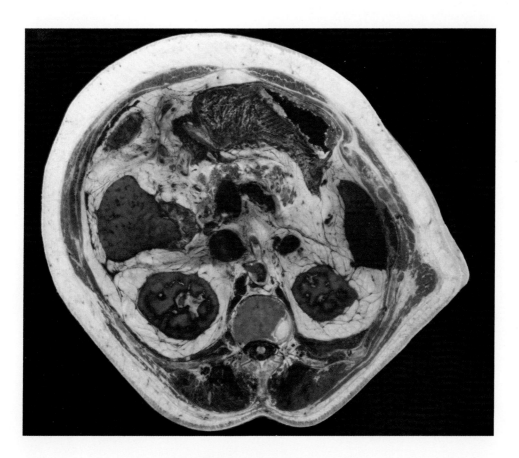

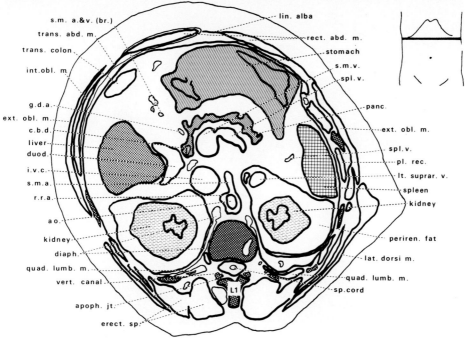

s.m. a.&v. (br.)
trans. abd. m.
trans. colon
int.obl. m
g.d.a.
ext. obl. m.
c.b.d.
liver
duod.
i.v.c.
s.m.a.
r.r.a.
ao.
kidney
diaph.
quad. lumb. m.
vert. canal
apoph. jt.
erect. sp.

lin. alba
rect. abd. m.
stomach
s.m.v.
spl. v.
panc.
ext. obl. m.
spl. v.
pl. rec.
lt. suprar. v.
spleen
kidney
periren. fat
lat. dorsi m.
quad. lumb. m.
sp.cord

L1

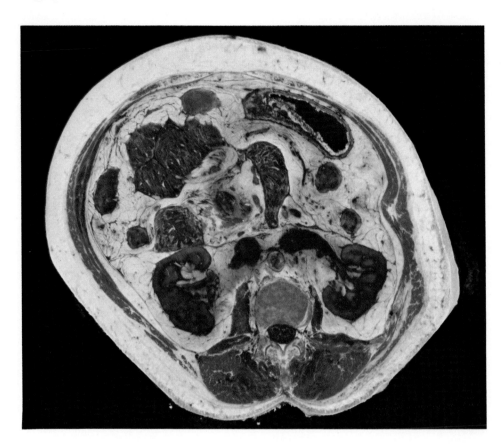

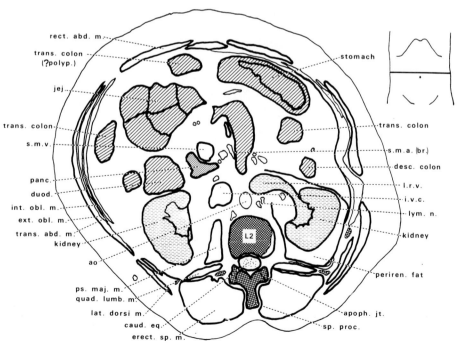

rect. abd. m.

trans. colon
(?polyp.)

jej.

trans. colon

s.m.v.

panc.

duod.

int. obl. m.

ext. obl. m.

trans. abd. m.

kidney

ao

ps. maj. m.

quad. lumb. m.

lat. dorsi m.

caud. eq.

erect. sp. m.

stomach

trans. colon

s.m.a. (br.)

desc. colon

l.r.v.

i.v.c.

lym. n.

kidney

periren. fat

apoph. jt.

sp. proc.

L2

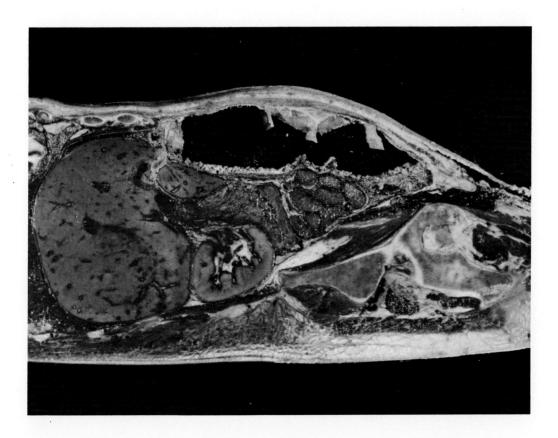

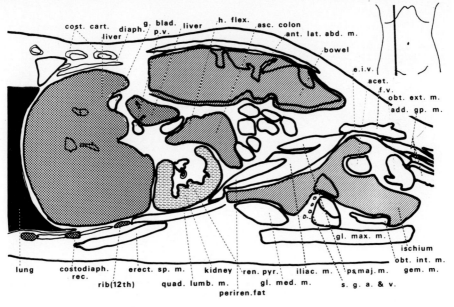

cost. cart.   diaph.   g. blad.   liver   h. flex.   asc. colon

liver   p.v.   ant. lat. abd. m.

bowel

e.i.v.

acet.

f.v.

obt. ext. m.

add. gp. m.

gl. max. m.

ischium

obt. int. m.

lung   costodiaph.   erect. sp. m.   kidney   ren. pyr.   iliac. m.   ps.maj. m.   gem. m.

rec.

rib(12th)   quad. lumb. m.   gl. med. m.   s. g. a. & v.

periren.fat

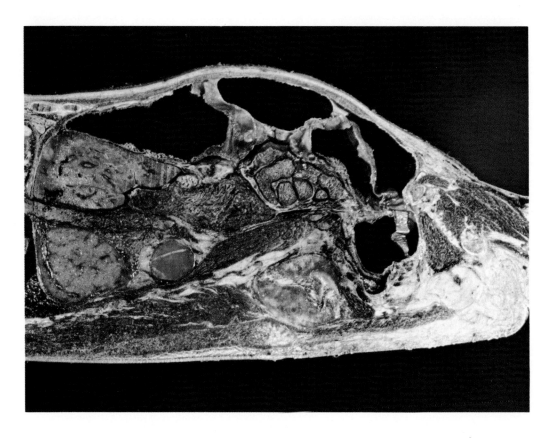

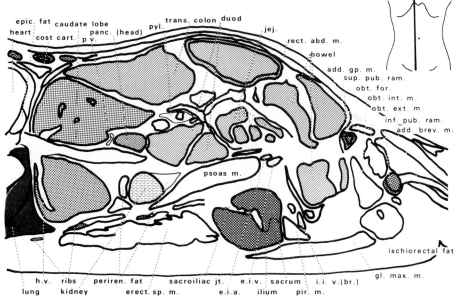

epic. fat caudate lobe trans. colon duod
heart cost cart. panc. (head) pyl. jej.
p v. rect. abd. m.
bowel
add. gp. m.
sup. pub. ram.
obt. for.
obt. int. m.
obt. ext. m.
inf. pub. ram.
add. brev. m.

psoas m.

ischiorectal fat
gl. max. m.

h.v. ribs periren. fat sacroiliac jt. e.i.v. sacrum i.i. v.(br.)
lung kidney erect. sp. m. e.i.a. ilium pir. m.

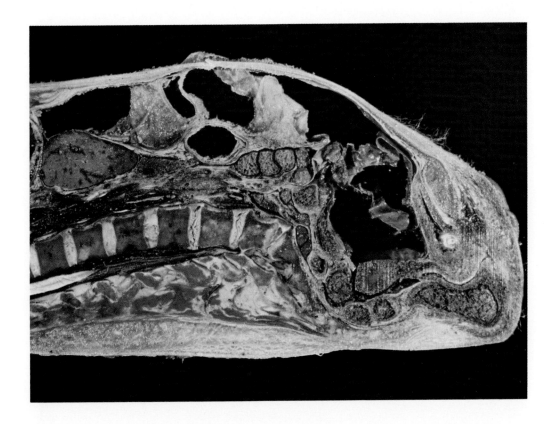

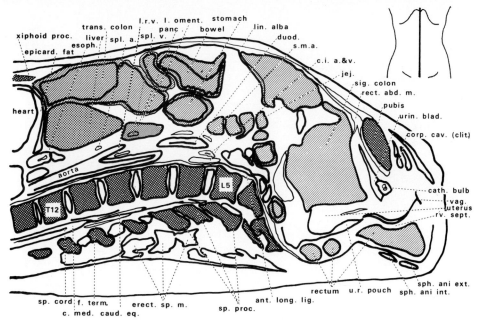

xiphoid proc.

trans. colon
liver   spl. a.   l.r.v. l. oment. stomach
esoph.   panc bowel   lin. alba
epicard. fat   spl. v.   duod.

s.m.a.

c.i. a.&v.

jej.

sig. colon
rect. abd. m.

heart   pubis
                                                urin. blad.

                                                corp. cav. (clit.)

aorta

L5   cath. bulb

T12   vag.
                                                uterus
                                                rv. sept.

                                                sph. ani ext.
rectum   u.r. pouch   sph. ani int.

sp. cord f. term.   erect. sp. m.   ant. long. lig.
c. med. caud. eq.   sp. proc.

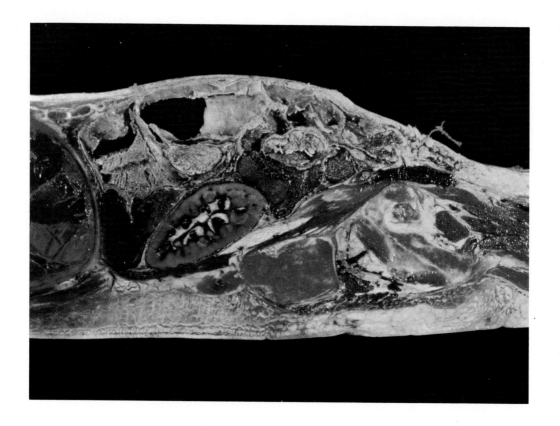

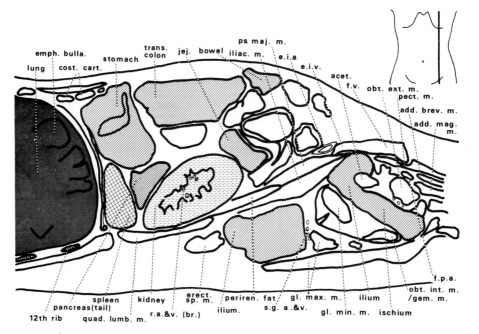

3

Liver

George R. Leopold

INTRODUCTION

As the largest soft tissue organ in the body, it has always seemed logical that the liver would be ideal for study by ultrasonography. Initial efforts, however, were hampered by its anatomic location. Since much of the liver is surrounded by ribs and air-filled lung, scanning was limited to the accessible subcostal portions. The alterations in acoustic impedance that occur with many types of pathologic processes were well beneath the recording threshold of early bistable devices. Although contour abnormalities were visible, meaningful information about the nature of parenchymal processes was obtained only in lesions that were cysts or cyst-like in composition.

Today, images of the liver are excellent, the result of a combination of improvements in technique and technology.[1,2] With increasing experience, the ultrasonographer has learned to image all portions of the liver with facility. Improvements in transducer technology and the introduction of gray scale capability have provided a wealth of new information about internal architecture of the liver. Additional information may be obtained in the future from more sophisticated signal processing. Research in this area seems quite promising.

SCANNING TECHNIQUES

Scanning the liver ordinarily begins with the patient in the supine position. The patient is asked to suspend respiration in deep inspiration. This brings the liver down from its subcostal position to a more accessible location. The vast majority of static scans are now performed with the single-pass, sectoring technique. This allows maximum resolution, since the image is not degraded by respiratory or vascular movement. Heavily compounded images, which were so common in bistable scanning, are no longer considered acceptable. The time-gain compensation of the instrument should be adjusted to provide uniform appearance of the parenchyma across the entire scan plane being studied (Fig. 3-1). The overall gain setting or sensitivity level should be the lowest that produces parenchymal echoes—allowing the detection of both echogenic and echolucent processes.

Transducer selection plays a major role in the quality of hepatic images obtained. While most early studies employed the 2.25-MHz transducer, design

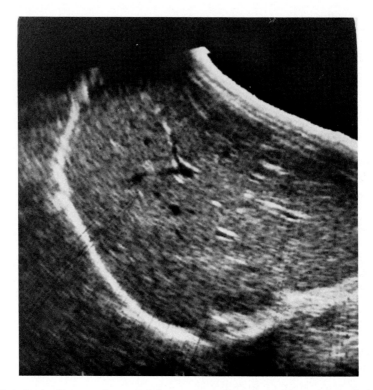

Figure 3-1 Sagittal scan of normal liver. Note the even echogenicity of the hepatic parenchyma interrupted only by hepatic veins.

improvements now make 3.5-MHz transducer the choice for routine scanning. For children and smaller adults, 5 MHz is perfectly adequate, and the increase in frequency produces striking improvement in resolution. Transducers may also be described in terms of their focal length. While medium focal length is usually chosen for routine scanning, there are situations where both short- and long-focus transducers are useful in studying specific areas of interest.

Excellent quality images may be obtained using either static or real-time equipment. Static images are usually obtained in a series of both transverse and sagittal planes. The scan planes should be separated by no more than 1 cm.

When only real time is used, the examiner visually inspects all areas of the liver and records only those images that are of interest. While linear array scans can be used, sector scanners are preferred since they allow better access to narrow areas such as the intercostal spaces. Unfortunately, these images are pie-shaped and frequently are difficult to explain to colleagues who have not actually witnessed the study.

While supine scanning is the usual approach, there are times when coronal scanning in the left lateral decubitus position produces better results. This is usually limited to obese patients or to those with considerable gaseous distension. Using one or both of these approaches, a complete study of the liver is possible in nearly all patients.

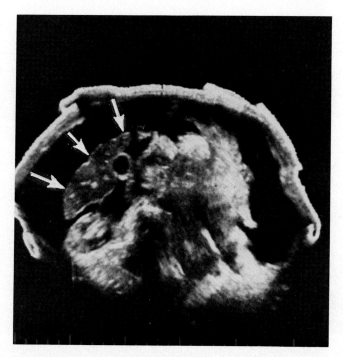

Figure 3-2 Transverse scan. The brightness of the capsular echo (arrowheads) is readily apparent in this patient with a large amount of ascites.

NORMAL ANATOMY

Surface Anatomy

The Capsule

The liver is completely invested with a dense fibrous capsule (Glisson's) that surrounds it and accompanies the portal vessels for a portion of their intrahepatic course. The capsule is a specular reflector, therefore producing a high-intensity echo that readily allows identification of the hepatic perimeter. It is the echo source that made a crude evaluation of the liver (size, shape) with bistable equipment possible. When significant ascites surrounds the liver and separates it from the abdominal wall and/or the right kidney, visualization of the liver is often improved (Fig. 3-2). Careful attention should be given to this structure since it may supply valuable diagnostic information. A smooth contour, for example, is seen in normals and patients with the usual alcoholic (micronodular type of cirrhosis, while a lumpy contour is seen in patients with postnecrotic (macronodular) cirrhosis or metastatic disease. The capsule is also helpful in assessing the location of fluid collections around the periphery of the liver. With extracapsular collections, the dense echo of the capsule is immediately adjacent to liver parenchyma. When the fluid collection lies beneath the liver capsule, no distinct bright echo can be identified separating it from the parenchyma—the edges of the fluid collection merge almost imperceptibly

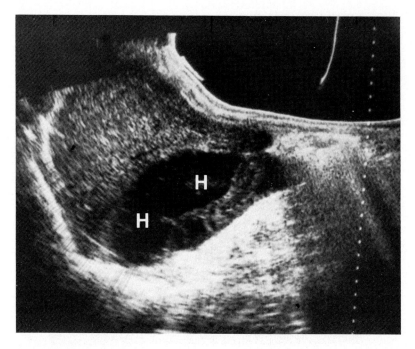

Figure 3-3 Sagittal scan. The posteriorly located fluid collection is a partially organized subcapsular hematoma (H).

with the liver parenchyma (Fig. 3-3). Such a distinction may have considerable clinical importance.

Diaphragmatic Surface
The diaphragmatic surface is usually easier to examine in sagittal scans. Like the capsule, it is a strong specular reflector and readily identified. In the normal patient, this echo blends with the capsule of the superior surface of the liver to produce an extremely echogenic structure. Identification of this echo usually permits ready distinction between supra and subdiaphragmatic fluid collections or masses. When the right hemidiaphragm is inverted by a pathologic process in the chest, this can be demonstrated on longitudinal scans. It should be noted that in such cases, transverse scans can be misleading, since the process itself may, at first glance, appear to be intrahepatic. This difficulty is well known to those doing computed body tomography, where analysis is primarily based on transverse sections.

The curved nature of the diaphragm causes an interesting effect on liver ultrasonograms. It is common for the initial reflections from the diaphragm to strike the transducer and reradiate into hepatic tissue. This phenomenon produces an appearance of hepatic parenchyma on the scan that is clearly supradiaphragmatic in location and may confuse the uninitiated (Fig. 3-4).[3] In some cases, cystic lesions near the dome of the liver actually appear as a mirror image on the lung side of the diaphragm. These effects are eliminated when a

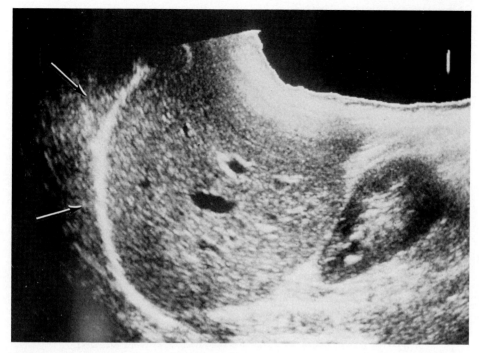

Figure 3-4 Sagittal scan. Apparent "parenchymal" echoes are seen in a supradiaphragmatic location (arrows).

thoracic mass or fluid collection is adjacent to the thoracic surface of the diaphragm (Fig. 3-5).

Attention should also be given to the diaphragmatic contour to detect unusual flattening, suggesting pulmonary emphysema, and localized bulges that may indicate the site of eventration or diaphragmatic hernia. Superimposed inspiration and expiration scans readily document the presence, direction, and magnitude of diaphragmatic excursion (Fig. 3-6). This is more easily done by direct observation with real-time scanning.

The appearance of the subdiaphragmatic space when considerable ascites is present deserves special comment. On sagittal scans performed far laterally, it is possible for fluid to separate completely the liver from the diaphragm. More medially, however, in the area between the right and left triangular ligaments of the liver lies the so-called "bare area"—the only portion of the organ not covered by peritoneum. Sagittal scans through this area therefore show the liver in contact with the diaphragm, since it is impossible for ascites to enter this space.

Falciform Ligament

The falciform ligament, an important surface anatomic feature of the liver, has great importance to the ultrasonographer. On opening the abdomen, this broad fold of the anterior parietal peritoneum may be seen extending from the region of the umbilicus upward and posteriorly to bisect the left lobe of the liver.

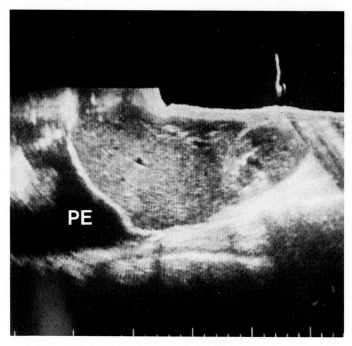

Figure 3-5 Sagittal scan. In this patient with a large right pleural effusion (PE), the spurious supradiaphragmatic echoes are not present.

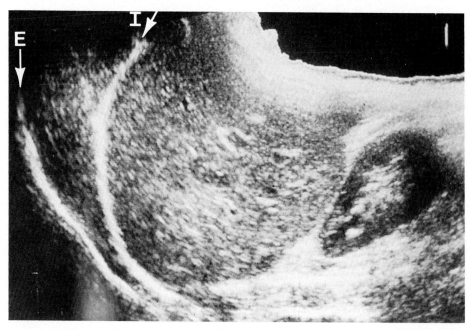

Figure 3-6 Sagittal scan. Inspiration (I) and expiration (E) superimposed. Motion of the diaphragm is clearly present.

Superiorly it is attached to the diaphragm. It is composed of two distinct layers of peritoneum, and within its posterior edge lies the umbilical vein—usually obliterated in adult life and referred to as the ligamentum teres (round ligament).

Early anatomists considered the falciform ligament the structure dividing the right and left lobes of the liver. More careful studies however, on the basis of blood supply, show that it, in fact, separates the medial and lateral segments of the left lobe.[4] Since the intrahepatic portion of the falciform (or a portion of it) is seen on many transverse scans of the left lobe, it is an important structure in describing the intrahepatic location of focal disease processes.

Ultrasonic scans show this segment of the falciform ligament as a highly echogenic focus within the left lobe (Fig 3-7). This echo is so strong that it was frequently visualized on bistable scanning. Older texts refer to this as the "left lobe artifact" and ascribe the appearance to a reverberation from the overlying rectus sheath. It is now known, primarily from CT scanning, that the echogenicity stems from the small collection of fat that surrounds the ligament at this point.[5] Being aware of the characteristic location and appearance of this structure prevents its misdiagnosis as a metastasis or other pathologic process. On many occasions, a discrete shadow can be seen emanating from the falciform (Fig. 3-8). This is believed to be due to the cord-like fibrous nature of the round ligament.

Anterior to the left lobe of the liver near the midline, an echolucent collection is seen in many heavier patients (Figs. 3-9, and 3-10). This was a source of confusion to early ultrasonographers, frequently being mistaken for a perihepatic fluid collection. Computed body tomography has been helpful in clarifying this situation and identifying it as a collection of fat into which the falciform ligament inserts.[5] As has been noted in other areas of the body, fat may be either echodense or echolucent—probably depending on the amount of water and fibrous tissue that it contains. Again, recognition of this characteristic appearance and location should preclude diagnostic difficulties.

In the normal person the extrahepatic portion of the falciform ligament is not visible ultrasonically, while it may be readily identified in patients with ascites (Fig. 3-11). Since it is a specular reflector and therefore, highly dependent upon correct scanning angle for demonstration, real-time study is usually the simplest way to demonstrate it. If portal hypertension is present, the venous structures within the falciform may be a route of collateral flow, and pulsation can often be recognized if real time is used. The ligament itself is usually very lax and can be observed to flap like a sail in the breeze.

Cardiac Confusion

Neophyte scanners are often startled by the appearance of a multiseptated cyst appearing in the center of the left lobe of the liver on transverse scans (Fig. 3-12). Sagittal scanning however, readily demonstrates that this is the heart, sitting in a depression on the top of the liver and clearly supradiaphragmatic in location (Fig. 3-13). Real-time scanning will, of course, demonstrate characteristic cardiac motion and help to prevent making this misinterpretation.

While performing sagittal scanning of the left lobe, one should pay attention to the relationship of the heart to the liver since it may be possible to recognize

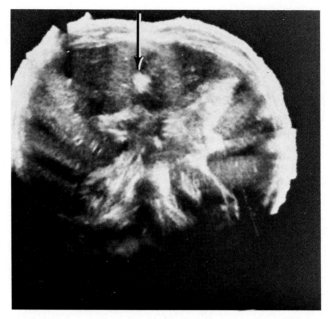

Figure 3-7 Transverse scan. The echogenic focus (arrow) dividing the medial and lateral segments of the left lobe is due to fat around the falciform ligament.

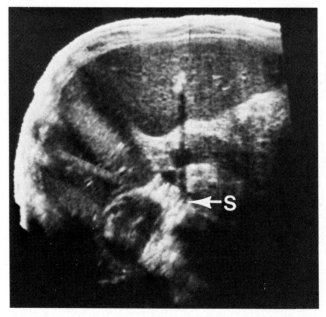

Figure 3-8 Transverse scan. Discrete shadowing (S) is noted from the fibrous ligamentum teres.

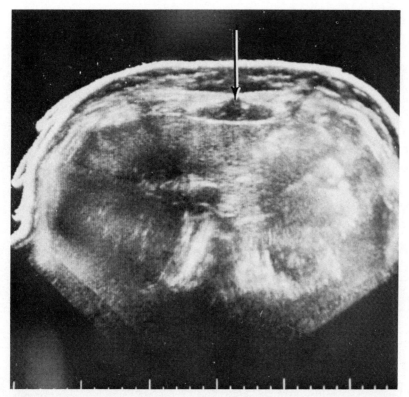

Figure 3-9 Transverse scan. An area of lucency (arrow) is seen anterior to the left lobe of the liver.

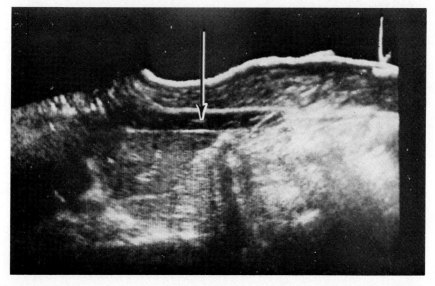

Figure 3-10 Sagittal scan. The same area (arrow) as in Figure 3-9 is seen and represents a collection of fat (into which the falciform ligament inserts).

89

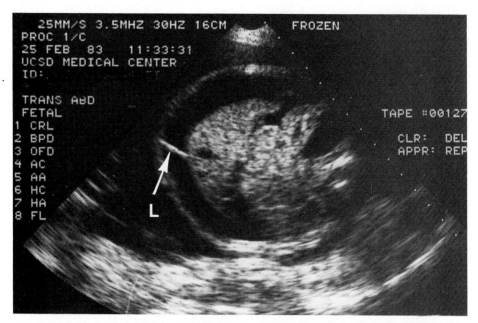

Figure 3-11 Transverse scan of fetal abdomen. In this fetus with marked ascites, the falciform ligament (arrow) attaching the liver (L) to the anterior abdominal wall is clearly seen.

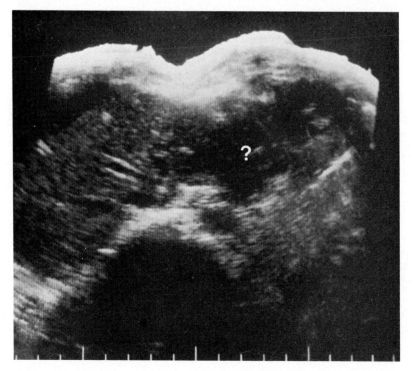

Figure 3-12 Transverse scan. A "cystic" area (?) is noted in the region of the left lobe of the liver.

90

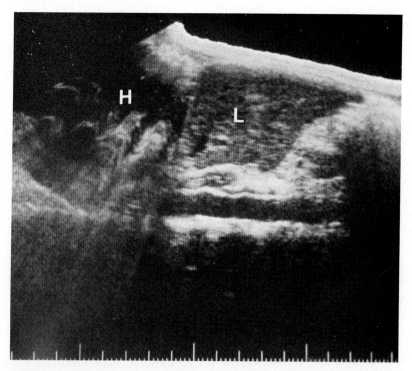

Figure 3-13 Sagittal scan of same patient as Figure 3-9. The cystic mass is seen to be the heart (H) (note pulsatile structures and supradiaphragmatic location).

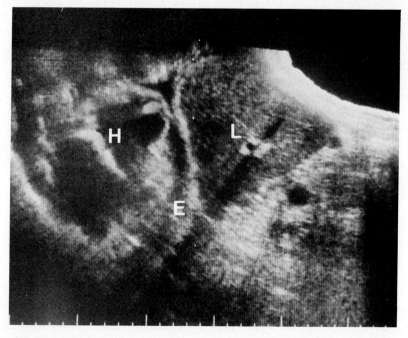

Figure 3-14 Sagittal scan. A pericardial effusion (E) separates the heart (H) and the liver (L).

pericardial effusion separating the two (Fig. 3-14). This can be done with either static or real-time scanning. In such instances, a complete echocardiographic study should be performed as the appearance of separation may occasionally be due to an abundance of either intra or extrapericardial fat.

The Liver Parenchyma

In contrast to the intrahepatic void seen on bistable scanning, current ultrasound images provide exquisite anatomic detail of the liver parenchyma. If the equipment functions properly, the background of the liver should appear as a low level shade of gray that is uniform throughout the liver. While most equipment produces discrete parenchymal echoes, other manufacturers lean toward a type of signal processing that produces a "softer" image that causes confluence of these echoes. Controversy exists as to which method is better for recognizing focal abnormalities. It is likely that both presentations have strengths and weaknesses. The sophisticated machines of the future will probably be able to extract considerably more information from these patterns than is currently possible.

Incorrect setting of the time-gain compensation of the instrument produces images that give undue emphasis to one portion of the liver. Care should be used in making this adjustment so that reflections of equal strength appear similar throughout the plane of the scan. In addition to this pitfall, focusing the transducer may also result in an artifactual appearance that may be confusing. Since within the focal zone of the transducer the beam is narrower, there is more sound energy per unit area, and the result is a swath of increased echogenicity through the midzone of the liver (Fig. 3-15). At times this may simulate a lesion. It can be avoided by making minor TGC adjustments in the regions of the beam that lie outside the focal zone of the transducer. As mentioned above, both short- and long-focus transducers may be helpful in specific cases to better characterize an abnormality.

Superimposed on the hepatic parenchymal pattern are the tubular systems that traverse the liver. Most workers feel that only the two venous networks (systemic and portal) are visible in normal patients. It is true, however, that the main right and left hepatic biliary ducts are frequently imaged where they parallel the corresponding branches of the portal vein. In most cases, a distinction between the two venous systems can be made with ease. Advantage is taken of the fact that the portal venous branches are accompanied by other structures such as the capsule, hepatic arteries, and bile ducts, which while not recognizable as individual entities, do succeed in producing bright echoes at the edge of the portal veins. Systemic hepatic veins, which travel unaccompanied, show no such boundary echoes (Fig. 3-16). Although this is a good general rule, it is apparent that some of the larger hepatic veins also demonstrate this finding near their entrance into the inferior vena cava (Fig. 3-17).[6] Differentiation is also simplified with real-time scanning, since the vessel in question may be easily traced to either the inferior vena cava or the portal vein. When dilatation of the bile ducts is present, an extra set of tubular structures appears within the liver. In most cases, they are readily differentiated from the intrahepatic veins by the acoustic enhancement posterior to the former. This

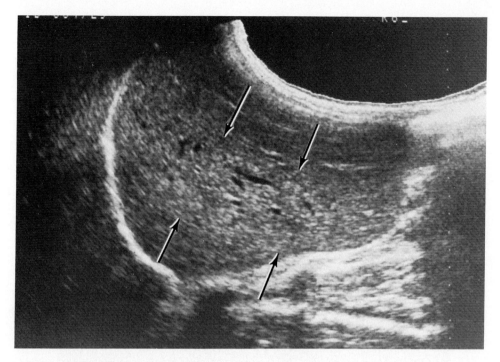

Figure 3-15 Sagittal scan. Increased echo intensity is seen in a wide band (arrows) through the liver in the location of the focal zone of the transducer.

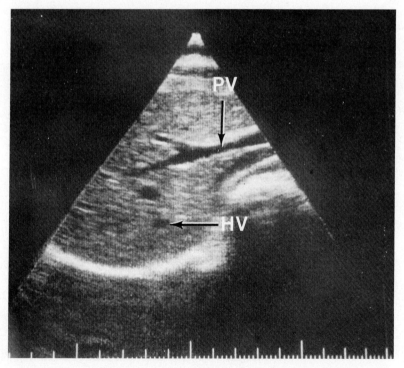

Figure 3-16 Transverse scan. Portal venous branches (PV) usually have strong echoes at their boundaries while hepatic veins (HV) do not.

93

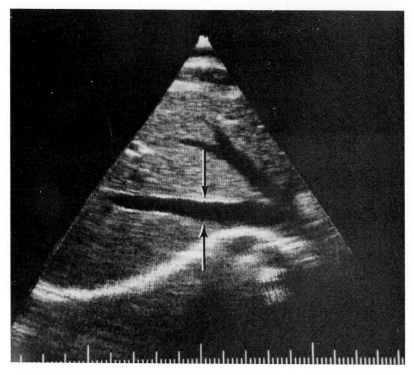

Figure 3-17 Transverse scan. Large systemic veins (arrows) near the inferior vena cava sometimes show echogenic borders.

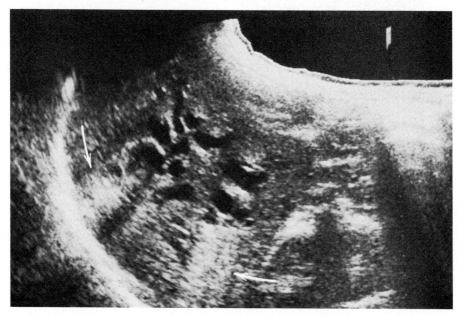

Figure 3-18 Sagittal scan. In this patient with dilated intrahepatic biliary radicles, posterior enhancement (arrows) is apparent behind the bile-filled tubes.

94

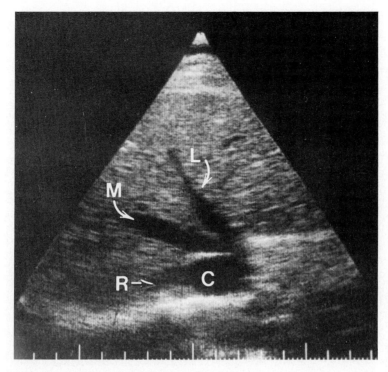

Figure 3-19 Transverse scan. The right (R), middle (M), and left (L) hepatic veins are seen entering the inferior vena cava (C).

finding results from the decreased absorption of sound in bile-filled tubes as compared to those filled with blood (Fig. 3-18).

Understanding the intrahepatic venous anatomy is the key to identifying the individual lobes and segments.[4] This has obvious clinical importance in assessing the resectability of a focal lesion within the liver. In general, it should be remembered that the portal venous branches enter the center of each segment, while the systemic veins lie within the fissures that divide lobes and segments.

Although some variability in the systemic venous anatomy exists, in most patients the inferior vena cava receives three major tributaries—the right, middle, and left hepatic veins. These are usually easiest to image in a transverse plane angled toward the patient's head (Fig. 3-19). It is often not possible to demonstrate all three within a single scan plane. The vein that appears to arise nearly vertically is the left hepatic vein. It lies in the plane that separates the medial and lateral segments of the left lobe. It should be clearly noted that the terms *medial* and *lateral* refer to the liver itself, not to the anatomic midline. In the older literature, the medial segment of the left lobe is usually referred to as the quadrate lobe. (More caudad in the liver, the falciform ligament also lies within this plane, as discussed above.)

The right hepatic vein usually enters the inferior vena cava from a direct lateral direction. This vessel divides the much larger right lobe of the liver into a ventral and dorsal division. Between the right and left hepatic veins, the

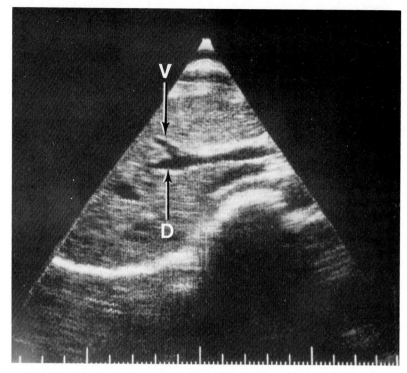

Figure 3-20 Transverse scan. The right portal vein divides into ventral (V) and dorsal (D) branches supplying the respective subsegments of the right lobe.

middle hepatic vein inserts into the inferior vena cava at an oblique angle. The middle hepatic vein delineates the plane of the intersegmental fissure, which divides the right and left lobes.

The main portal vein usually courses at an oblique angle of about 45 degrees toward the hilum of the liver and is easily imaged on both transverse and sagittal scans. At its point of bifurcation, the larger right portal vein continues in a lateral direction for 4 to 5 cm before dividing into ventral and dorsal branches, which are the major blood supply to those segments of the right lobe. Transverse scans are used to demonstrate this bifurcation (Fig. 3-20). The right hepatic biliary duct may be visualized as a slit-like structure coursing parallel to the right portal vein on its ventral aspect (Fig. 3-21). While the right portal vein appears to be intrahepatic in location, actual perforation of liver substance does not occur until the division into its ventral and dorsal branches.

The left portal vein is easier to recognize in transverse scan. Smaller than the right portal vein, it courses ventrally for several centimeters and then gives off medial and lateral branches to supply those segments of the left lobe. This results in a T-shaped configuration that aids identification (Fig. 3-22).

The caudate lobe, while usually considered to be a segment of the right lobe, has a variable blood supply and might be thought of as a completely separate lobe.[7] It arises from the medial aspect of the right lobe by an attachment known as the caudate process of the caudate lobe. This portion of the lobe is bounded

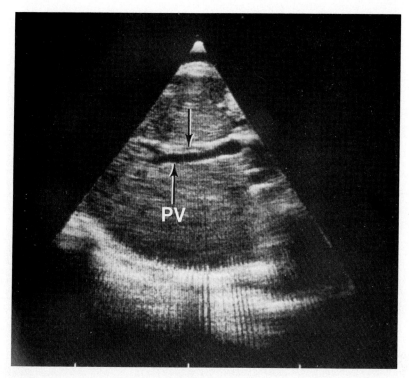

Figure 3-21 Transverse scan. The slit-like structure (arrow) anterior and parallel to the right portal vein (PV) is the right hepatic bile duct.

by the main portal vein anteriorly, and posteriorly often abuts on the right lateral edge of the inferior vena cava. Enlargement often produces separation of the portal vein and vena cava and may render portacaval shunt technically more difficult to perform. More importantly for imagers, enlargement of this portion of the caudate may be mistaken for an extrinsic mass in the porta hepatis if careful attention is not paid to sagittal scans (Fig. 3-23).

The remainder of the caudate lobe is a vertically oriented bar of parenchyma that extends cephalad to the diaphragm and lies dorsal to the left lobe of the liver. Recognizing the L-shaped nature of this lobe is helpful in analyzing liver ultrasonograms. This portion of the caudate is best recognized on sagittal scans in the area of the aorta and inferior vena cava (Fig. 3-24). The highly echogenic line separating the caudate and left lobe represents a combination of capsule, ligamentum venosum (obliterated ductus venosus), and at its caudad extent infolding of a small amount of peritoneum from the lesser omental sac.

Anatomic Variants

Although the principles outlined above provide a framework for recognizing liver anatomy, remember that considerable variation exists in normal subjects. One of the most common variations is the thin left lobe. Such patients may be referred after having had a radionuclide liver scan showing "decreased uptake"

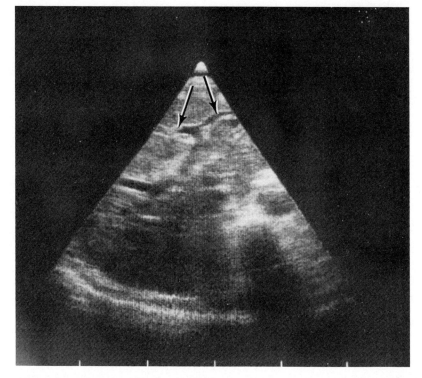

Figure 3-22 Transverse scan. The T-shaped configuration of the left portal vein is seen. The limbs of the T (arrows) pierce the medial and lateral segments of the left lobe.

in the left lobe.[8] Ultrasonography can be useful in these cases by showing the actual amount of parenchyma present.

Another region of variability is the porta hepatis. In some patients the main portal vein and surrounding connective tissue structures are deeply embedded in the liver; in others, they seem relatively superficial. In the former case, radionuclide examination may again be confusing.[9] This problem is also easily solved by ultrasonography (Fig. 3-25).

Variation in shape of the right lobe is also common. The term *Riedel's lobe* by corruption has come to mean almost any unusual downward extension of the right lobe, but more properly is reserved for those situations in which there is a waist-like narrowing and a bulbous expansion of the inferior aspect of the liver (Fig. 3-26). Such patients are frequently referred for ultrasound studies because a right midabdominal "mass" has been found on physical examination.

Liver Size

Since hepatomegaly is a common finding in many disease states, it would be useful to have a quantitative measure of size that could be obtained noninvasively. Some have approached this problem by summating the areas from multiple ultrasound scans at known intervals into a liver volume, but this method is too cumbersome for routine clinical work. More recently, interest

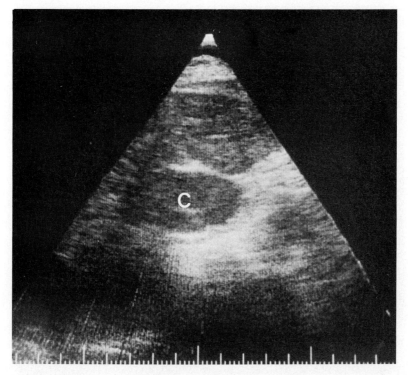

Figure 3-23 Transverse scan. This patient shows an enlarged caudate lobe (C), which could be mistaken for an extrahepatic mass if careful scanning is not done.

has been shown in looking at a single longitudinal measurement in the midportion of the liver as a predictor of hepatomegaly. Using this measurement, livers over 15.5 cm in length (in adults) were proven to be enlarged in 75% of cases, while measurements of less than 13 cm showed no hepatomegaly in 93% of cases.[10] While these measurements may be useful, the experienced observer, looking at both transverse and sagittal scans, soon becomes adept at making this assessment by inspection.

ULTRASONOGRAPHY OF LIVER PATHOLOGY

Many liver disorders produce textural changes that can be recognized using ultrasound. In general, these disorders may be divided into those that produce focal defects and others that indicate abnormality by parenchymal echo alteration without discrete borders. Although this latter category is sometimes termed *diffuse* liver disease, it seems more precise to use the term *nonfocal*, since focal disease is at times so widespread (metastases, polycystic disease) that it too, is diffuse.

Nonfocal Disorders

Increased Echogenicity
By far, the most common parenchymal change seen is an overall increase in echogenicity. Since this phenomenon can also be a technical artifact produced

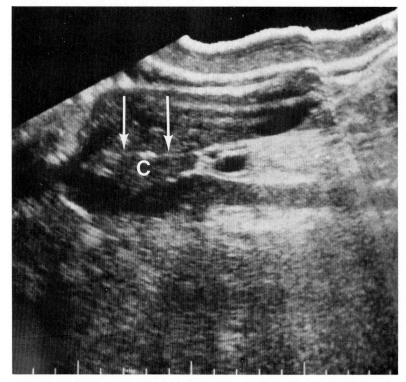

Figure 3-24 Sagittal scan. The caudate lobe (C) is separated from the more anteriorly located left lobe by the fissure for the ligamentum venosum (arrows).

by scanning with too much overall system gain, steps must be taken to ensure that it is a real finding. Various authors have used both A-mode and B-scan methods in an attempt to quantify this change. While these methods have met with some success, they are still impractical for the ordinary clinical ultrasound laboratory. In practice, it is easier to compare the echogenicity of the liver with that of the right kidney. Such an analysis assumes a normal renal parenchyma. It is essential that the portions of the two organs that are immediately adjacent to each other are compared, since failure to do so ignores effects that can be produced by sampling different distances from the transducer and different position referable to the focal zone of the transducer. In most normal patients, the liver and kidney parenchyma are very similar in their gray-scale texture. In others, the echogenicity of the liver slightly exceeds that of the kidney. A definite mismatch of the two tissues is strong evidence for parenchymal disease of the organ showing greater echogenicity (Fig. 3-27).

In the vast majority of these cases, the changes observed are due to replacement of normal parenchyma by either fat (fatty metamorphosis) or fibrosis (cirrhosis). Currently it is impossible to distinguish between the two by ultrasonic methods. Other findings frequently present are a paucity of intra-hepatic vessels and difficulty in penetrating the liver with the usual gain settings. At times, it is necessary to use lower frequency transducers to overcome this difficulty.

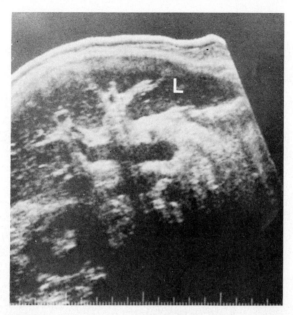

Figure 3-25 Transverse scan. In this patient with a thin left lobe (L) and deep porta hepatis, it is easy to understand why a radionuclide examination might be confusing.

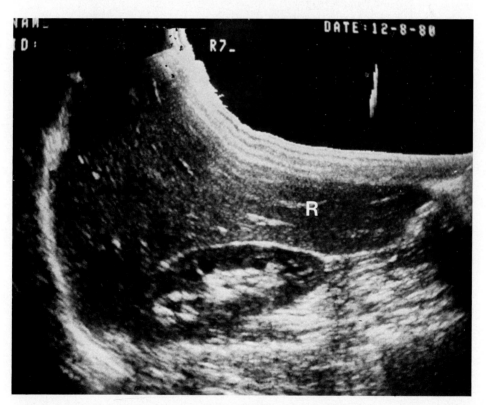

Figure 3-26 Sagittal scan. This patient shows a tendency toward Riedel's lobe (R) (bulbous expansion of the lower pole of the right lobe).

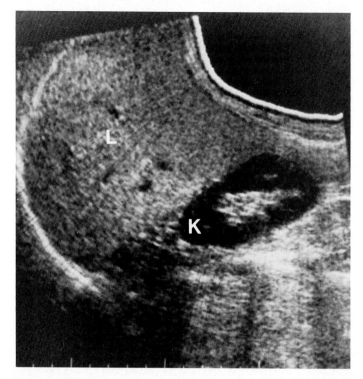

Figure 3-27 Sagittal scan. There is gross mismatch in echogenicity between the liver (L) and right kidney (K) in this patient with fatty metamorphosis.

If the changes seen are secondary to fatty liver, there are many possible causes. Alcohol abuse is by far the most common, but diabetes, chemotherapy, intestinal bypass operations, and changes from other toxic substances are also seen with some frequency. Not all of the patients with these disorders exhibit characteristic changes. At least two recent series indicate that 25 to 35 percent of patients with biopsy-proven fatty metamorphosis or cirrhosis have normal liver ultrasonograms.[11,12] It seems likely that radionuclide liver scans are more sensitive than ultrasonography in detecting early changes, but the nonspecificity of these findings on the former are widely recognized.

In addition to these difficulties, some authors have recently pointed out that fatty infiltration may involve only portions of the liver rather than the entire organ.[13,14] This situation produces discrete areas of increased echogenicity alternating with normal parenchyma, and the potential for confusion with metastatic disease is great. Similar difficulties exist in the interpretation of computed tomographic scans.

When fibrosis is the cause of increased echogenicity (Fig. 3-28), this is generally a result of cirrhosis that may also result from multiple causes. Unlike fatty liver, these changes are not considered reversible. Although alcohol abuse again heads the list, chronic viral hepatitis, schistosomiasis, other parasitic diseases, and storage diseases are occasionally responsible.[15,16] In the presence of this pattern careful sagittal scans of the left lobe should be performed to

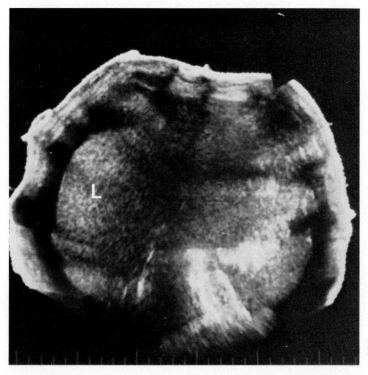

Figure 3-28 Transverse scan. Gross increase in echogenicity of the liver (L) is present in this patient with cirrhosis. Note the difficulty in penetrating to the spine and other posteriorly located structures.

detect the recanalized umbilical vein—an indicator of portal hypertension (Fig. 3-29)[17]

Confusion exists in the ultrasound literature as to the appearance of regenerating nodules that frequently accompany cirrhosis. While some authors contend that such nodules are hypoechoic with reference to surrounding parenchyma, others report texture similar to that of adjacent liver. Most note, however, that these nodules can be quite large and frequently distort the external contour of the liver.[18] For reasons that are unknown, marked enlargement of the caudate lobe is commonly encountered.

Decreased Echogenicity
Decreased echogenicity, an abnormal pattern, is confined almost exclusively to situations where the liver is infiltrated diffusely with a cellular process such as lymphoma, leukemia, amyloid, etc. Lymphoma is by far the most common of this group, and the diffuse appearance may be seen in both the Hodgkin's and non-Hodgkin's variety (Fig. 3-30).[19] Focal lesions, both hypoechoic and echogenic have also been reported with lymphoma.

Hepatitis
In many cases of acute viral hepatitis the liver parenchyma appears normal; however, some authors contend that recognizable changes in some patients do

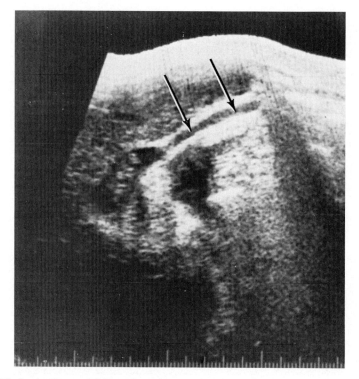

Figure 3-29 Sagittal scan. This patient demonstrates recanalization of the umbilical vein (arrows) secondary to portal hypertension.

exist.[20] There is said to be brightening of the periportal echoes thought to result from the lucency of the surrounding parenchymal cells (Fig. 3-31). As the process becomes more chronic, the periportal echoes fade and may become invisible. The validity of this observation and hypothesis needs to be confirmed in larger patient series.

Passive Congestion of the Liver

Patients with right heart failure and elevated systemic venous pressure develop marked dilatation of the intrahepatic veins, which produce significant liver function test abnormalities. These patients are frequently referred for ultrasound evaluation. While parenchymal texture is usually normal, the number of vessels visualized within the liver is much increased. In addition, the diameter and length of the vessels visualized is greater than normal. If real-time imaging is used, it will be noted that these vessels are persistently dilated, rather than showing phasic collapse with respiration. The ultrasonographer should be alert to this situation, since on occasion this may be the first indication that the problem is cardiac rather than hepatic in origin.

Utility of Ultrasound in Nonfocal Liver Disease

Although radionuclide liver scanning is usually the preferred screening test in patients suspected of having nonfocal liver disease, a large number of these

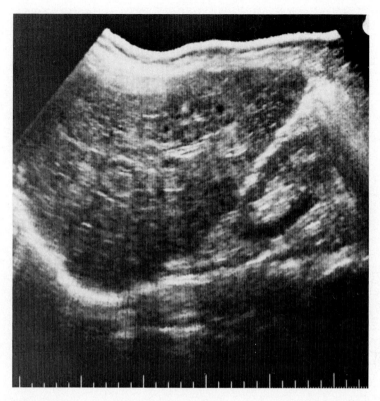

Figure 3-30 Sagittal scan. Diffuse infiltration by echolucent lymphoma is responsible for this unusual appearance.

people also have an ultrasound study. For this reason, the ultrasonographer needs a good working knowledge of the possible appearances of the liver. Frequently, it is not clear whether the patient's liver function aberrations are on the basis of parenchymal disease or obstruction of the biliary tree. Ultrasonography can differentiate these possibilities with a high degree of accuracy.

In cases where radionuclide uptake in the liver is much reduced, the question of superimposed focal disease (hepatoma, metastases) is often raised. Since ultrasonography is independent of liver function, it is well suited to perform this evaluation.

In many ways, ultrasonography and computed tomography are complementary in the study of nonfocal disease. While fatty metamorphosis and cirrhosis have quite similar ultrasonic appearances, CT is easily able to distinguish fatty infiltration by its characteristic attenuation numbers. The cirrhotic parenchyma (with the exception of hemochromatosis), however, looks quite normal on CT, but is definitely abnormal on sonography. It has quickly become apparent to those involved in both ultrasonography and CT that the two imaging techniques are measuring quite different parameters of tissue. It is predictable that each will be superior in selected clinical situations.

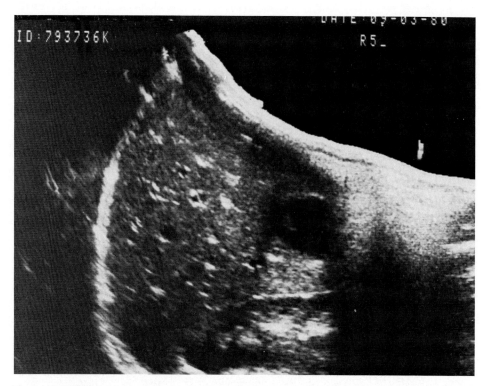

Figure 3-31 Sagittal scan. Accentuation of the periportal echoes is seen in this patient with hepatitis.

Focal Disorders

General Principles

Without question, one of the most valuable applications for ultrasonography is the detection of focal lesions within the liver (as well as other solid organs). The presence of focal lesions is of obvious clinical importance in both inflammatory and neoplastic disorders.

Although the question of resolution capability of ultrasonography is often asked, there is no simple answer. Recognition of a lesion is dependent on the difference in acoustic property (impedance) between the lesion and the medium in which it is situated. If the target is quite different in acoustic property from the medium, then a very small target may be imaged. If, on the other hand, the target has an acoustic impedance that is similar to that of the medium, even sizeable lesions may escape detection. In the liver, cystic lesions (as well as some solid ones) as small as 1 cm in diameter are readily apparent.

As mentioned previously, transducer selection is important in ensuring maximum possible resolution. It is apparent, however, that the transducer is no longer the limiting factor in recognizing abnormalities. Administration of a nontoxic material that could alter the acoustic impedance of the liver would be of obvious clinical benefit in recognizing lesions that are difficult to see with current technology. This research in imaging is currently being shared by both ultrasonography and computed body tomography.

Shadowing Lesions

In some clinical situations, focal processes having a distinct posterior acoustic shadow are noted within the liver. These are usually more evident on single-pass sector scan, since compounding tends to obliterate them. Although there are multiple possible causes for this finding, their ultrasonic appearance is usually quite similar.

NORMAL SHADOW.   On sagittal scans near the neck of the gallbladder in normal patients, it is frequently possible to see a discrete shadow projected on the posterior aspect of the liver. Various explanations have been offered for this, which include the thick fibrous tissue surrounding the right portal vein and the spiral valve of Heister within the gallbladder neck. More recently, this phenomenon has been explained as a refractive effect caused by tangential incidence of the ultrasound beam to the interface between the liver and gallbladder.[21] When the finding is present, decubitus scans are mandatory to search for tiny biliary calculi that may be lodged in the cystic duct and produce a similar appearance. If such calculi are not gravity dependent, it may be impossible to distinguish them from physiologic shadowing.

CALCIFICATIONS.   Calcification may be the end result of several processes within the liver. In the majority of cases, a previous inflammatory process (usually granulomatous or parasitic) is responsible for the appearance of these bright foci and discrete shadows. The width of the shadow(s) is dependent on the size of the calcification and may vary considerably in size.

Calcification is also present in a small number of metastatic malignancies involving the liver. In children, this is most frequently seen with neuroblastoma; in adults, mucinous tumors of the gastrointestinal tract are the most common source. As with inflammatory calcification, the size of individual foci is quite variable. The total number of metastases seen in the liver containing calcifications is quite small.

AIR IN THE LIVER.   When air enters the tubular systems within the liver, shadowing is produced mimicking the appearance of multiple calcifications. In most cases, the cause is a surgical connection between the biliary tree and the gut, usually performed for relief of malignant obstruction of the ducts. If there has been no surgery, gallstone ileus and penetrating duodenal ulcer disease must be considered in the differential diagnosis.

The other possibility for entrance of air within the liver is the portal venous system (Fig. 3-32). Much less common than biliary air, it is generally related to a suppurative process involving the bowel which has eroded into a branch of the portal vein. The presence of shadowing lesions in the periphery of the liver may be helpful in distinguishing portal venous air from biliary air which is ordinarily more central in location.

Cysts and Cyst-Like Lesions

The presence of fluid within a focal lesion of the liver can be detected accurately with sonographic techniques, but unfortunately the specificity of such a finding is not great. As with cystic disorders elsewhere in the body, the criteria are absence of internal echoes, sharp posterior margin, and acoustic enhancement posterior to the lesion.

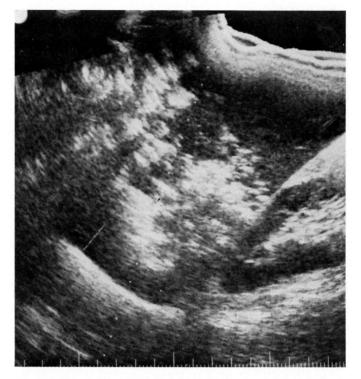

Figure 3-32 Sagittal scan. This confusing appearance was caused by extensive intrahepatic portal venous air in a patient with Crohn's disease.

CONGENITAL CYSTS. Once considered unusual, ultrasonography and CT have established that congenital cysts are relatively common.[22,23] Although usually single (Fig. 3-33), cases of multiple cysts unassociated with renal disease are also being reported with increasing frequency. Congenital cysts usually meet the criteria listed above, but on occasion possess echogenic internal structure (Fig. 3-34). This may be in the form of septations or a small peripheral focus that represents debris or infolding of epithelium. Because the malignant potential of such lesions cannot be established on the basis of ultrasonic appearance alone, percutaneous aspiration of the cyst and cytologic examination of its contents is recommended.[24]

Polycystic disease of the liver is a well known clinical entity seen in about one-third of the patients who have adult-type polycystic renal disease. Involvement can range from minimal to virtually complete replacement of the hepatic parenchyma by cystic lesions (Fig. 3-35). Surprisingly, even patients with extensive involvement often have normal liver function as measured by laboratory parameters. Although polycystic liver disease is usually asymptomatic, there are occasional complications in which ultrasound may provide additional information. Malignant transformation of cysts has been reported, so that nodularity lining a cyst should probably be followed by needle aspiration of the lesion in question. Hemorrhage into a cyst and infection occasionally occur and may produce varying degrees of internal echogenicity. Finally, obstructive

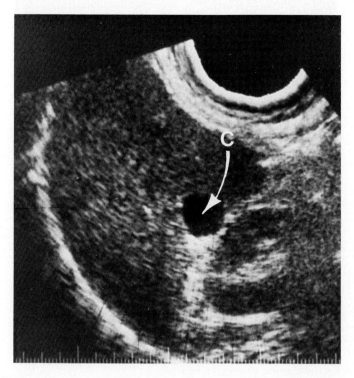

Figure 3-33 Sagittal scan. A single congenital cyst (C) is seen on the surface of the right lobe of the liver.

jaundice may be caused by pressure from cysts on the biliary system, and the resultant pattern of dilated bile ducts then appears superimposed on that of the polycystic disease.

Communicating cavernous ectasia of the biliary tree (Caroli's disease) may also appear as multiple focal cystic collections throughout the liver.[25] While the appearance superficially resembles that of polycystic disease, careful scanning usually demonstrates that these collections communicate with the biliary tree, unlike the isolated cysts of polycystic disease.

ACQUIRED CYSTS. Cystic masses identical to those of the congenital variety are occasionally encountered in patients whose history reveals a previous episode of trauma or localized inflammatory process of the liver. These are much less common than the congenital variety, and percutaneous aspiration is again considered necessary to exclude cystic neoplasm.

Patients who have segmental obstruction of the biliary tree may also appear to have focal cysts that cause confusion with other cystic entities within the liver. In most cases, the origin is a stricture from previous surgery, infection, or cholangiocarcinoma.

COMPLICATED CYSTIC LESIONS. Cysts that have irregular internal contour and/or internal echogenicity of significant amount can result from a variety of disorders. Statistically, liver abscesses of either bacterial or amebic origin are the most common (Fig. 3-36).[26-28] When bacterial abscess is suspected clinically, percu-

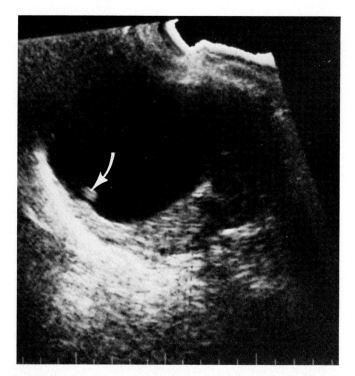

Figure 3-34 Sagittal scan. This congenital cyst shows a small peripheral solid nodule (arrow). Cytology was negative on cyst aspirate.

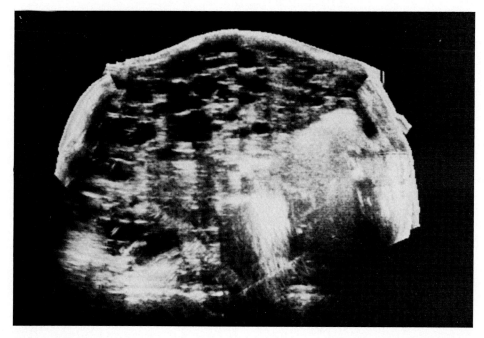

Figure 3-35 Transverse scan. Massive liver involvement by cysts in patient with adult type polycystic renal disease.

110

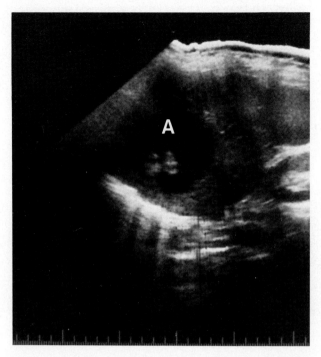

Figure 3-36 Sagittal scan. This complicated cystic mass is an amebic abscess (A).

taneous aspiration is helpful in identifying the responsible organism. In areas where amebiasis is endemic, needle aspiration is generally not performed since it is unusual to recover the organism from the aspirate. In addition, there is the potential danger of converting the abscess into a life-threatening bacterial infection. In such cases, antiamebic therapy is begun empirically, and symptomatic response usually occurs within hours of its initiation. If the patient does not respond, aspiration may become necessary to exclude bacterial abscess or necrotic tumor. The amount of echogenic material within an abscess is quite variable. Ultrasonography is valuable in following the therapy of these lesions. Serial scans on patients with amebic abscesses may show either a return to normal or evolution to a well-defined cyst. When radionuclide scans are employed in such patients, the defect persists much longer than on sonograms, indicating that while the lesion fills in, it takes some time for the area to develop functioning hepatic parenchyma.

Complex cystic lesions are seen in patients with hepatic echinococcal (hydatid) disease. These masses are usually multiseptated, and the daughter cysts, or scolices, are sometimes demonstrable. Needle aspiration of these lesions is said to be contraindicated, since peritoneal spread of the disorder is often fatal. An appearance similar to that of hydatid disease may be produced by biliary cystadenoma—a rare benign tumor of the bile ducts that morphologically resembles the cystadenomas seen in the pancreas and ovary.[29]

The increased use of ultrasound and CT scanning has resulted in the discovery of a large number of cavernous hemangiomas.[30,31] Although these

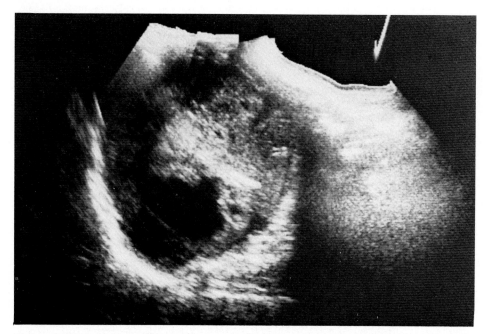

Figure 3-37 Sagittal scan. Necrosis within metastatic tumor has resulted in this complex cystic appearance.

fluid-filled lesions are usually 4 to 6 cm in size, they can be huge and involve an entire lobe of the liver. Hepatic arteriography is usually diagnostic (pooling of contrast on films late in the venous phase of the injection). More recently, dynamic CT scanning has proven to be of benefit. Scans performed rapidly after a bolus injection show a peripheral enhancement of the hemangioma, while those obtained 20 to 30 minutes later show complete fill-in of the lesion with contrast material. Many consider such a sequence to be diagnostic of this entity, and further workup is thought unnecessary.

When there has been liver trauma, fluid collections that represent accumulations of blood or bile may present an appearance similar to that of an abscess.[32] In the case of hematoma, its internal appearance is very dependent on the age of the hemorrhage. As with bleeding observed elsewhere, there is a period following the hemorrhage (several days to several weeks) where the blood is quite echogenic. This presumably results from clot organization. Following this, an echo-free appearance returns, representing the seroma phase of evolution.

When tumor in the liver undergoes liquefactive necrosis, the pattern of a complex cystic lesion again results (Fig. 3-37).[33] This can occur either from rapid growth, in which the tumor outgrows its blood supply, or from the effects of antitumor therapy on the mass. As has been pointed out by many authors, the former is most commonly seen in sarcomas that have metastasized to the liver, but it does occasionally occur with more common tumors. Patients who are successfully treated for liver neoplasms may be left with a fluid-filled cavity that is devoid of tumor cells and, therefore, quite indistinguishable from many of the other lesions previously discussed.

Solid Lesions

A variety of solid pathologic abnormalities may be present within the liver and can be visualized on ultrasonic scans. In comparison to normal hepatic parenchyma, these range from strongly echogenic to echo-poor lesions. Given this variability, it is not surprising that some lesions are very similar in texture to normal liver and are therefore difficult or impossible to detect.

CAPILLARY HEMANGIOMA. As stated repeatedly in this chapter, very few ultrasonic appearances are highly specific. One lesion that is probably the exception to the rule is the small (1–3 cm) capillary hemangioma that nearly always appears as a highly echogenic focus superimposed on the background of normal liver parenchyma (Fig. 3-38). Such lesions are common, but are difficult to demonstrate by most other diagnostic methods (including CT). Some advocate percutaneous thin-needle biopsy to confirm the diagnosis, while others say that this is contraindicated by the risk of hemorrhage and frequent failure of the pathologist to make the diagnosis on the aspirate. At present, our policy is to observe such findings with serial examinations if the patient has no clinical or laboratory evidence of tumor elsewhere. If tumor is known or suspected, however, it is usually necessary to expand the diagnostic workup to include needle aspiration and/or angiography since metastatic lesions occasionally produce echogenicity of this magnitude.

ABSCESSES. Although not strictly solid lesions, it is well recognized that abscesses may have so much debris within that they appear solid on ultrasonic scanning (Fig. 3-39).[34] This is true for both the large abscesses seen in amebiasis and bacterial sepsis, as well as the smaller foci seen in the diffuse spread of infection that occurs in patients who are immune suppressed. Clues to the true cystic nature of the lesion may be posterior acoustic enhancement and refractive edge shadowing of the lesion. In many cases, the clinical history is sufficiently clear so that differentiation is possible. Serial scans may also be helpful, since echogenic abscesses invariably evolve toward a more cystic appearance.

METASTASES. Hepatic metastases, because of their prognostic import, are a subject of great importance to ultrasonographers. Initially, it was hoped that some tumors would have a characteristic appearance, but experience has shown that this is not the case. Metastases can be large, small, echogenic, echolucent, partially cystic, focal, or diffuse (Figs. 3-40, 3-41, and 3-42).[35] As mentioned earlier, the ability of ultrasound to show these lesions depends on the differences in acoustic impedance that exist. While these findings mean that ultrasound is quite nonspecific, it does not mean that it is without value in these patients. Since ultrasound frequently is one of the earliest imaging tests employed, there is ample opportunity to be the first to suggest that liver lesions are present, whether there is a clinical history of tumor or not. Using the ultrasound image as a guide, even very small lesions may be localized for thin-needle aspiration biopsy.

Ultrasound is also of value in following patients to evaluate therapy (or lack of it). It is common to see central cystic changes develop within metastatic deposits.[36] While this may be due to the effects of chemotherapy, it can also be the result of a rapidly growing tumor that has outgrown its blood supply. If such a lesion is to be biopsied, it is important that the aspirate be taken from the more peripheral solid component of the mass to maximize diagnostic accuracy.

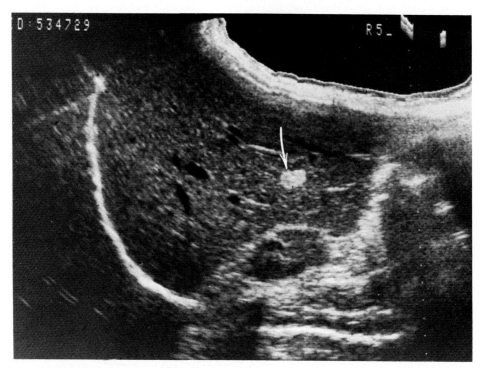

Figure 3-38 Sagittal scan. This small, extremely echogenic focus (arrow) is a typical appearance for capillary hemangioma.

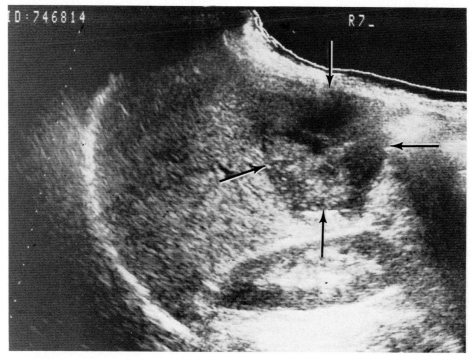

Figure 3-39 Sagittal scan. Although this focal lesion (arrows) contains many echoes, it is actually a complicated fluid-filled abscess. Note the posterior acoustic enhancement.

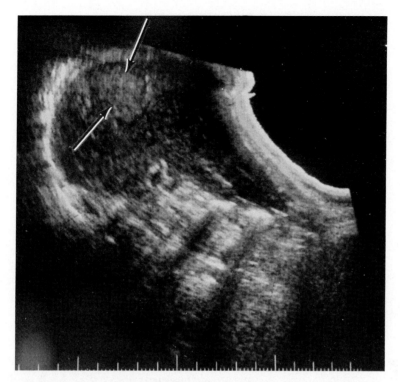

Figure 3-40 Solid focal lesion (arrows) of hepatic metastasis.

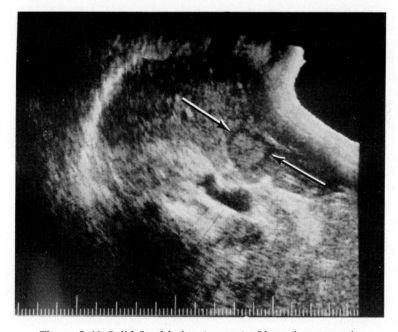

Figure 3-41 Solid focal lesion (arrows) of hepatic metastasis.

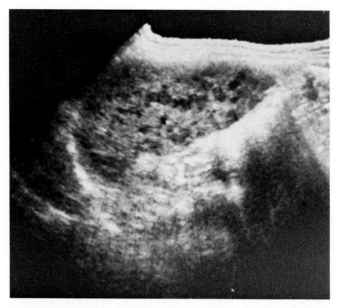

Figure 3-42 Solid focal lesion of hepatic metastasis.

It is impossible to make a categorical statement about the overall accuracy of ultrasound in the detection of these lesions. Studies in the literature that claim to make comparisons between methods of detection, are usually flawed by types of equipment used, technique variations, patient population, or observer bias. In addition, a considerable amount of time frequently elapses between the imaging diagnosis (either positive or negative) and autopsy examination.[37,38] Given these vagaries, most observers estimate that state of the art ultrasound has a detection rate of 85 to 90 percent, similar to that estimated for computed body tomography.

HEPATOMA. Primary hepatic carcinoma usually (but not always) arises on a background of underlying liver disease, such as cirrhosis or parasitic infections. In this situation, the area(s) of tumor usually appear echolucent (Fig. 3-43) when contrasted to the remainder of the liver.[39] When hepatoma arises in otherwise normal liver, it may appear echogenic. Multifocal origin of this tumor is well known, so that multiplicity of lesions cannot be relied on to differentiate between primary and secondary tumor.

Although it is usually not possible to make such a differentiation, there is a feature of hepatoma, which when identified, is highly specific. Frank invasion of the portal venous system by hepatoma is common (Fig. 3-44), but is rare with metastatic lesions.[40] Therefore, if tumor thrombus can be visualized within the portal venous radicles, the diagnosis of hepatoma should be strongly suspected. Invasion of the inferior vena cava also occurs, but with much lesser frequency.

Other findings that may help to identify the ultrasonic abnormality as hepatoma include an elevated serum alpha-feto protein, avidity for gallium

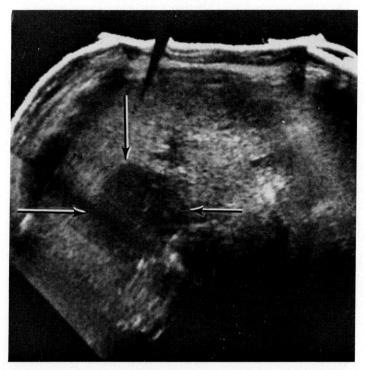

Figure 3-43 Transverse scan. The echolucent focus (arrows) in this cirrhotic liver proved to be a primary hepatocellular carcinoma.

(gallium[67] citrate)[41] on radionuclide examination, and the characteristic appearance of abnormal blood vessels as seen with hepatic angiography.

HEPATIC ADENOMA AND FOCAL NODULAR HYPERPLASIS (FNH). These benign lesions are being encountered with increasing frequency now that ultrasound and CT are being employed more routinely.[42,43] As with other tumors, their appearance is quite variable and cannot be diagnosed with certainty by ultrasound alone.

One recent report indicates that FNH may show a strong central echo that is believed to be the fibrous scar found at the center of such lesions pathologically.[44] Further evaluation of this finding is necessary.

Since the prognosis with the two lesions is quite different, it is important to use additional methods such as radionuclide scanning and angiography to arrive at a definitive diagnosis. Even with these aids, it is not always possible to make this distinction.

Hepatic adenomas are frequently seen in women taking oral contraceptives. Less commonly, they arise in patients with type I glycogen storage disease (von Gierke's)[45] or in patients with no predisposing facotrs. Although benign, such lesions have a propensity to rupture, and surgery is indicated when they can be definitively diagnosed.

Focal nodular hyperplasia is a benign tumor of unknown pathogenesis that has a much less clear-cut relationship with contraceptives, and is not known to rupture. Therefore, no specific therapy is necessary.

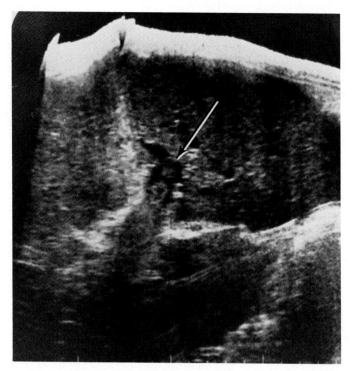

Figure 3-44 Transverse scan. Thrombus (arrow) is seen within the left portal vein in this patient, a finding highly specific for hepatoma.

Radionuclide scanning can be helpful in making this distinction. Since the lesions of FNH contain Kupffer cells and hepatic adenomas do not, uptake of technetium sulfur colloid indicates the former. Unfortunately, only 40 percent of patients with FNH exhibit this finding, so that failure to accumulate the radioactive material is nonspecific.

REFERENCES

1. Pertcheck L, Mack L, Johnson M: Ultrasound evaluation of the liver. *Appl Radiol* ‹ 139–150 Sept/Oct, 1978.
2. Yeh H, Rabinowitz J: Ultrasonography and computed tomography of the liver. *Radiol Clin North Am* 18:321–338, 1980.
3. Taylor K, Carpenter D, McCready V: Grey scale echography in the diagnosis of intrahepatic disease. *J Clin Ultrasound* 1:284–288, 1972.
4. Marks W, Filly R, Callen P: Ultrasonic anatomy of the liver: A review with new applications. *J Clin Ultrasound* 7:137–146, 1979.
5. Prando A, Goldstein H, Bernardino M, Green B: Ultrasonic pseudolesions of the liver. *Radiology* 130:403–407, 1979.
6. Chafetz N, Filly R: Portal and hepatic veins: Accuracy of margin echoes for distinguishing intrahepatic vessels. *Radiology* 130:725–728, 1979.

7. Brown B, Filly R, Callen P: Ultrasonographic anatomy of the caudate lobe. *J Ultrasound Med* 1:189–192, 1982.

8. Sullivan D, Taylor K, Gottschalk A: The use of ultrasound to enhance the diagnostic utility of the equivocal liver scintigraph. *Radiology* 128:727–732, 1978.

9. Sample W, Gray R, Poe N, et al: Nuclear imaging, tomographic nuclear imaging, and gray scale ultrasound in the evaluation of the porta hepatis. *Radiology* 122:773–779, 1977.

10. Gosink B, Leymaster C: Ultrasonic determination of hepatomegaly. *J Clin Ultrasound* 9:37–41, 1981.

11. Gosink B, Lemon S, Scheible W, Leopold G: Accuracy of ultrasonography in diagnosis of hepatocellular disease. *AJR* 133:19–23, 1979.

12. Taylor K, Gorelick F, Rosenfield A, et al: Ultrasonography of alcoholic liver disease with histological correlation. *Radiology* 141:157–161, 1981.

13. Scott W, Sanders R, Siegelman S: Irregular fatty infiltration of the liver: Diagnostic dilemmas. *AJR* 135:67–71, 1980.

14. Halvorsen R, Korobkin M, Ram P, Thompson W: CT appearance of focal fatty infiltration of the liver. *AJR* 139:277–281, 1982.

15. Miller J, Stanely P, Gates G: Radiography of glycogen storage disease. *AJR* 132:379–387, 1979.

16. Henschke C, Goldman H, Teele R: The hyperechogenic liver in children: Cause and sonographic appearance. *AJR* 138:841–846, 1982.

17. Saddekni S, Hutchinson D, Cooperberg P: The sonographically patent umbilical vein in portal hypertension. *Radiology* 145:441–443, 1982.

18. Laing F, Jeffrey B, Federle M, et al: Noninvasive imaging of unusual regenerating nodules in the cirrhotic liver. *Gastrointest Radiol* 7:245–249, 1982.

19. Ginaldi S, Bernardino M, Jing B, et al: Ultrasonographic patterns of hepatic lymphoma. *Radiology* 136:427–431, 1980.

20. Kurtz A, Rubin C, Cooper H, et al: Ultrasound findings in hepatitis. *Radiology* 136:717–723, 1980.

21. Sommer F, Filly R, Minton M: Refractive and reflective acoustic shadowing. *AJR* 132:973–977, 1979.

22. Weaver R, Goldstein H, Green B, et al: Gray scale ultrasonographic evaluation of hepatic cystic disease. *AJR* 130:849–852, 1978.

23. Spiegel R, King D, Green W: Ultrasonography of primary cysts of the liver. *AJR* 131:235–238, 1978.

24. Roemer C, Ferrucci J, Mueller P, et al: Hepatic cysts: Diagnosis and therapy by sonographic needle aspiration. *AJR* 136:1065–1070, 1981.

25. Mittelstaedt C, Volberg F, Fischer G, et al: Caroli's disease: Sonographic findings. *AJR* 134:585–587, 1980.

26. Sukov R, Cohen L, Sample W: Sonography of hepatic amebic abscesses. *AJR* 134:911–915, 1980.

27. Kuligowska E, Connors S, Shapiro J: Liver abscess: Sonography in diagnosis and treatment. *AJR* 138:253–257, 1982.

28. Ralls P, Colletti P, Quinn M, Halls J: Sonographic findings in hepatic amebic abscess. *Radiology* 145:123–126, 1982.

29. Forrest M, Cho K, Shields J: Biliary cystadenomas: Sonographic-angiographic-pathologic correlations. *AJR* 135:723–727, 1980.

30. Wiener S, Parulekar S: Scintigraphy and ultrasonography of hepatic hemangioma. *Radiology* 132:149–153, 1979.

31. Freeny P, Vimont T, Barnett D: Cavernous hemangioma of the liver: Ultrasonography, arteriography, and computed tomography. *Radiology* 132:143–148, 1979.

32. Froelich J, Simeone J, McKusick K, et al: Radionuclide imaging and ultrasound in liver/spleen trauma: A prospective comparison. *Radiology* 145:457–461, 1982.

33. Federle M, Filly R, Moss A: Cystic hepatic neoplasms: Complementary roles of CT and sonography. *AJR* 136:345–348, 1981.

34. Kressl H, Filly R: Ultrasonographic appearance of gas-containing abscesses in the abdomen. *AJR* 130:71–73, 1978.

35. Scheible W, Gosink B, Leopold G: Gray scale echographic patterns of hepatic metastatic disease. *AJR* 129:983–987, 1977.

36. Bernardino M, Green B: Ultrasonographic evaluation of chemotherapeutic response in hepatic metastases. *Raiology* 133:437–441, 1979.

37. Kemeny M, Sugarbaker P, Smith T, et al: A prospective analysis of laboratory tests and imaging studies to detect hepatic lesions. *Ann Surg* 195:163–167, 1982.

38. Smith T, Kemeny M, Sugarbaker P, et al: A prospective study of hepatic imaging in the detection of metastatic disease. *Ann Surg* 195:486–491, 1982.

39. Kamin P, Bernardino M, Green B: Ultrasound manifestations of hepatocellular carcinoma. *Radiology* 131:459–461, 1979.

40. Pauls C: Ultrasound and computed tomographic demonstration of portal vein thrombosis in hepatocellular carcinoma. *Gastrointest Radiol* 6:281–283, 1981.

41. Broderick T, Gosink B, Menuck L, et al: Echographic and radionuclide detection of hepatoma. *Radiology* 135:149–151, 1980.

42. Casarella W, Knowles D, Wolff M, Johnson P: Focal nodular hyperplasia and liver cell adenoma: Radiologic and pathologic differentiation. *AJR* 131:393–402, 1978.

43. Rogers J, Mack L, Freeny P, et al: Hepatic focal nodular hyperplasia: Angiography CT, sonography, and scintigraphy. *AJR* 137:983–990, 1981.

44. Scatarige J, Fishman E, Sanders R: The sonographic "scar sign" in focal nodular hyperplasia of the liver. *J Ultrasounf Med* 1:275–278, 1982.

45. Grossman H, Ram P, Coleman R, et al: Hepatic ultrasonography in Type I glycogen storage disease (von Gierke's disease). *Radiology* 141:753–756, 1981.

4

Gallbladder and Bile Ducts

Peter L. Cooperberg

INTRODUCTION

In the last few years, ultrasound has become the imaging modality of choice for the diagnosis of disorders of the gallbladder and biliary tract.[1] Whereas in other areas of the body, ultrasound has been used as a modality that supplemented the existing armamentarium including CT, nuclear medicine, and contrast radiographic studies, ultrasound has become the primary technique in the diagnosis of gallstones and the evaluation of the jaundiced patient. This trend commenced with conventional static gray scale ultrasound, but it is high-resolution real-time ultrasound, particularly when using sector-scan techniques, that has given ultrasound its present preeminent role.

CLINICAL ASPECTS

Approximately 600,000 cholecystectomies are performed per year in the United States. For every patient who eventually undergoes cholecystectomy, it is estimated that there are three to five who have symptoms of right upper quadrant pain that require gallbladder evaluation and in whom some imaging technique is needed to diagnose the presence or absence of gallstones. Chronic cholecystitis is a widespread condition characterized by right upper quadrant pain that may vary from vague dyspepsia to repeated acute attacks of gallbladder colic. There is frequently a history of fatty food intolerance but generally no physical findings. The presence of gallstones in such a patient usually provides a surgical justification for cholecystectomy. Although gallstones may in fact be "silent," pathologic examination of the gallbladder reveals a few lymphocytes per high-power field in virtually all patients over the age of 40. Therefore, any patients with gallstones and right upper quadrant pain have pathologic confirmation of the diagnosis of chronic cholecystitis to justify the surgical procedure.

If a calculus becomes impacted in the neck of the gallbladder, gallbladder colic results. The patient has severe right upper quadrant pain, most commonly beginning after a meal containing fatty foods. By the time these patients come

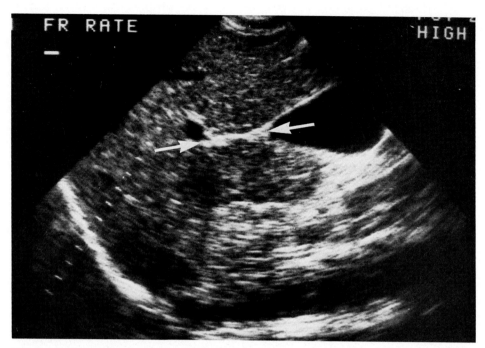

Figure 4-1 Normal gallbladder. Longitudinal image demonstrates a normal gallbladder with its relationship to the interlobular fissure (arrows) of the liver clearly seen.

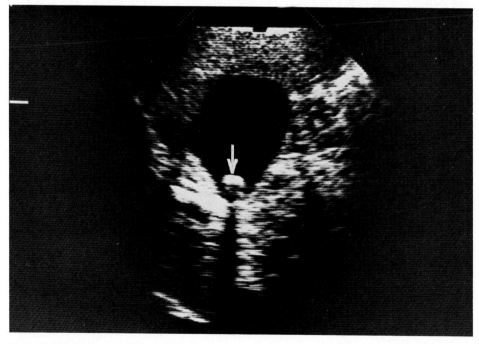

Figure 4-2 Gallstone. Longitudinal real-time sector scan image in the right upper quadrant showing a gallstone (arrow) in the gallbladder. Note the curvilinear echo at the near surface of the gallstone and the acoustic shadow deep to the echo. These are the characteristic findings of cholelithiasis.

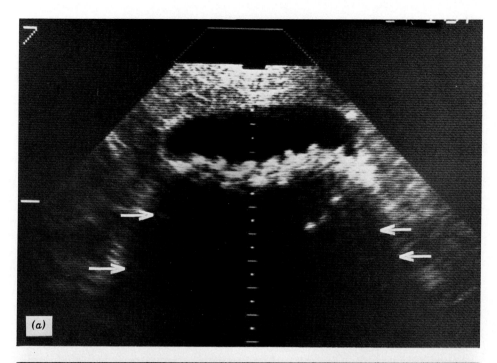

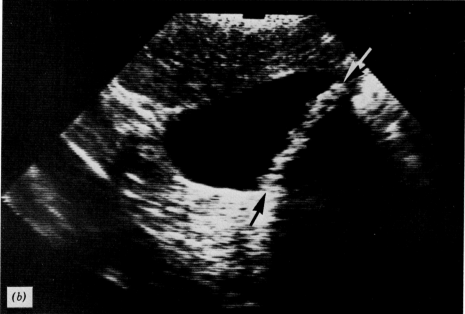

Figure 4-3 Longitudinal image from a real-time ultrasonogram in the right upper quadrant showing the dependent portion of the gallbladder containing numerous tiny (2 to 3 mm) calculi clumped together. Here we can see not only the echoes from the proximal aspect of the stones, but the individual calculi themselves. The clumping of these small calculi blocks out enough sound to produce an acoustic shadow (arrows). (*b*) Imaging the gallbladder with the patient in the erect position shows movement of the stones dependently (arrows).

123

for ultrasound, the stone has usually become disimpacted, either falling back into the gallbladder or passing forward into the common bile duct and duodenum. Even if the obstructing stone has moved, the demonstration of stones in the gallbladder is an indication for cholecystectomy. Most patients seen in the emergency room with such a constellation of findings are frequently offered the choice of surgery during that admission rather than discharging the patient for elective admission at some later date.

If the stone remains impacted in the cystic duct, acute cholecystitis almost invariably results, and, in addition to the right upper quadrant pain and tenderness, there should be a positive Murphy's sign. In the full-blown case, fever and an elevated white blood cell count with a shift to the left may also occur. Although the characteristic findings of acute cholecystitis may be definite, they may merge imperceptibly with those of gallbladder colic. We therefore prefer to call this situation acute gallbladder disease rather than acute chole-

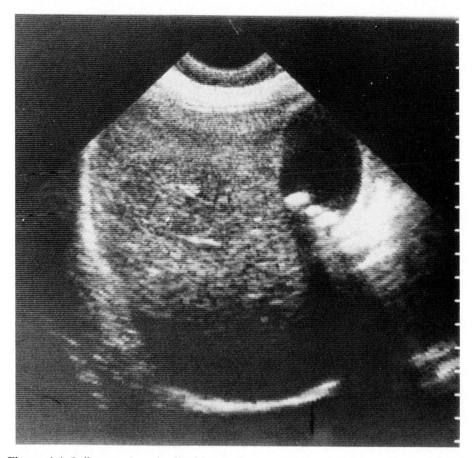

Figure 4-4 Gallstones. Longitudinal image from a real-time ultrasonogram in the right upper quadrant showing the echoes arising from three calculi within the gallbladder. Note that only the most superior calculus blocks out enough sound to produce a strong acoustic shadow. The middle calculus is just infringing on the side of the ultrasound beam and does not block out enough sound to produce a noticeable shadow.

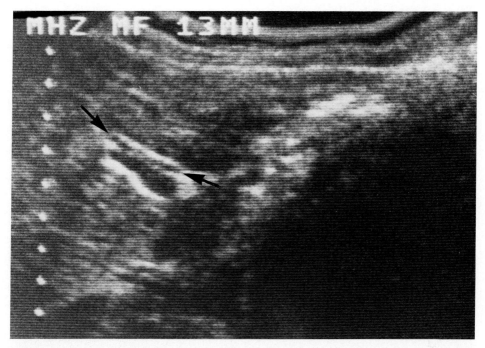

Figure 4-5 Normal CHD. Longitudinal static scan image showing the long axis of the common hepatic duct (arrows) anterior to the oval view of the short-axis segment of the right portal vein. Since the scale markers indicate 10 mm, this lumen measures approximately 3 mm in internal diameter.

cystitis. Generally, if the patient has acute gallbladder disease and gallstones can be demonstrated by ultrasound, this is sufficient indication for surgery during that admission.[1-5] If no stones are demonstrated in the gallbladder by ultrasound, or if there is a relative contraindication to surgery, a biliary isotope (HIDA) scan can be helpful. Nonvisualization of the gallbladder will provide further proof that the cystic duct is obstructed.

A totally normal ultrasound and nuclear scan in the current clinical setting still does not rule out the relatively rare acalculous cholecystitis. Even less common is the situation in which there are gallstones, but the acute findings are actually caused by problems elsewhere, for example in the kidney, liver, or duodenum.

Although it is possible to have dilated bile ducts before the onset of jaundice,[9,10] patients are most frequently referred for ultrasound of the biliary tract after jaundice has occurred. The ultrasound examination is performed to differentiate intrahepatic from extrahepatic obstruction and, in the latter case, to define the level and origin of the obstruction. In theory, it is easy to differentiate the two biochemically by the proportion of direct (conjugated) versus indirect (unconjugated) serum bilirubin. However, some hepatocellular diseases, especially hepatitis and drug-induced causes of jaundice, can cause swelling of the hepatocytes which will block the intrahepatic biliary canaliculi resulting in an obstructive picture with high direct bilirubin in a patient with

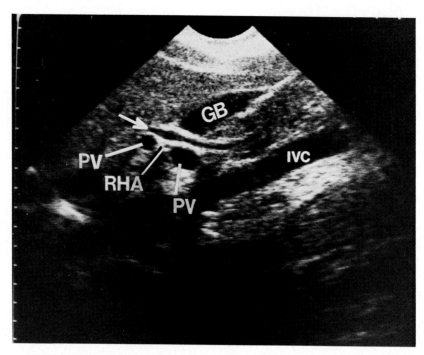

Figure 4-6 Normal CHD. Longitudinal real-time sonogram in the right upper quadrant showing the common hepatic duct (arrow) passing anterior to the right portal vein (RPV) and the right hepatic artery (RHA). GB = gallbladder; PV = portal vein; IVC = inferior vena cava.

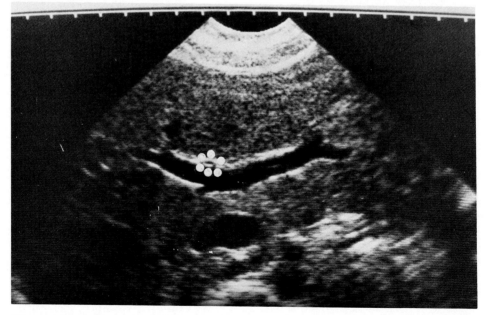

Figure 4-7 Normal CHD. Transverse scan demonstrates the common hepatic duct (dots) anterior to the long axis of the portal vein.

126

hepatocellular disease. Since it is important to diagnose biliary obstruction as quickly as possible so that the obstruction may be relieved either surgically or radiologically,[11] the patient should undergo ultrasound early in the course of jaundice if there is the slightest suspicion of obstruction.

Although classically the patient with a pancreatic tumor may have painless jaundice with a palpable "Courvoisier" gallbladder, this is certainly not always true. Similarly, every patient with a common duct stone need not have had a history of previous stones or have had intermittent episodes of acute pain.

ANATOMY

The gallbladder is a teardrop-shaped structure that lies in the fossa formed by the junction of the right and left lobes of the liver. Although the position of the fundus of the gallbladder is variable and can extend as low as the right lower quadrant and as far to the left as the left anterior axillary line, the neck

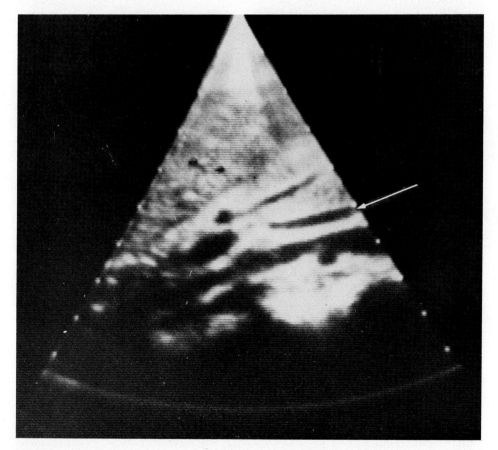

Figure 4-8 Normal CBD. Longitudinal image from a real-time sonographic study of the head of the pancreas showing the common bile duct (arrow) in the posterolateral aspect of the head of the pancreas. Note the gastroduodenal artery in the anterolateral aspect.

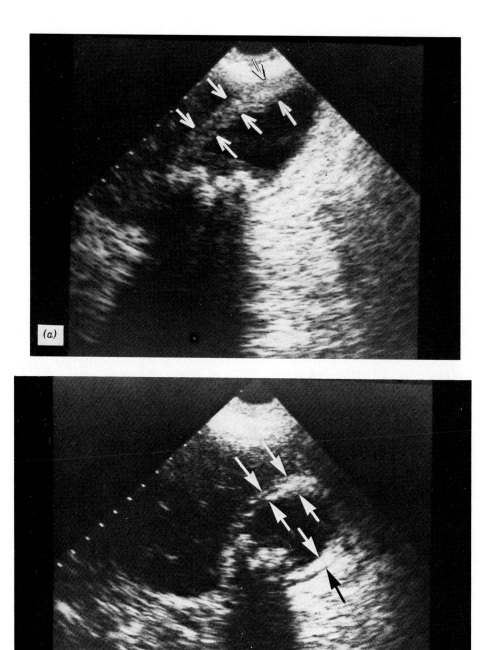

Figure 4-9 Acute cholecystitis. (*a* and *b*) Longitudinal images from a real-time ultrason-ogram of the right upper quadrant show marked gallbladder wall thickening (arrows), as well as associated sludge and calculii.

128

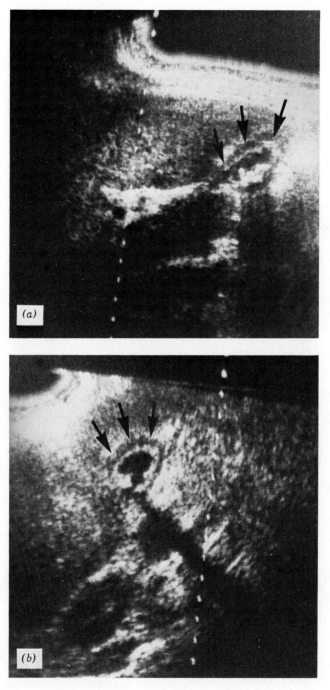

Figure 4-10 Chronic cholecystitis. Longitudinal (*a*) and transverse (*b*) static scan images show grossly thickened gallbladder walls (arrows) with stones.

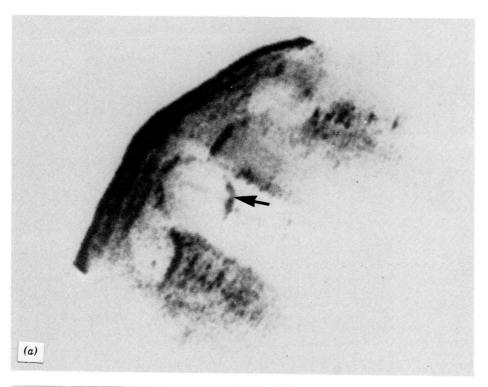

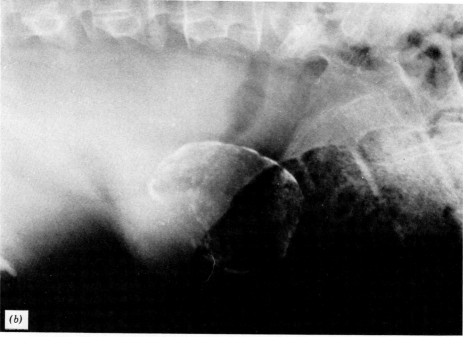

Figure 4-11 (*a*) Porcelain gallbladder. Transverse scan showing a proximal curvilinear echo with shadowing, but the distal wall of the gallbladder can be seen (arrow). (*b*) Radiograph of the right upper quadrant showing the calcified gallbladder wall. The calcification is spotty, accounting for the slight degree of through transmission to allow the distal wall to be seen. This can differentiate a porcelain gallbladder from a contracted gallbladder full of stones.

130

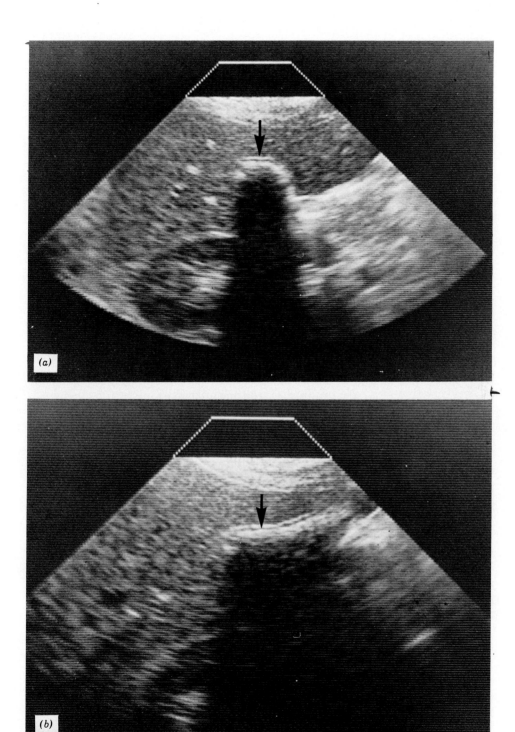

Figure 4-12 WES triad. Transverse (*a*) and longitudinal (*b*) real-time sonogram images in the right upper quadrant showing a contracted gallbladder with stones as indicated by the echo-poor *w*all, the *e*cho of the proximal aspect of the calculi (arrows), and the acoustic *s*hadow.

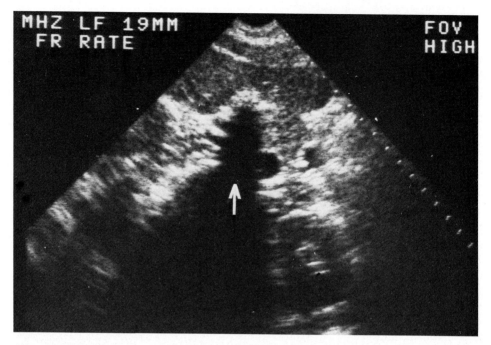

Figure 4-13 WES triad. Transverse static image showing the WES triad of the contracted gallbladder with stones. Note the distal acoustic shadowing (arrow).

and body of the gallbladder are invariably related to the region of the porta hepatis and the major interlobar fissure of the liver (Fig. 4-1).[10] The gallbladder may appear to be folded on itself, giving it the appearance of having a septum.[13] There may, however, be a true gallbladder septum. If there is a fold or septum toward the fundus, it is called a *phrygian cap*. A Hartman's pouch may be due to a fold or septum near the neck of the gallbladder, or there may be just a slight narrowing between the neck and body. While the gallbladder can become overly distended with biliary obstruction (Courvoisier gallbladder), there can be great overlap between a large normal gallbladder and a small obstructed gallbladder, so that size by itself is not a useful indication of pathology. If the gallbladder is distended, the walls will be very thin measuring approximately 1 to 2 mm in thickness.

The intrahepatic bile ducts are situated in the portal triads with the portal veins and hepatic arteries. They are normally too small to be visualized by ultrasound. The main right and left hepatic ducts accompany the main right and left portal veins into the porta hepatis. They join to form the extrahepatic common hepatic duct and pass anterior to the straight segment of the right portal vein, which is its proximal portion just to the right of the main portal vein bifurcation.[14] Inferiorly, the common hepatic duct continues anterior to the main portal vein in the gastrohepatic ligament, the anterior border of the foramen of Winslow. The cystic duct joins the common hepatic duct at a variable level to become the common bile duct. Since the cystic duct is not normally identified on ultrasound, it does not show where the common hepatic duct becomes the common bile duct. We therefore refer to the more proximal portion as the common hepatic duct and to the more distal portion as the common bile duct. The common bile duct then continues posterior to the first portion of the duodenum and directly anterior to the inferior vena cava before entering the posterolateral aspect of the head of the pancreas. It ends in the ampulla of Vater in the medial aspect of the second portion of the duodenum.

ULTRASOUND TECHNIQUE

Although conventional static ultrasound is acceptable to visualize the gallbladder[15–24] and biliary tract,[25–34] it is simpler, quicker and probably more accurate to use real-time techniques.[35–39] Furthermore, real time is easier to learn and there is less dependence on operator skill and enthusiasm. The main drawbacks of real time that have been cited, namely poor resolution and poor

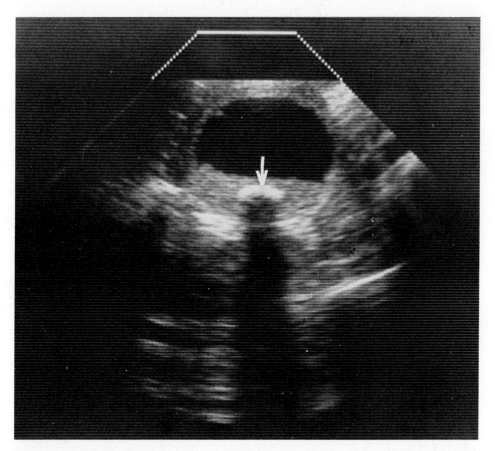

Figure 4-14 Sludge and stone. Transverse real-time image of the gallbladder showing echogenic sludge in the dependent portion of the gallbladder with a fluid-fluid level. Note that the coexistent calculus (arrow) in the gallbladder can be seen and clearly differentiated from the sludge by the curvilinear echo and the acoustic shadow.

hard copy images, are no longer a problem with the newer units. The only possible remaining disadvantage of real time is the relatively small field of view but, to demonstrate gallstones in the gallbladder or dilatation of the bile ducts, a large field of view is not necessary. With practice, a person can easily identify the internal anatomy even with those sector scanners having the smallest formats.[40]

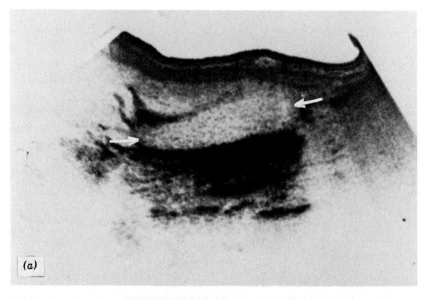

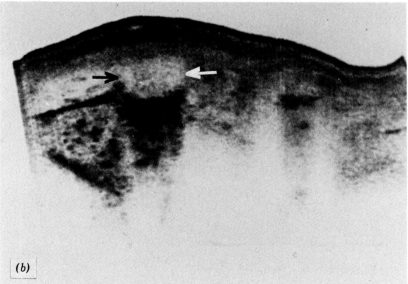

Figure 4-15 Sludge. Longitudinal (*a*) and transverse (*b*) static scan images showing total bile sludging. The smooth deep border and enhanced through transmission belie the true cystic nature of the gallbladder despite its internal echogenicity. Arrows define the gallbladder.

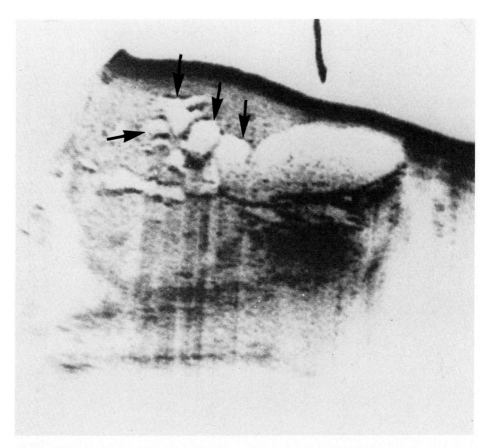

Figure 4-16 Sludge in biliary obstruction. Longitudinal static scan image in a patient with carcinoma of the pancreas showing dilated bile ducts (arrows) in the liver and a grossly dilated gallbladder with sludge in the dependent position. With a longstanding biliary obstruction, the sludge frequently does not layer out and can even have a fluffy appearance, suggesting a primary and secondary tumor in the gallbladder.

Despite the clinical indication for the examination, we do not perform an ultrasound study of a single organ in isolation. Rather, all of the structures of the upper abdomen are visualized in every patient sent for an upper abdominal problem, be it right upper quadrant pain, jaundice, or even trauma. The techniques for this standard examination of the upper abdomen are described elsewhere,[40] and we limit the discussion here to that portion of the examination directly concerned with the gallbladder and biliary ducts.

Using conventional articulated-arm static scanners, the bile-filled gallbladder should be found on longitudinal section, if possible, and the orientation of the gallbladder determined. The examiner should then perform slices through the long axis of the gallbladder at closely spaced intervals. Next, the examiner turns the gantry to produce closely spaced slices through the short axis of the gallbladder. This procedure should then be repeated with the patient in a left-side-down oblique or decubitus position. This change in position may be

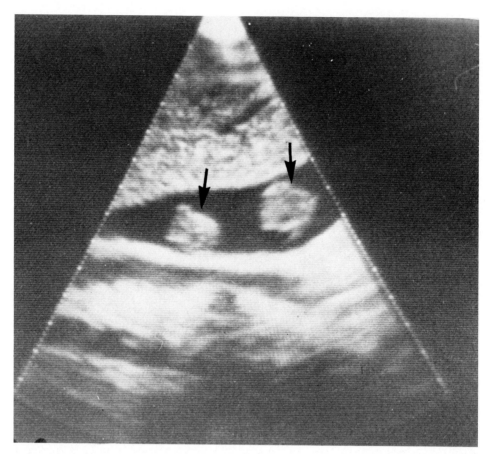

Figure 4-17 Sludge balls. Longitudinal real-time sector scan image of the gallbladder in a patient with Crohn's disease showing two nonshadowing, mobile structures (arrows). These have been seen on repeated examinations, but we have no proof as to the nature of this material.

necessary to bring the liver and gallbladder out from behind the costal margin. Even if the gallbladder is visualized in the supine position, stones which may be hidden in the region of the neck of the gallbladder, are more easily visualized if they roll into the body or fundus.

With a real-time sector scanner, the procedure is simplified by sweeping the transducer starting from a stationary point of contact in the right upper quadrant. Although a subcostal space is most frequently used, occasionally, the gallbladder is better visualized using a lower intercostal space with the patient in expiration, or in shallow respiration. Most commonly, the left-side-down position with the patient in deep inspiration is optimal. Once the gallbladder is found, the transducer is again swept through the gallbladder in long axis. A slow sweep along this axis allows a very thorough examination of the entire internal aspect of the gallbladder to rule out even tiny calculi. The short-axis view may be used if necessary, but is generally not needed.

It is most important to examine the dependent portion of the gallbladder, no matter what the patient's position. Almost without exception, calculi have a higher specific gravity than bile and sink to the dependent portion.[41] It is also important to have a vertical plane of section. If the patient is in a left-side-down decubitus position and the long axis of the gallbladder is shown by having the transducer horizontal, the far wall will not be the dependent position. The image produced in this plane will, in fact, pass over the dependent portion of the gallbladder, and small stones will be missed.

After a thorough examination of the gallbladder, if no calculi are identified, only a few hard-copy images through the long axis of the gallbladder are necessary. Calculi are generally easier to see during the examination and, if none are identified, there is no point in producing several dozen images. If calculi are identified, several images should be taken to prove their presence (Fig. 4-2). While it is most important to attempt to show acoustic shadowing deep to the calculi, to confirm their identification as stones, demonstrating an acoustic shadow can be difficult with small calculi (Fig. 4-3). It is most important

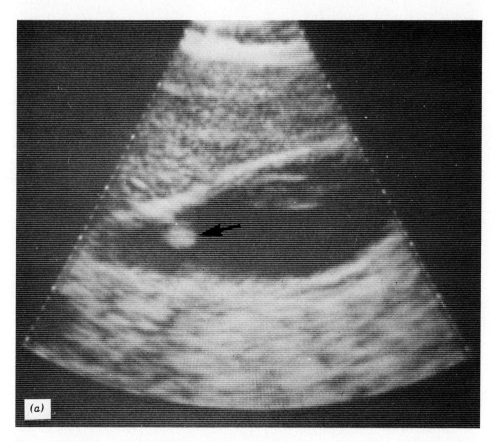

(a)

Figure 4-18 Polyp. Longitudinal (a) and transverse (b) real-time sonographic images showing an adenomatous polyp (arrows) attached to the nondependent, medial wall of the gallbladder. Note the strong echogenicity of the benign polyp.

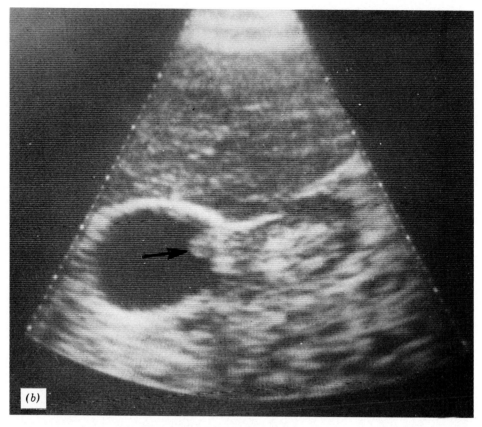

Figure 4-18 (*continued*)

to use the appropriate transducer frequency and diameter so that the calculi are in the focal zone of the beam.[42] Virtually all stones over 2 to 3 mm show acoustic shadowing,[43,44] although it is possible to demonstrate the echo from the calculus and yet fail to demonstrate the shadow if the stone is not within the central portion of the focused part of the beam (Fig. 4-4). Using real time, another definite sign of calculi is mobility while having the patient change position—the "rolling stone sign."[46]

In over 99 percent of patients, a bile-filled gallbladder can be well demonstrated, especially using real time, almost regardless of body habitus. Since the gallbladder usually sits in a relatively superficial position even in large people, it is sometimes surprising how well it can be seen in the very obese patient. If the gallbladder is contracted and full of stones, it can still be identified in the majority of people. It is important to have a patient fast so that the gallbladder is well distended. However, even if the patient is not fasting, if the gallbladder lumen can be clearly identified stones can be ruled out. The examination need not be repeated.

To evaluate the state of the biliary tree, we generally focus attention on the common hepatic duct, both because it is the most reliably visualized portion of the extrahepatic duct system and because dilatation of the extrahepatic ducts can be detected before the intrahepatic segments. To find the common hepatic duct the examiner must identify the straight segment of the right portal vein. By using a right subcostal or lower intercostal window with the patient in the supine, left-side-down oblique, or decubitus position and usually with a deeply held inspiration, the transducer head is swept back and forth along the right portal vein in longitudinal plane. When a small tubular structure is identified anterior to the right portal vein, the obliquity of the transducer is rotated slightly to show the long axis of this tubular structure, which is the common hepatic duct (Fig. 4-5). The right hepatic artery generally passes posterior to the common hepatic duct, either inferior or superior to the right portal vein. Therefore, on a longitudinal or nearly longitudinal plane of section, the long axis of the common hepatic duct should be seen anterior to the oval short axis of the right portal vein. The small circle between or just anterior to the two, is the right hepatic artery (Fig. 4-6). If the transducer head is turned 90 degrees,

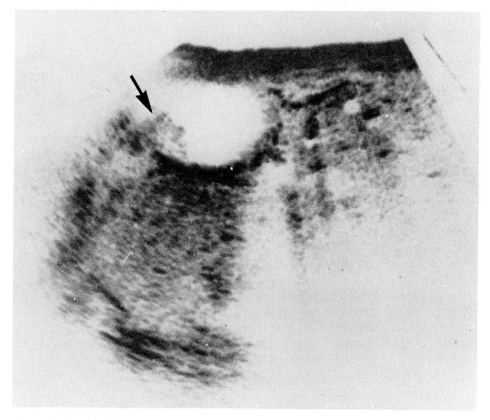

Figure 4-19 Carcinoma. Transverse static scan image of the gallbladder showing a polypoid mass (arrow) that was not mobile and was subsequently proven to be a gallbladder carcinoma. This appearance can mimic a clump of sludge within the gallbladder, but the lack of mobility (if the patient is sufficiently cooperative to roll over) can help in the differentiation.

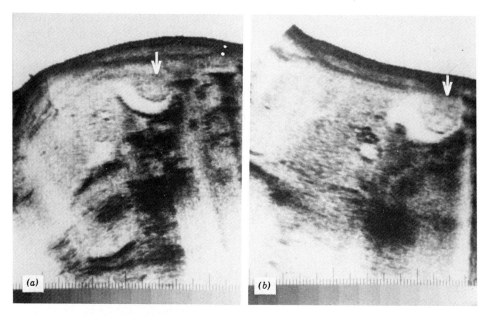

Figure 4-20 Metastasis to gallbladder from malignant melanoma. Longitudinal (*a*) and transverse *b*) scans showing a large soft tissue mass (arrow) arising from the fundus of the gallbladder.

the examiner can then obtain a long-axis view of the right portal vein showing a small circle (the common hepatic duct) anterior to it (Fig. 4-7). This is important if an accessory duct was visualized on the longitudinal view. The examiner could conceivably miss a more dilated main duct medial or lateral to the accessory duct, except that the transverse view should absolutely rule out any biliary dilatation.

It is then important to follow the duct more distally. This can be done in a longitudinal plane by changing the obliquity and position slightly to show continuity as the duct passes anterior to the right portal vein. Frequently, the midportion of the duct is obscured by overlying gas in the duodenum and hepatic flexure of the colon. Occasionally, the duct can be visualized again in the head of the pancreas, especially in thin people (Fig. 4-8). It is frequently helpful also to follow the duct inferiorly by looking transversely. With an eye fixated on the small circle of the duct, the transducer is moved inferiorly, maintaining visualization of the small circle and making it easier to differentiate the duct from the portal vein more inferiorly. This is especially useful when a pancreatic tumor is present, as this will distort the position and orientation of the duct. With a pancreatic carcinoma, the distal common bile duct frequently deviates medially, occasionally crossing the midline. If there is a stone in the duct, the normally echo-free circle of the lumen of the duct will become filled with an echogenic structure, and an acoustic shadow is also seen distal to it when the level of the stone is reached. By sweeping the transducer superiorly and inferiorly over the level of the stone, the examiner can have more confidence that this shadow is not an artifact. This image would be difficult to obtain in a hard-copy static image, but is generally very obvious during the real-time scan.

It is also important to evaluate the intrahepatic ducts. Although dilatation of the intrahepatic ducts generally occurs significantly after the extrahepatic portions, there may be an obstruction at the porta hepatis. If so, there will be intrahepatic ductal dilatation without extrahepatic dilatation.

Cholelithiasis

With the classic appearance of an echo arising from the near surface of the calculus and an accompanying acoustic shadow, the diagnosis of gallstones is highly specific (Fig. 4-2). It is possible to miss small calculi in the neck of the gallbladder. If the patient is very large and the gallbladder is situated deep beneath the costal cartilage, slight changes in position make it possible to miss calculi entirely. Nonetheless, false-negative results are relatively rare, especially

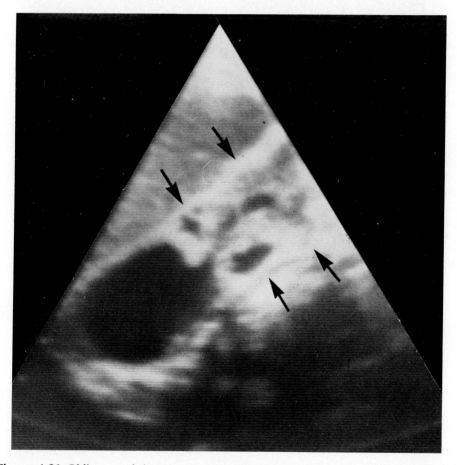

Figure 4-21 Oblique real-time sector scan through the long axis of the gallbladder showing the bile-filled proximal gallbladder region and the thickened walls (arrows) containing small cystic areas in the midportion of the gallbladder.

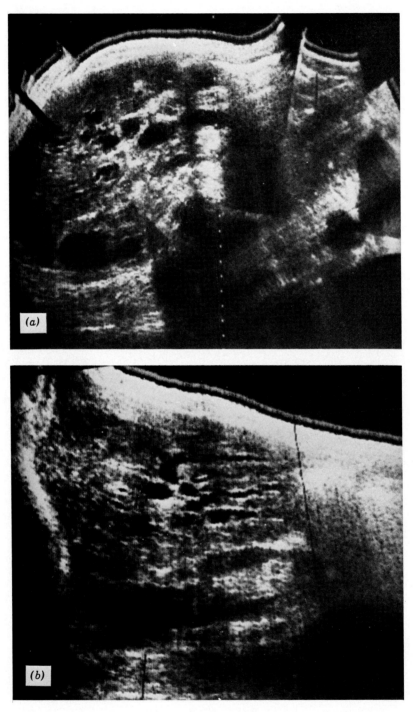

Figure 4-22 Dilated intrahepatic bile ducts. Longitudinal (*a*) and transverse (*b*) static scan images showing dilated, branching, irregular bile ducts in a jaundiced patient with pancreatic carcinoma.

142

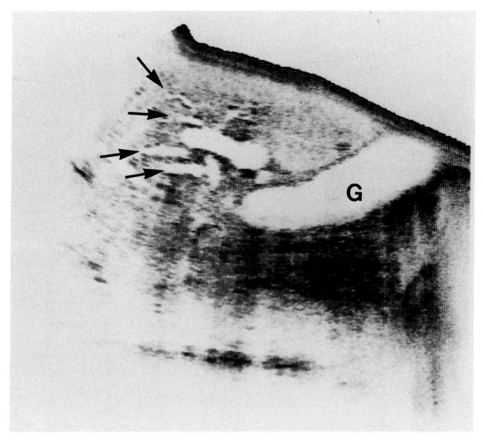

Figure 4-23 Dilated intrahepatic bile ducts and gallbladder. Note the confluence of dilated bile ducts (arrows) in the region of the porta hepatis and the large "Courvoisier" gallbladder (G) in the same patient as Figure 4-21.

using real-time techiques. The examiner must be wary not to diagnose gallstones by seeing only the acoustic shadow since acoustic shadows can occur near the neck of the gallbladder in the absence of calculi. A fold in the gallbladder can produce both an echo and a distal shadow,[13] as can a loop of bowl indenting the gallbladder. It is important, however, to err on the false-negative side. Less damage to the patient, and to the ultrasonologist's reputation, occurs with a false-negative diagnosis than with a false-positive one.

Although ultrasound is extremely accurate in the diagnosis of cholelithiasis, it is important to point out that ultrasound cannot specifically diagnose acute cholecystitis. The examiner may see thickening of the wall of the gallbladder and even a calculus impacted in the Hartman's pouch (Fig. 4-9). However, these are non-specific signs. Gallbladder wall thickening may occur in a variety of other conditions including ascites, hypoproteinemia,[47] right-sided congestive cardiac failure, and hepatitis.[48,49] Chronic cholecystitis may also appear with thickened walls (Fig. 4-10). A stone may appear to be impacted in the cystic duct if the patient is not rotated far enough to get the stone to fall into the

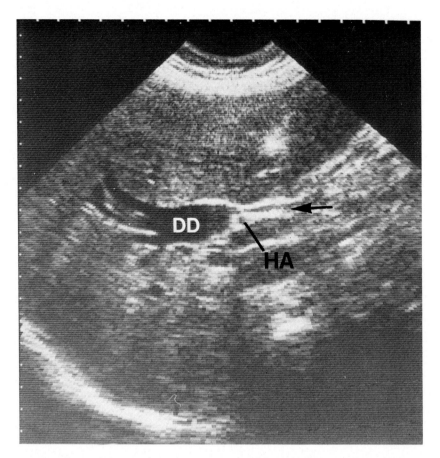

Figure 4-24 Cholangiocarcinoma (Kaltskin tumor). Longitudinal real-time sector scan image through the porta hepatis showing the dilated intrahepatic ducts (DD) and right hepatic duct down to the level of the porta hepatis where the common hepatic duct is seen to continue at normal caliber (arrow). The obstruction is at the level of the small circle representing the short-axis view of the right hepatic artery (HA:cp. This in turn is anterior to the oblique view of the portal vein. This places the level of obstruction at the carina—that is, the junction of the right and left hepatic ducts. At surgery, there was an infiltrating cholangiocarcinoma (Klatskin tumor).

body. The most definite ultrasound finding in acute cholecystitis is the "specific Murphy's sign," a complaint of pain by the patient as the transducer passes over the gallbladder. The sign is particularly useful when there is a clinical suspicion of acute cholecystitis and, although no gallstones are seen, the tenderness is directly related to the gallbladder. In this case the surgeon should be alerted to the possibility of either acute acalculous cholecystitis or the presence of a small stone in the cystic duct even though none is visible. In this situation, a HIDA scan can be useful, although occasionally the cystic duct is not blocked in acute acalculous cholecystitis. In advanced cases, corrections may develop around or within the gallbladder walls.

    If there is chronic cholecystitis and the gallbladder is contracted and full of calculi, the diagnosis can be more difficult. If the patient is fasting and no bile-filled gallbladder is seen, nonvisualization provides suggestive evidence of a contracted gallbladder full of calculi.[50,51] This diagnosis is more likely if the patient has had a previous nonfunctioning oral cholecystogram and is almost definite if a curvilinear echo with accompanying acoustic shadowing can be demonstrated arising from the region of the gallbladder bed.[52] A similar echo may be seen with emphysematous cholecystitis[53] or a porcelain gallbladder (Fig. 4-11). To differentiate from gas in the duodenal bulb or colon in that region, the examiner must repeat the scan after a few minutes and try to change the position of any gas bubble present by rolling the patient into different positions. We have noted a specific sign to indicate a contracted gallbladder with calculi; that is the demonstration of the echo-poor wall of the gallbladder superficial to the echo of the calculi. We have called this the *WES* triad, for the *W*all, the *E*cho of the calculi, and the accompanying acoustic *S*hadow (Figs. 4-12 and 4-13).[54]

It is important not to mistake gallbladder sludge for gallbladder calculi or to ascribe any other pathologic significance to the appearance of sludge.[55] Sludge, or echogenic bile, is due to the presence of cholesterol crystals and calcium bilirubinate granules in the bile.[56,57] It occurs when there is biliary stasis due to prolonged fasting as in such cases as a patient who is sick and vomiting for several days or a postoperative patient being fed intravenously. In this situation

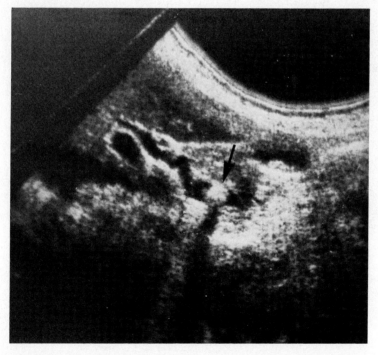

Figure 4-25 Choledocholithiasis. Longitudinal static scan image showing a calculus in the common bile duct (arrow) located in the region of the pancreas. Note the right hepatic artery anterior to the common hepatic duct and the right portal vein.

the echogenic material generally layers out in the dependent portion of the gallbladder (Fig. 4-14). A confusing picture may be found if there is total bile sludging, in which case the usually identifiable horizontal fluid-fluid level is not detected (Fig. 4-15).[58] In prolonged extrahepatic biliary obstruction, the bile tends not to layer out as easily and may have a fluffy appearance that might be confused with a solid lesion in the gallbladder such as a metastasis (Fig. 4-16). Longstanding cystic duct obstruction (hydrops of the gallbladder) may also give rise to echogenic bile. In this situation, the echoes completely fill the gallbladder and are nonhomogeneous with some echoes brighter than others. It is certainly possible to miss tiny gallstones in the presence of echogenic bile.[59] The examiner should not diagnose gallstones unless they can be seen. It is usually possible to visualize the gallstones separately in the presence of echogenic bile. Other causes of echogenic bile include hemobilia[60] and empyema[61] of the gallbladder. Rarely, nonshadowing sludge-balls may be found (Fig. 4-17).

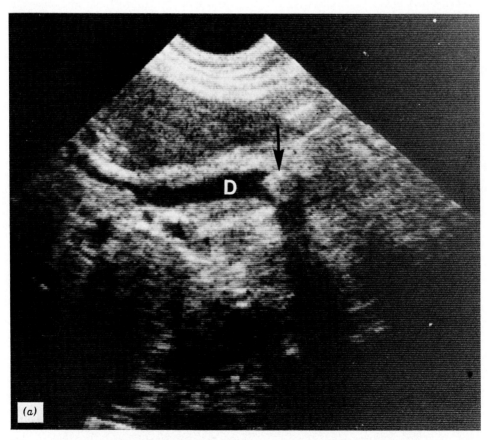

Figure 4-26 Choledocholithiasis. Longitudinal (*a*) and transverse (*b*) images showing the calculus (arrow) in the distal end of the common bile duct (D). The transverse scan through the head of the pancreas shows the dilated common duct (D) above the level of the calculus.

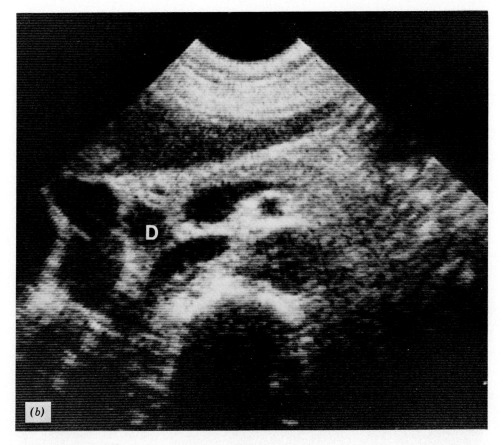

(b)

Figure 4-26 (*continued*)

Other Abnormalities of the Gallbladder

Although patients are referred for ultrasound evaluation of the gallbladder to demonstrate calculi, other abnormalities may be detected by the examination. These abnormalities include adenomatous polyps,[62] which are differentiated predominantly by their fixation to the wall, frequently the nondependent portion, and their lack of acoustic shadowing. They tend to be strongly echogenic (Fig. 4-18). Carcinomas of the gallbladder can be visualized in several ways.[63-66] They may appear as a slightly larger than usual polyp, generally having less echogenicity than does a benign adenomatous polyp (Fig. 4-19). They may appear only as irregular thickening of the wall. They most commonly appear late in their course as a large poorly defined mass in the right upper quadrant that has already invaded the region of the porta hepatis, the liver, and the other surrounding structures. At this stage, it is difficult to distinguish a gallbladder carcinoma from a lesion arising from the hepatic flexure of the colon or the liver. The one feature that helps in the diagnosis is the demonstration of gallstones, which are almost invariably present in association with gallbladder carcinoma. Metastases to the gallbladder are exceedingly rare, but can occur with malignant melanoma (Fig. 4-20). Occasionally, a mound of sludge can simulate the appearance of gallbladder carcinoma; however, sludge should be distinguishable by its mobility. We have seen one case of adenomyomatosis of the gallbladder in which there was a segmental thickening of the wall containing small cystic areas which were the Rokitansky-Aschoff sinuses (Fig. 4-21).[67] Since this condition is said to be relatively common, we must be missing most of them.

Jaundice

If the intrahepatic bile ducts are grossly dilated, there is no problem making the diagnosis. The large, branching, tortuous, irregular tubular structures (Fig. 4-22) that are seen heading to a confluence (Fig. 4-23) at the region of the porta hepatis can be easily identified by even an inexperienced ultrasonologist or ultrasonographer.[25,26,28,30–34] This pattern is most aptly described as the "too many tubes" sign.[68] However, if there is only mild dilatation, the findings may be more subtle. In such cases, the normally nonvisualized bile ducts

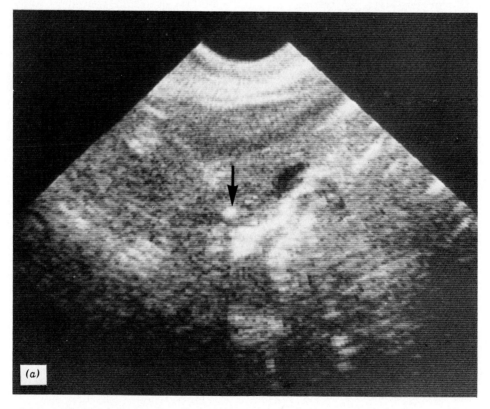

(a)

Figure 4-27 Choledocholithiasis. Transverse (a) and longitudinal (b) real-time images through the head of the pancreas showing a small calculus (arrows) in the position of the distal common bile duct in the posterolateral aspect of the head of the pancreas in a nonjaundiced patient with right upper quadrant pain; and (c) subsequent operative cholangiogram showing the nondilated ducts with the calculus (arrow) in the distal common bile duct.

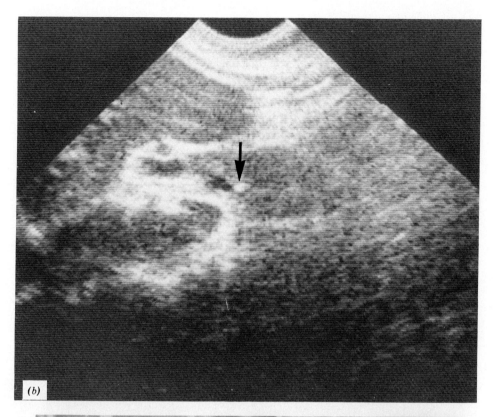

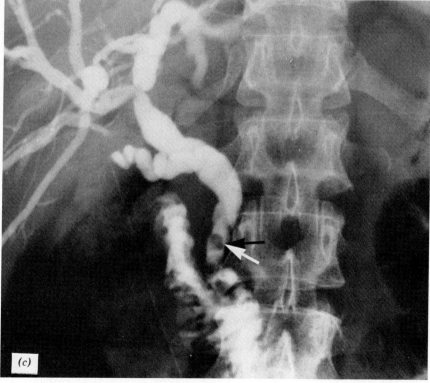

Figure 4-27 (*continued*)

accompanying the major branches of the portal veins are identified and the appearance is that of the "double channel"[69] or "double-barreled shotgun" sign.[39] This sign is easiest to identify in the left lobe of the liver, but the right ducts should be searched for as well. Although dilatation of the intrahepatic ducts can occur in the absence of extrahepatic ductal dilatation due to porta hepatis obstruction, the converse is more often true since extrahepatic ducts dilate first in cases of early, mild, or partial obstruction.[70–72]

When examining the extrahepatic bile ducts, the intraluminal diameter should be measured. Various authors have measured different portions of the duct and reported different upper limits of normal. Kazam has used 7 mm as the upper limit of normal for the largest part of the duct he could see.[73] We have used 4 mm measuring the common hepatic duct as it crosses anterior to the

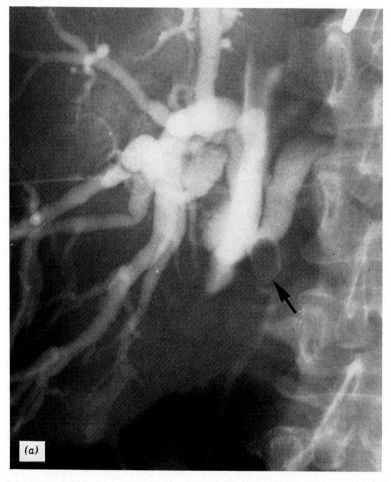

(a)

Figure 4-28 Nonshadowing common duct stone. (a) Transhepatic cholangiogram shows a calculus (arrows) in the proximal common hepatic duct. (b) Longitudinal real-time image showing the slightly dilated right hepatic duct and normal-sized common hepatic duct with the nonshadowing calculus (arrow). (c) A scan of the calculus (arrow) in a waterbath postoperatively showing no evidence of acoustic shadowing. This calculus was very porous and looked like a lava rock, presumably accounting for the lack of shadowing.

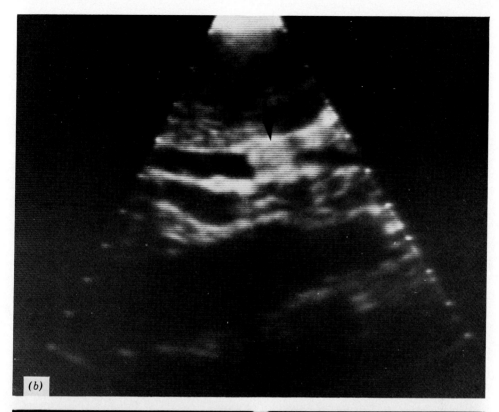

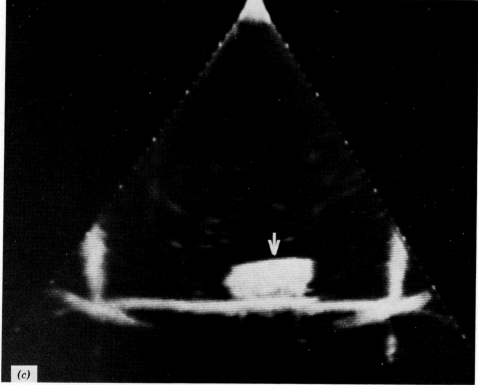

Figure 4-28 (*continued*)

151

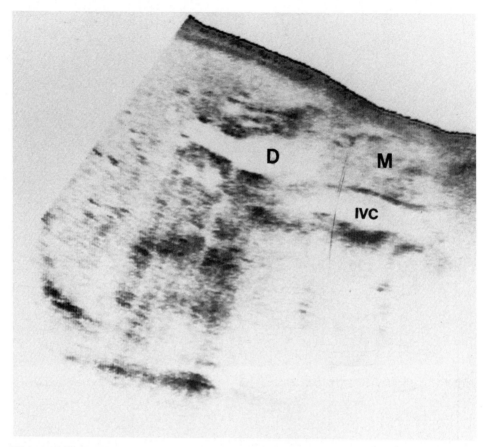

Figure 4-29 Carcinoma of the pancreas. Longitudinal static scan showing the dilated common hepatic and common bile duct (D) down to the level of the mass in the head of the pancreas (M). IVC = inferior vena cava.

right portal vein.[35] Sample evaluated the false-negative and false-positive rates using 6 mm, 8 mm, and 10 mm as the upper limits of normal.[74] In his series of 129 patients there were 4 false-positive and 10-false-negative studies for obstruction using 6 mm. At 10 mm, the false-positive rate dropped to 0, but there were 21 false-negative cases. His conclusion was that 6 mm should be considered the upper limit of normal in the patient with no previous biliary tract surgery.

Four millimeters would seem small as compared to other studies and certainly in comparison to the values obtained with radiographic techniques.[75] We did another study in our institution comparing the size of common hepatic ducts using ultrasound before and following intravenous cholangiography.[76] We

Figure 4-30 Pancreatitis. (*a*) Longitudinal real-time sector scan image shows a dilated bile duct (arrows) ending in a mass in the head of the pancreas (P). (*b*) Transverse scan shows the generalized enlargement of the pancreas (arrowheads) indicating that it is pancreatitis.

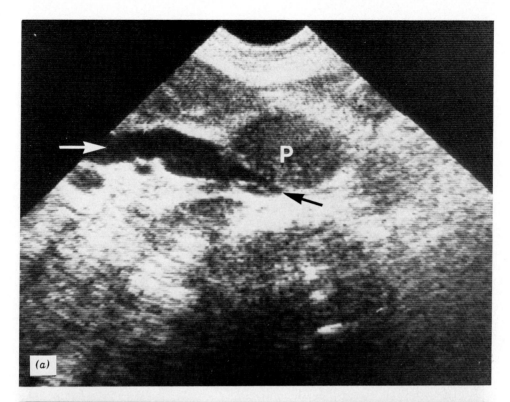

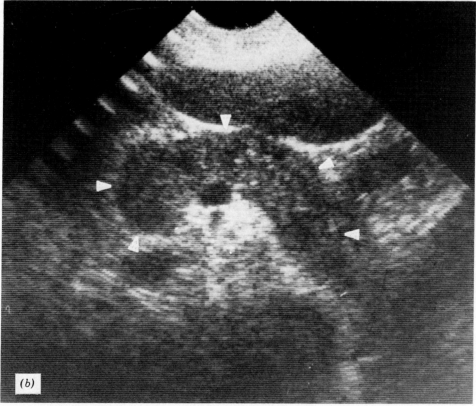

153

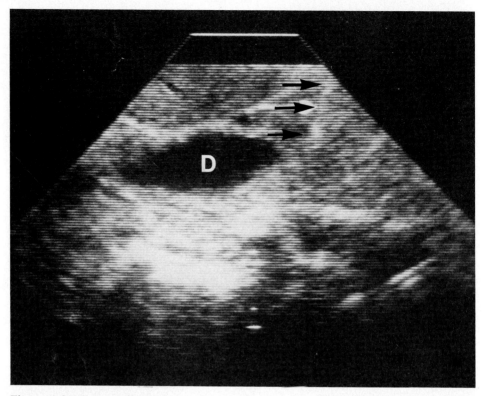

Figure 4-31 Fine-needle aspiration biopsy of a carcinoma in the head of the pancreas. A longitudinal real-time sector scan image shows the dilated common bile duct (D) ending irregularly in the head of the pancreas. The arrows indicate the echoes arising from the shaft of the needle introduced for the percutaneous aspiration biopsy.

determined that the discrepancy in size was due to a combination of several factors. There is a radiographic magnification factor, an ultrasonographic wall reverberation minifying factor, and a choleretic effect of contrast material on intravenous cholangiography (and most likely a direct mechanical dilatation due to the pressure effect of direct injection studies). However, the most important cause for the discrepancy between our limit and other ultrasound figures, as well as radiographic limits, is the different place of measurement. The common hepatic duct is usually smaller than the common bile duct.

We conducted another study to evaluate 4 mm as the upper limit of normal in 170 patients.[37] Fourteen of 98 patients had common hepatic ducts larger than 4 mm without evidence of obstruction on the subsequent radiographic imaging study. Seven of these patients had a clinical suspicion of a recently passed calculus. We,[77] and others,[78,79] have shown that the ducts can return to normal size very rapidly following passage of a calculus. Thus, if the radiographic "proof" is obtained too long after the sonogram, there may be a discrepancy in the results. Another 7 patients, with unobstructed bile ducts larger than 4 mm, had a previous cholecystectomy. There has long been controversy regarding the potential of the common bile duct to dilate without obstruction following cholecystectomy.[80] In 57 asymptomatic patients 4 to 16 months following cholecystectomy, with or without common bile duct exploration, we found that 86 percent had common hepatic ducts measuring 4 mm or less.[81] In 4 patients the duct measured 5 mm, and in 7 the duct measured 6 to 10 mm. Similarly, Mueller et al showed that 38 of 40 asymptomatic patients did not have dilatation of the extrahepatic bile ducts 6 months or more after cholecystectomy.[82] We also reviewed our data on 56 patients who were referred for ultrasound following cholecystectomy to evaluate possible bile duct obstruction.[83] There were 13 out of 36 false-positive examinations, but some did have common bile ducts that were considered dilated on the subsequent radiographic contrast studies. Thus, although it is possible to have a duct larger than 4 mm following cholecystectomy without evidence of obstruction, this is relatively uncommon. It is also possible to have a retained common duct stone in a duct of normal caliber. Nonetheless, we feel it is worthwhile to evaluate the size of the common hepatic duct in patients following cholecystectomy. If it measures significantly over 4 mm, further studies such as intravenous cholangiography or transhepatic cholangiography may be indicated if clinical suspicions are high. If the duct size is normal and there is a mild suspicion of choledocholithiasis, nothing further should be done. If there is a strong suspicion, a further study should be attempted.

Level and Cause of Obstruction

Although ultrasound is highly accurate in differentiating extrahepatic from intrahepatic causes of jaundice,[74,84-88] the ability to detect the level of obstruction is not as great and the ability to detect its cause is even lower. It is generally easy to differentiate a high level of obstruction from those at a lower level. The examiner may detect a tumor in the liver around the porta hepatis or masses within the porta hepatis causing obstruction. If the examiner can visualize dilated intrahepatic ducts with normal caliber extrahepatic ducts, he or she can accurately assess the level of obstruction (Fig. 4-24). Finding that the intrahepatic ducts are dilated and the gallbladder is small usually indicates a level of obstruction above the cystic duct. If the examiner can visualize the dilated ducts more distally, a pancreatic tumor on distal calculus may be seen. (Figs. 4-24–4-27) However, there is sometimes overlying bowel gas covering the region of the distal common bile duct. If biliary dilatation is apparent and the distal bile duct is obscured (Fig. 4-28), it is not acceptable to guess at the cause of obstruction based on the presence or absence of gallstones in the gallbladder. In a recent study from our institution,[89] gallbladder calculi were present in 40 percent of 32 patients with noncalculous obstruction, and no gallbladder stones were present in 25 percent of 28 patients with choledocholithiasis. If a dilated bile duct can be seen in the head of the pancreas and no mass or stone is apparent, the likely cause, especially if the pancreatic duct can be shown to be dilated, is an ampullary carcinoma or a very small periampullary pancreatic carcinoma. This is the type of case most likely resectable by a Whipple's procedure and should be pursued vigorously. Virtually all other tumors are unresectable at the time of diagnosis. If a pancreatic mass is visualized, it is not possible by ultrasound alone to differentiate between a pancreatic cancer (Fig.

4-29) and a localized area of chronic pancreatitis (Fig. 4-30). In this situation, a fine-needle aspiration biopsy (Fig. 4-31) should be done. We generally do this, after consultation with the referring physician, at the time of the first ultrasound examination.

If the bile ducts are not dilated in a jaundiced patient, the diagnosis is "medical" or intrahepatic jaundice. Ultrasound is not successful in differentiating between different causes of hepatocellular abscess,[90,91] although there may be some signs to suggest hepatitis[92] or cirrhosis.[93] Liver tumors can be seen easily, but these usually cause hyperbilirubinemia by intrahepatic obstruction rather than hepatocellular destruction.

Other Abnormalities

A *biloma* may appear as an upper abdominal fluid collection.[94-96] There is nothing specific about the appearance, but the clinical story and, especially, the results of fine-needle aspiration, should be helpful in making the distinction from other fluid collections. Choledochal cysts[97] also appear as localized fluid collections in the region of the porta hepatis, generally in jaundiced children. Biliary cystadenomas appear as septated intrahepatic cysts.[98,99] Caroli's disease (communicating cavernous ectasia of the intrahepatic ducts) shows up as segmental tubular fluid collections in the liver.[100]

OTHER IMAGING TECHNIQUES

With the possible exception of the patient who has undergone a previous biliary-enteric anastomosis, ultrasound should be the first imaging technique in the jaundiced patient. Although transhepatic cholangiography can be done despite finding normal-sized bile ducts, it is exceedingly rare to find an obstructing lesion causing jaundice in the presence of normal-sized intrahepatic and extrahepatic bile ducts. (This is not true with ball-valve calculi, which certainly can be present within normal-sized bile ducts, but the bilirubin in these situations is not elevated.) If dilated bile ducts are apparent without evidence of a cause, a transhepatic cholangiogram should be done.[101] If a tumor is identified by ultrasound, whether or not the lesion was biopsied percutaneously by ultrasound, a transhepatic cholangiogram should be done if percutaneous biliary external or internal drainage is considered. If surgical resection is considered in a patient where no mass is demonstrated by ultrasound and only a small tumor is seen by transhepatic cholangiogram, a CT scan should be done to determine the extent of the tumor and to obtain information regarding inoperability. If a pancreatic tumor was not identified on the ultrasound examination, a percutaneous biopsy can be done under CT control. Although the accuracy of CT in the detection of dilated bile ducts is similar to that of ultrasound, there is no particular benefit to CT unless the previously performed ultrasound has been inadequate, a rare situation in this diagnostic area, especially with real time.[100-104] A biliary HIDA scan may be useful in a patient following a biliary-enteric anastomosis when gas within the biliary tree can prevent evaluation by ultrasound.[105] There is less and less use for intravenous cholangiography now.[106] It is specifically used for postcholecystectomy patients in whom the likelihood of a common duct stone is considered too low to justify transhepatic cholangiography. ERCP is generally reserved for further evaluation of patients without demonstrable intrahepatic ductal dilatation or for pancreatic abnormalities.[107]

There have also been reports on the use of ultrasound to complement or even replace operative cholangiography.[108,109] This could be a somewhat cumbersome technique. There has also been a report of the use of ultrasound to guide percutaneous transhepatic bile drainage.[110] The authors of the report feel that the ultrasound method is preferrable to radiologic techniques for several reasons, but predominantly to reduce radiation to the operator.

In summary, ultrasound and particularly real-time ultrasound, is an important imaging technique in the patient with right upper quadrant symptoms to identify gallstones and, in the jaundiced patient, to differentiate intrahepatic from extrahepatic causes of jaundice.

REFERENCES

1. Margulis AR: Radiologic imaging: Changing costs, greater benefits. *AJR* 136:657–665, 1981.

2. Clintora I, Ben-Ora A, MacNeil R, et al: Cholecystosonography for the decision to operate when acute cholecystitis is suspected. *Am J Surg* 138:818–820, 1979.

3. Dillon E, Parkin GJS: The role of upper abdominal ultrasonography in suspected acute cholecystitis. *Clin Radiol* 31:175–179, 1980.

4. Sherman M, Ralls PW, Quinn M, et al: Intravenous cholangiography and sonography in acute cholecystitis: Prospective evaluation. *AJR* 135:311–313, 1980.

5. Stoller JL, Cooperberg PL, Simpson WM: Diagnostic ultrasonography in acute cholecystitis. *Can J Surg* 22:374–376, 1979.

6. Fonseca C, Greenberg D, Rosenthall L, et al: Assessment of the utility of gallbladder imaging with ^{99m}Tc-IDA. *Clin Nuc Med* 3:437–441, 1978.

7. Weissmann HS, Badia J, Sugarman LA, et al: Spectrum of 99m-Tc IDA cholescintigraphic patterns in acute cholecystitis. *Radiology* 138: 167–175, 1981.

8. Weissmann HS, Frank MS, Bernstein, LH, et al: Rapid and accurate diagnosis of acute cholecystitis with 99mTc-HIDA cholescintigraphy. *AJR* 132:523–528, 1979.

9. Weinstein BJ, Weinstein DP: Biliary tract dilatation in the nonjaundiced patient. *AJR* 134:899–906, 1980.

10. Zeman R, Taylor KJW, Murrell MI, et al: Ultrasound demonstration of dilatation of the biliary tree. *Radiology* 134:689–692, 1980.

11. Harbin WP, Ferrucci JR Jr: Nonoperative management of malignant biliary obstruction: A radiologic alternative. *AJR* 135:103–107, 1980.

12. Callen PW, Filly RA: Ultrasonographic localization of the gallbladder. *Radiology* 133:687–691, 1979.

13. Sukov RJ, Sample WF, Sarti DA, et al: Cholecystosonography—The junctional fold. *Radiology* 133:435–436, 1979.

14. Filly RA, Laing FC: Anatomic variation of portal venous anatomy in the porta hepatis: Ultrasonographic evaluation. *J Clin Ultrasound* 6:83–89, 1978.

15. Arnon S, Rosenquist CJ; Gray scale cholecystosonography: An evaluation of accuracy. *AJR* 127:817–818, 1976.

16. Bartrum RJ Jr, Crow HC, Foote SR: Ultrasonic and radiographic cholecystography. *N Engl J Med* 296:538–541, 1977.

17. Bartrum RJ Jr, Crow HC, Foote SR: Ultrasound examination of the gallbladder: An alternative to "double-dose" oral cholecystography. *JAMA* 236:1,147–1,148, 1976.

18. Crade M, Taylor KJW, Rosenfield AT, et al: Surgical and pathologic correlation of cholecystosonography and cholecystography. *AJR* 131:227–229, 1978.

19. Dempsey PJ, Phillips JR, Warren DL, et al: Cholecystosonography for the diagnosis of cholecytolithiasis. *Ann Surg* 187:465–472, 1978.

20. Goldberg BB, Harris K, Broocker W: Ultrasonic and radiographic cholecystography. *Radiology* 111:405–409, 1974.

21. Hublitz UF, Kahn PC, Sell LA: Cholecystosonography: An approach to the nonvisualized gallbladder. *Radiology* 103:645–649, 1972.

22. Lawson TL: Gray scale cholecystosonography: Diagnostic criteria and accuracy. *Radiology* 122:247–251, 1977.

23. Leopold GR, Amberg J, Gosink BB, et al: Gray scale ultrasonic cholecystography: A comparison with conventional radiographic techniques. *Radiology* 121:445–448, 1976.

24. McKay AJ, Duncan JG, Imrie CW, et al: A prospective study of the clinical value and accuracy of gray scale ultrasound in detecting gallstones. *Br J Surg* 65:330–333, 1978.

25. Cooperberg PL, Ayre-Smith G, Garrow DG: Gray-scale ultrasound of biliary tract disease: A correlative study with percutaneous transhepatic cholaniography. *J Can Assoc Radiol* 28: 237–242, 1977.

26. Dewbury KC, Joseph AEA, Hayes S, et al: Ultrasound in the evaluation and diagnosis of jaundice. *Br J Radiol* 52:276–280, 1979.

27. Goldberg BB: Ultrasonic cholangiography. *Radiology* 118:401–404, 1976.

28. Isikoff MB, Diaconis JN: Ultrasound: A new diagnostic approach to the jaundiced patient. *JAMA* 238:221–223, 1977.

29. Lee T, Henderson SC, Ehrlich T: Ultrasound diagnosis of common bile duct dilatation, *Radiology* 124:793–797, 1977.

30. Malini S, Sabel J: Ultrasonography in obstructive jaundice, *Radiology* 123:429–433, 1977.

31. Neiman HL, Mintzer RA: Accuracy of biliary duct ultrasound: comparison with cholangiography. *AJR* 129:979–982, 1977.

32. Stone LB, Ferrucci, JT Jr, Warshaw AL, et al: Gray scale ultrasound diagnosis of obstructive biliary disease. *AJR* 125:47–50, 1975.

33. Taylor KJW, Carpenter DA, McCready VR: Ultrasound and scintigraphy in the differential diagnosis of obstructive jaundice. *J Clin Ultrasound* 2:105–116, 1974.

34. Taylor KJW, Rosenfield AT: Grey-scale ultrasonography in the differential diagnosis of jaundice. *Arch Surg* 112:820–825, 1977.

35. Cooperberg PL: High-resolution real-time ultrasound in the evaluation of the normal and obstructed biliary tract. *Radiology* 129:477–480, 1978.

36. Cooperberg PL, Burhenne HJ: Real-time ultrasonography: A diagnostic technique of choice in calculous gallbladder disease. *N Engl J Med* 302:1,277–1,279, 1980.

37. Cooperberg PL, Li D, Wong P, et al: Accuracy of common hepatic duct size in the evaluation of extrahepatic biliary obstruction. *Radiology* 135:141–144, 1980.

38. Krook PM, Allen FH, Bush WH Jr, et al: Comparison of real-time cholecystoson- ography and oral cholecytography. *Radiology* 135:145–148, 1980.

39. Weill F, Eisencher A, Zeltner F: Ultrasonic study of the normal and dilated biliary tree. *Radiology* 127:221–224, 1978.

40. Cooperberg PL, Li DKB, Sauerbrei EE: Abdominal and peripheral applications of real-time ultrasound. *Radiol Clin North Am* 18:59–77, 1980.

41. Scheske GS, Cooperberg PL, Cohen MM, et al: Floating gallstones: The role of contrast material. *J Clin Ultrasound* 8:277–231, 1980.

42. Taylor KJW, Jacobson P, Jaffe CC: Lack of an acoustic shadow on scans of gallstones: A possible artifact. *Radiology* 131:463–464, 1979.

43. Carroll BA: Gallstones: In vitro comparison of physical, radiographic, and ultrasonic characteristics. *AJR* 131:223–226, 1978.

44. Good LI, Edell SL, Soloway RD, et al: Ultrasonic properties of gallstones: Effect of stone size and composition. *Gastroenterology* 77:258–263, 1979.

45. Filly RA, Moss AA, Way LW: In vitro investigation of gallstone shadowing with ultrasound tomography. *J Clin Ultrasound* 7:255–262, 1979.

46. Cooperberg PL, Pon MS, Wong P, et al: Real-time resolution ultrasound in the detection of biliary calculi, *Radiology* 131:789–790, 1979.

47. Fiske CE, Laing FC, Brown TW: Ultrasonographic evidence of gallbladder wall thickening in association with hypoalbuminemia. *Radiology* 135:713–716, 1980.

48. Sanders RC: The significance of sonographic gallbladder wall thickening. *J Clin Ultrasound* 8:143–146, 1980.

49. Shlaer WJ, Leopold GR, Scheible FW: Sonography of the thickened gallbladder wall: A nonspecific finding. *AJR* 136:337–339, 1981.

50. Harbin WP, Ferrucci JR Jr, Wittenberg J, et al: Nonvisualized gallbladder by cholecystosonography. *AJR* 132:727–728, 1979.

51. Laing FC, Gooding GAW, Herzong KA: Gallstones preventing ultrasonographic visualization of the gallbladder. *Gastrointest Radiol* 1:301–303, 1977.

52. Raptopoulos V, D'Orsi C, Smith E, et al: Dynamic cholecystosonography of the contracted gallbladder: The double-arc-shadow sign. *AJR* 138:275–278, 1982.

53. Hunter ND, Macintosh PK: Acute emphysematous cholecystitis: An ultrasonic diagnosis, *AJR* 134:592, 1980.

54. MacDonald FR, Cooperberg PL, Cohen MM: The WES traid. A specific sonographic sign of gallstones in the contract gallbladder. *Gastrointest Radiol* 6:39–41, 1981.

55. Conrad MR, Janes JO, Dietchy J: Significance of low-level echoes within the gallbladder. *AJR* 132:967–972, 1979.

56. Filly RA, Allen B, Minton MJ, et al: In vitro investigation of the origin of echoes within biliary sludge. *J Clin Ultrasound* 8:193–200, 1980.

57. Thurber LA, Cooperberg PL, Clement JG, et al: Echogenic fluid: A pitfall in the ultrasonographic diagnosis of cystic lesions. *J Clin Ultrasound* 7:273–278, 1979.

58. Weeks LE, McCune BR, Martin JF, et al: Unusual echographic appearance of a Courvoisier gallbladder. *J Clin Ultrasound* 5:341–342, 1977.

59. Simeone JF, Mueller PR, Ferrucci JT Jr, et al: Significance of nonshadowing focal opacities at cholecystosonography. *Radiology* 137:181–185, 1980.

60. Grant EG, Smirniotopoulos JG: Intraluminal gallbladder hematoma: Sonographic evidence of hemobilia. *J Clin Ultrasound* 11:507–509, 1983.

61. Kane RA: Ultrasonographic diagnosis of gangreous cholecystitis and empyema of the gallbladder. *Radiology* 134:191–194, 1980.

62. Carter SJ, Rutledge J, Hirsch JH, et al: Papillary adenoma of the gallbladder: Ultrasonic demonstration. *J Clin Ultrasound* 6:433–435, 1978.

63. Olken SM, Bledsoe R, Newmark H III: The ultrasonic diagnosis of primary carcinoma of the gallbladder. *Radiology* 129:481–482, 1978.

64. Raghavendra BN: Ultrasonographic features of primary carcinoma of the gallbladder: Report of five cases. *Gastrointest Radiol* 5:239–244, 1980.

65. Yeh H-C: Ultrasonography and computed tomography of carcinoma of the gallbladder. *Radiology* 133:167–173, 1979.

66. Yum HY, Fink AH: Sonographic findings in primary carcinoma of the gallbladder. *Radiology* 134:693–696, 1980.

67. Rice J, Sauerbrei EE, Semogas P, et al: The sonographic appearance of adenomyomatosis of the gallbladder. *J Clin Ultrasound* 9:336–337, 1981.

68. Laing FC, London LA, Filly RA: Ultrasonographic identification of dilated intrahepatic bile ducts and their differentiation from portal venous structures. *J Clin Ultrasound* 6:90–94, 1978.

69. Conrad MR, Landay MJ, Janes JO: Sonographic "parallel channel" sign of biliary tree enlargement in mild to moderate obstructive jaundice. *AJR* 130:279–286, 1978.

70. Shanser JD, Korobkin, Goldberg HI, et al: Computed tomographic diagnosis of obstructive jaundice in the absence of intrahepatic ductal dilatation. *AJR* 131:389–392, 1978.

71. Shawker TH, Jones BL, Girton ME: Distal common bile duct obstruction: An experimental study in monkeys. *J Clin Ultrasound* 9:77–82, 1981.

72. Zeman RK, Taylor KJW, Rosenfield AT, et al: Acute experimental biliary obstruction in the dog: Sonographic findings and clinical implications. *AJR* 136:965–967, 1981.

73. Behan M, Kazam E: Sonography of the common bile duct: Value of the right anterior oblique view. *AJR* 130:701–709, 1978.

74. Sample WF, Sarti DA, Goldstein LI, et al: Gray-scale ultrasonography of the jaundiced patient. *Radiology* 128:719–725, 1978.

75. Wise RE, O'Brien RG: Intravenous cholangiography: A preliminary report. *Lahey Clin Found Bull* 9:52, 1954.

76. Sauerbrei EE, Cooperberg PL, Gordon P, et al: The discrepancy between radiographic and sonographic bile-duct measurements. *Radiology* 137:751–755, 1980.

77. Scheske GA, Cooperberg PL, Cohen MM, et al: Dynamic changes in the calibre of the major bile ducts, related to obstruction. *Radiology* 135:215–216, 1980.

78. Gooding GAW: Acute bile duct dilation with resolution in 43 hours: An ultrasonic demonstration. *J Clin Ultrasound* 9:201–203, 1981.

79. Sullivan FJ, Eaton SB Jr, Ferrucci JT Jr, et al: Cholangiographic manifestations of acute biliary colic. *N Engl J Med* 228:33–35, 1973.

80. Wise RE, O'Brien RG: Interpretation of the intravenous cholangiogram. *JAMA* 160:819–827, 1956.

81. Graham MF, Cooperberg PL, Cohen MM, et al: The size of the normal common hepatic duct following cholecystectomy: An ultrasonographic study. *Radiology* 135:137–139.

82. Mueller PR, Harbin WP, Ferrucci JT Jr, et al: Fine-needle transhepatic cholangiography: Reflections after 450 cases. *AJR* 136:85–90, 1981.

83. Graham MF, Cooperberg PL, Cohen MM, et al: Ultrasonographic screening of the

common hepatic duct in symptomatic patients after cholecystectomy. *Radiology* 138:137–139, 1981.

84. Hadidi A: Distinction between obstructive and nonobstructive jaundice by sonography. *Clin Radiol* 31:181–187, 1980.

85. Koenigsberg M, Wiener SN, Walzer A: The accuracy of sonography in the differential diagnosis of obstructive jaundice: A comparison with cholangiography. *Radiology* 133:157–165, 1979.

86. Salem S, Vas W: Ultrasonography in evaluation of the jaundiced patient. *J Can Assoc Radiol* 31:30–34, 1981.

87. Taylor KJW, Rosenfield AT, Spiro HM: Diagnostic accuracy of gray scale ultrasonography for the jaundiced patient: A report of 275 cases. *Arch Intern Med* 139:60–63, 1979.

88. Vallon AG, Lees WR, Cotton RB: Grey-scale ultrasonography in cholestatic jaundice. *Gut* 20:51–54, 1979.

89. Gordon P, Cooperberg PL, Cohen MM: Presence of gallstones is a poor indicator of the cause of obstructive jaundice. *Surg Gyn Obstet* 151:635–636, 1980.

90. Gosink BB, Lemon SK, Scheible W, et al: Accuracy of ultrasonography in diagnosis of hepatocellular disease. *AJR* 133:19–23, 1979.

91. Joseph AEA, Dewbury KC, McGuire PG: Ultrasound in the detection of chronic liver disease (the bright "liver"). *Br J Radiol* 52:184–188, 1979.

92. Kurtz AB, Rubin CS, Cooper HS, et al: Ultrasonic findings in hepatitis. *Radiology* 136:717–723, 1980.

93. Harbin WP, Robert NJ, Ferrucci JT Jr: Diagnosis of cirrhosis based on regional changes in hepatic morphology. *Radiology* 135:273–283, 1980.

94. Gould L, Patel A: Ultrasound detection of extrahepatic encapsulated bile: "Biloma". *AJR* 132:1,014–1,015, 1979.

95. Reuter K, Raptopoulos VD, Cantelmo N, et al: The diagnosis of a choledochal cyst by ultrasound. *Radiology* 136:437–438, 1980.

96. Weissman HS, Chun KJ, Frank M, et al: Demonstration of traumatic bile leakage with cholescintigraphy and ultrasonography. *AJR* 133:843–847, 1979.

97. Kangarloo H, Sarti DA, Sample WF, et al: Ultrasonographic spectrum of choledochal cysts in children. *Pediatric Radiol* 9:15–18, 1980.

98. Carroll BA: Biliary cystadenoma and cystadenocarcinoma: Gray scale ultrasound appearance. *J Clin Ultrasound* 6:337–340, 1978.

99. Forrest ME, Cho KJ, Shields JJ, et al: Biliary cystadenomas: Sonographic-angiographic-pathologic correlations. *AJR* 135:723–727, 1980.

100. Mittelstaedt CA, Volberg FM, Fischer GJ, et al: Caroli's disease: Sonographic findings. *AJR* 134:585–587, 1980.

101. Harbin WP, Mueller PR, Ferrucci JT Jr: Transhepatic cholangiography: Complications and use patterns of the fine-needle technique. *Radiology* 135:15–22, 1980.

102. Goldberg HI, Filly RA, Korobkin M, et al: Capability of CT body scanning and ultrasonography to demonstrate the status of the biliary ductal system in patients with jaundice. *Radiology* 129:731–737, 1978.

103. Raskin MM: Hepatobiliary disease: A comparative evaluation by ultrasound and computed tomography. *Gastrointest Radiol* 3:267–271, 1978.

104. Baron RL, Stanley RJ, Lee JKT: A prospective comparison of the evaluation of biliary obstruction using computed tomography and ultrasonography. *Radiology* 145:91–98, 1982.

105. Rosenthall L: Directions in radionuclide hepatobiliary imaging. *J Can Assoc Radiol* 31:220–224, 1980.

106. Goodman MW, Ansel JH, Vennes JA, et al: Is intravenous cholangiography still useful? *Gastroenterology* 79:642–645, 1980.

107. Gregg JA, McDonald DG: Endoscopic retrograde cholangiopancreatography and gray-scale abdominal ultrasound in the diagnosis of jaundice. *Am J Surg* 137:611–615, 1979.

108. Lane RJ, Crocker EF: Operative ultrasonic bile duct scanning. *Aust NZ J Surg* 49:454–458, 1979.

109. Sigel B, Coelho JCU, Spigos DG, et al: Real-time ultrasonography during biliary surgery. *Radiology* 137:531–533, 1980.

110. Makuuchi M, Bandai Y, Ito T, et al: Ultrasonically guided percutaneous transhepatic bile drainage. *Radiology* 136:165–169, 1980.

5

Pancreas

Alfred B. Kurtz
Barry B. Goldberg

NORMAL ANATOMY

General Characteristics

The pancreas is a nonencapsulated, multilobulated retroperitoneal gland, measuring 12.5 to 15 cm in length.[1] It is difficult to make general statements about the anatomy of the normal pancreas due to the wide variations that exist in size and shape. The pancreas is, however, usually long and irregularly prismatic in shape, extending transversely across the upper abdomen with its tail at a slightly more cranial level than its head. In addition, it is closely related to the major abdominal arteries, veins, and adjacent organs.[1]

The pancreatic head is the largest part with the uncinate process, a triangular prolongation, extending off the caudal and left lateral border. The head is lodged within the curvature of the duodenum; the cranial border is overlapped by the superior portion, the caudal border by the horizontal portion, and the right and left borders by the descending and ascending portions respectively. The gallbladder lies immediately lateral to the descending portion of the duodenum.[2] Superior to the pancreatic head are the portal vein and hepatic artery, while directly posterior is the inferior vena cava. Two structures enter the pancreas on its right lateral border; the gastroduodenal artery, the first branch of the hepatic artery, inserts on the superior edge, and the common bile duct enters on the inferior edge. The uncinate process projects medially between the superior mesenteric vein anteriorly and the inferior vena cava posteriorly and, on occasion, extends still further toward the midline to lie between the superior mesenteric artery and the aorta.

The pancreatic neck, the smallest portion of the pancreas, is about 2.5 cm long. Its anterior surface supports the floor of the stomach while its posterior surface lies at the commencement of the portal vein, the confluence of the superior mesenteric and splenic veins.[1]

The body of the pancreas is rectangular. It is covered on its anterior surface by the dorsum of the stomach and is separated from it by the omental bursa or lesser peritoneal sac. This bursa is a potential space between the stomach and pancreas, normally ultrasonically invisible.[2] The posterior surface is in

163

direct contact with the splenic vein. The pancreatic body is anterior to the aorta and the superior mesenteric artery.

The tail of the pancreas extends to the left as far as the spleen. It is usually in close relationship to the anterior caudal surface of the spleen and the anterior cranial surface of the adjacent left kidney. Posteriorly, it is in direct contact with the splenic vein. The tail is anterior to the left adrenal gland.

Normal Variations

Normal variations in the pancreas may be divided into changes in position, shape, form, and size.

Position

While in most patients the pancreas is at the level of the first and second lumbar vertebral body, in thin and elderly patients it may be low-lying, even extending caudad to the sacral promontory.[3] Infrequently, the pancreatic body may be caudad to the splenic vein, the pancreatic head may be located directly anterior to the aorta and spine, and rarely the entire pancreas may be left-sided.[2] In addition, the anteroposterior position of the pancreas is related to the amount of retroperitoneal fat; therefore, in thin patients the pancreas drapes across the spine with the body most anterior and the head and tail more posterior, while in heavier patients the pancreas is nearly uniform in depth, lying approximately half way between the anterior abdominal wall and the anterior surface of the spine.[2] While most pancreases are obliquely situated with the head at a slightly lower level than the tail, infrequently the pancreas may lie transversely across the abdomen.[2]

Shape

Three types of shapes of pancreases have been described: sausage-shaped in 23%, dumbbell-shaped in 33%, and tadpole-shaped in 44% of cases.[4]

Form

The most common forms of pancreases are linear and L-configurations. Less frequently, sigmoid, horseshoe, and rarely U-shaped pancreases have been seen.[2,4]

Size

In general, the pancreases in young children are proportionately larger, decreasing in relative size with age.[2,4-7] Actual dimensions as determined by measurements are discussed in the next section.

NORMAL ULTRASOUND FINDINGS

Technique

Ultrasound scans of the pancreas are performed routinely in the longitudinal and transverse axes. In addition, oblique scans are attempted along the long axis of the pancreas. To avoid the bowel, maneuvers such as angling the transducer cephalad or caudad, or placing the patient in the left-side-down posterior-oblique position may be of value.[8] A single-pass scanning technique, thus avoiding the possibility of image degradation caused by overwriting or by gas pseudotumors, is to be used whenever possible.[9,10] Gas pseudotumors are created when gas is imaged from the anterior, posterior, and lateral surfaces during compound scanning. The bright echo produced at each boundary of the gas leads to the artificial creation of the appearance of a mass.

Several of the previously mentioned anatomic landmarks are commonly used in localizing different parts of the pancreas. The pancreatic head is identified by its relationship to the inferior vena cava and portal vein (Figs. 5-1 and 5-2a). If the duodenal sweep is fluid-filled or if the gastroduodenal artery and common bile duct are imaged, the lateral margin of the pancreatic head will be accurately defined (Figs. 5-2b, c, and d). When overlying bowel gas persists, however, parts of the pancreatic head remain obscured (Fig. 5-2e). The neck of the pancreas is identified by its position anterior to the superior mesenteric vein and the commencement of the portal vein (Figs. 5-1 and 5-3). The pancreatic body and tail are best localized by their anterior relationship to the splenic vein (Figs. 5-1 and 5-4).[6,11] Frequently only part of the tail is identified during routine supine scanning (Figs. 5-1 and 5-5).

Criteria for Ultrasound Analysis

Once imaged, the pancreas may be analyzed for echogenicity, size, and contour. If the pancreas is to be considered normal, it must be normal by all three of these criteria.

Echogenicity

While the pancreas is uniformly bright throughout its substance, the degree of echogenicity is related to the extent of pancreatic fatty infiltration.[12] Older people usually have pancreases that are brighter than those in younger patients, and this ultrasonic characteristic is consistent with the finding that when older people have bright pancreases, fatty infiltration is found (Figs. 5-4 and 5-5).[13] Since most scans of the pancreas are performed through the liver, with frequent simultaneous imaging of the right kidney, it is possible to establish a series of relative echogenicities: renal sinus > pancreas ≥ liver > spleen > renal parenchyma.[4,11,14,15,16] When compared, the echo brightness of the normal pancreas is equal to or greater than that of the liver (Figs. 5-4 and 5-5). In addition, the pancreatic texture or dot size is usually coarser and more inhomogeneous than that of the liver (Figs. 5-1, 5-4, and 5-5).[2,8] It is important to compare the echo patterns of the liver and pancreas at the same tissue depth since echo amplitude and dot size are closely related to the transducer beam profile.[10] It is similarly important to avoid evaluating the liver posterior to the gallbladder or to fibrous tissue; distortion of the normal liver echo pattern can occur since the gallbladder may enhance and fibrous tissue may attenuate the ultrasound beam (Fig. 5-5).[10] In addition, since the pancreas is adjacent to the stomach and duodenum, gas within these structures may occasionally cause shadowing, decreasing the echogenicity of the underlying pancreas (Fig. 5-2e).

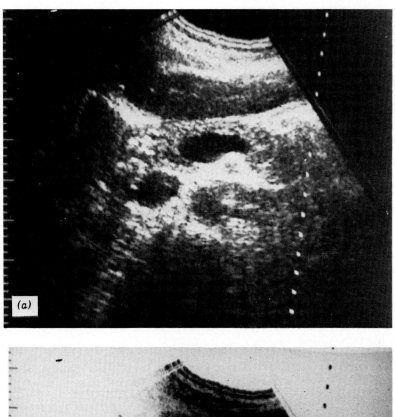

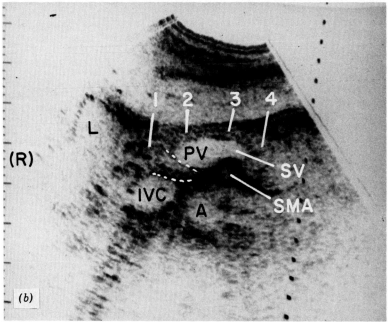

Figure 5-1 Normal pancreas. (*a*) Transverse supine ultrasound scan of the pancreas. (*b*) The reverse image of (*a*) with labels. 1 = pancreatic head; 2 = pancreatic neck; 3 = pancreatic body; 4 = partially imaged pancreatic tail. Dots outline uncinate process of the pancreatic head. A = aorta; IVC = inferior vena cava; PV = portal vein; SV = splenic vein; SMA = superior mesenteric artery; L = liver; (R) = toward right side of patient.

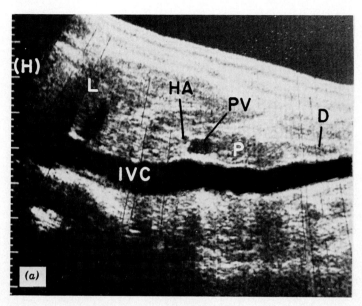

Figure 5-2 Normal pancreatic head (different patients). (*a*) Longitudinal ultrasound scan 2 cm to the right of the midline, showing the pancreatic head (P) anterior to the long axis of the inferior vena cava (IVC). Note the portal vein (PV) cephalad and the horizontal portion of the duodenum (D) caudad. The echogenicity of the pancreas is the same as the adjacent liver (L). HA = hepatic artery; (H) = toward head of patient. (From Kurtz, AB: Ultrasound of the pancreas. *Belgium Journal of Radiology* 64:13–24, 1981). (*b*) Transverse ultrasound scan after water ingestion with the patient right side down, showing a fluid-filled duodenal sweep (D) outlining the pancreatic head (P). Note the common bile duct (CBD) at the inferior and the gastroduodenal artery (GDA) at the superior margins of the pancreatic head. Also note the variation in position with the pancreatic head directly anterior to the aorta (A) rather than anterior to the inferior vena cava (IVC). PD = pancreatic duct; GB = gallbladder; RK = right kidney; L = liver; (R) = toward right side of patient. (*c*) Longitudinal ultrasound scan 2 cm to the right of the midline showing the lateral margin of the pancreatic head (P), the main portal vein (MPV) immediately cephalad and the gastroduodenal artery (GDA) extending over the superior lateral pancreatic border. HA = hepatic artery; IVC = inferior vena cava; L = liver; D = horizontal portion of duodenum; (H) = toward head of patient. (*d*) Oblique long-axis ultrasound scan of the pancreatic head (arrows), scanned from the right shoulder toward the left hip. Note the common bile duct (CBD) extending into the inferior lateral margin of the pancreatic head. MPV = main portal vein; IVC = inferior vena cava; (H) = toward head of patient. (From Kurtz, AB: Ultrasound of the pancreas, *Belgium Journal of Radiology* 64:13–24, 1981). (*e*) Oblique long-axis ultrasound scan of the pancreatic head (P), scanned from the right shoulder toward the left hip. Note the common bile duct (CBD) is obscured as it enters the pancreatic head due to gas in the region of the duodenal bulb (D). MPV = main portal vein; L = liver; IVC = inferior vena cava; A = aorta; HA = hepatic artery; (H) = toward head of patient.

167

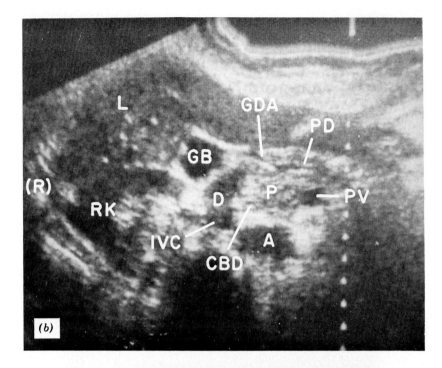

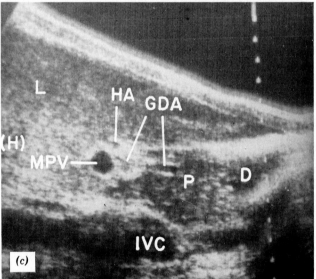

Figure 5-2 (*continued*)

Therefore, care must be taken when evaluating the pancreas in regions where bowel gas is present. Within the liver, the ligamentum teres may also cause an acoustic shadow obscuring small sections of the pancreas (Fig. 5-6). Rarely, a false pancreatic mass may be created by reverberation artifacts from an overlying gas-filled loop of bowel.[10]

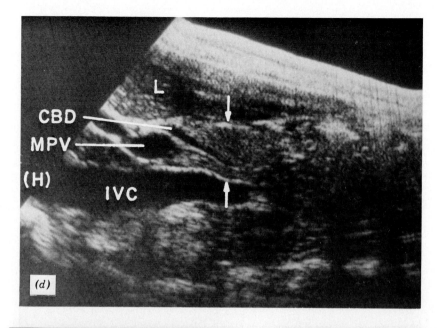

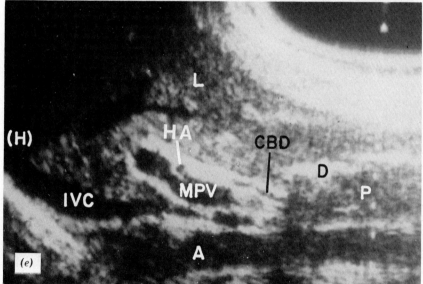

Figure 5-2 (*continued*)

Size

Ultrasound measurements of the overall anterior-posterior dimensions of the pancreas have been previously reported by several authors (Table 5-1).[4,5,13,14,17–20] In these studies, the measurements for the pancreatic head, neck, and body were performed using supine longitudinal and transverse views immediately anterior to the inferior vena cava, superior mesenteric vein, and superior

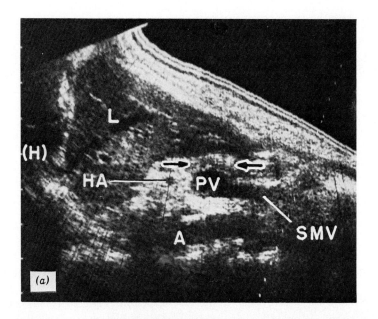

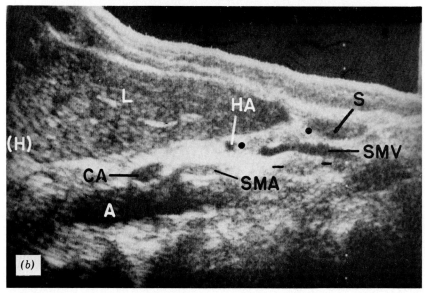

Figure 5-3 Normal pancreatic neck (different patients). (*a*) Longitudinal ultrasound scan 0.5 cm to the right of the midline showing the pancreatic neck (arrows) immediately anterior to the portal vein (PV). SMV = superior mesenteric vein; A = aorta; L = liver; HA = hepatic artery; (H) = toward head of patient. (From Kurtz, AB: Ultrasound of the pancreas. *Belgium Journal of Radiology* 64: 13–24, 1981). (*b*) Longitudinal midline ultrasound scan showing the superior mesenteric vein (SMV) surrounded by the pancreatic neck (dots) anteriorly and the uncinate process of the pancreatic head (lines) posteriorly. Note their proximity to the aorta (A), celiac axis (CA), hepatic artery (HA), and superior mesenteric artery (SMA). L = liver; S = stomach (antrum); (H) = toward head of patient.

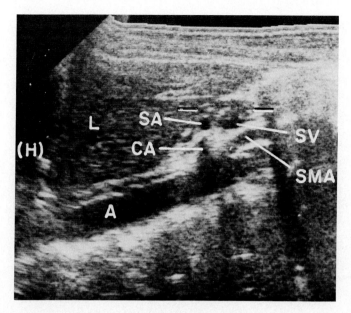

Figure 5-4 Normal pancreatic body in a teenage girl. Longitudinal midline supine ultrasound scan showing the pancreatic body (lines) immediately anterior to the splenic vein (SV). Note that the pancreas, while equal in echogenicity, is coarser in texture than the adjacent liver (L). A = aorta; CA = celiac axis; SMA = superior mesenteric artery; (H) = toward head of patient.

mesenteric artery respectively. The pancreatic tail, however, was measured either from supine or prone images, at either the distal tail or mid-left-prerenal area. In addition, there was variation in the way the measurements were obtained. While not specifically stated in all studies, the pancreatic head, neck, and body were probably measured directly anterior to posterior and the tail

Table 5-1   Maximum Normal Ultrasound Pancreatic Measurements

Studies and Year	Type of B-mode Imaging	Pancreas[a]			
		Head	Neck	Body	Tail
Doust and Pearce, 1976	Gray scale	15	—	15	15
Haber et al., 1976	Gray scale	34	—	29	28
Weill et al., 1977	Bistable	30	—	24	31 to 32
deGraaff et al., 1978	Gray scale	24	13	15.4	—
Goldstein and Katragadda, 1978	Gray scale	—	—	—	25
Lawson, 1978	Gray scale	25	—	20	15
Arger et al., 1979	Gray scale	25	—	20	20
Katz et al., 1980	Gray scale	35 25[b]	—	25 20[b]	—

[a] Anteroposterior in millimeters.
[b] Lower measurement if pancreatic contours irregular.

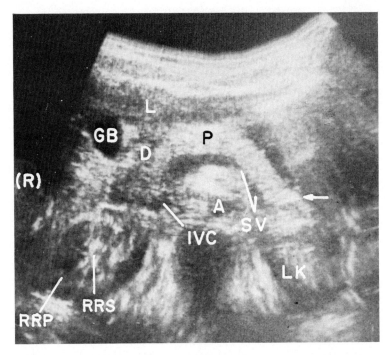

Figure 5-5 Normal pancreas in a man in his late seventies. Transverse supine ultrasound scan of the pancreas (P), descending portion of the duodenum (D), and gallbladder (GB). Note the increased pancreatic echogenicity relative to the adjacent liver (L), right renal parenchyma (RRP), and right renal sinus (RRS). The liver echo pattern is falsely enhanced posterior to the gallbladder. The incompletely seen pancreatic tail (arrow) is imaged only to the middle of the left kidney (LK). SV = splenic vein; IVC = inferior vena cava; (R) = toward right side of patient.

measured perpendicular to its long axis. In one study, however, the pancreatic head was instead evaluated perpendicular to the tangent of its posterior aspect.[4]

Nevertheless, when these different studies are compared, a pancreatic head less than 25 mm and a body and tail less than 20 mm were always within normal limits (Table 5-1). It is possible, however, for the pancreatic head to be normal up to 35 mm, for the body to be up to 30 mm in a sausage-shaped pancreas, and for the tail to approach 35 mm when the pancreas is dumbbell-shaped.[4] In addition, the measurement variations did not appear to be affected by the type of B-mode scanner used to image the pancreas (Table 1). In children, smaller measurements were obtained.[21] The maximum anteroposterior dimensions in the 0 to 6 age group was 1.9 cm for the head, 1.0 cm for the body, and 1.6 cm for the tail. The sizes remained the same for the 7 to 12 age group, increasing slightly up to age 18 to 2.2 cm, 1.0 cm and 1.8 cm for the pancreatic head, body, and tail respectively. It must be remembered that each ultrasound scan has three dimensions, with an approximate beam width of 10 mm for each slice. Since, for example, the pancreatic head has a usual cranial-caudad extent of 30 mm (Fig. 5-2a), one transverse scan would not be adequate to visualize the entire pancreatic head, and at least three overlapping transverse images would be necessary. On occasion, the cranial-caudad extent of the pancreatic head may be quite elongated, up to 60 mm.[5] Therefore, to ensure complete pancreatic head visualization, overlapping transverse scans should be started superior to the pancreatic head at the main portal vein and continued inferiorly through the head until the horizontal portion of the duodenum is encountered. This same technique should be applied to all areas of the pancreas.

Contour

In general, the borders of the pancreas are smooth, particularly early in life, but may become somewhat more irregular with age.[4,10] When marked irregularity or "lumpiness" occurs, pathology must be considered. These contour changes are probably easier to evaluate with computed tomography, but can be frequently appreciated on ultrasound examination.[5,10] The uncinate process, in particular, is an important indicator of disease since any enlargement or rounding implies abnormality (Fig. 5-1).[8]

Positioning for Optimal Imaging

Head

The pancreatic head is imaged most commonly with the patient in a supine position and with the scans performed over the anterior abdominal wall. When the left lobe of the liver is prominent, it serves as an excellent acoustic window

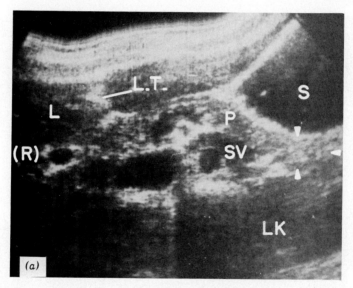

Figure 5-6 Normal pancreas with fluid distension of stomach. (*a*) Transverse erect ultrasound scan of the pancreas (P) through a water distended stomach (S) showing the entire pancreatic tail (arrowheads) between the stomach and the left kidney. Note the incomplete visualization of the pancreatic head caused by shadowing from the brightly echogenic ligamentum teres (LT) within the liver (L). SV = splenic vein; (R) = toward right side of patient. (*b*) Longitudinal erect ultrasound scan 4 cm to the left of the midline showing a fluid-filled stomach anterior to the pancreatic tail (P). SV = splenic vein; SA = splenic artery; (H) = toward head of patient. (*c*) Transverse computed tomographic image of the upper abdomen in another patient with intravenous contrast opacifying the left kidney (LK) and oral contrast filling the stomach (S). The pancreatic head (1), neck (2), body (3), and tail (4) are seen. Note the pancreatic tail (arrow) extends to the spleen (Sp) similar to the views obtained on ultrasound with water distension of the stomach (*a*).

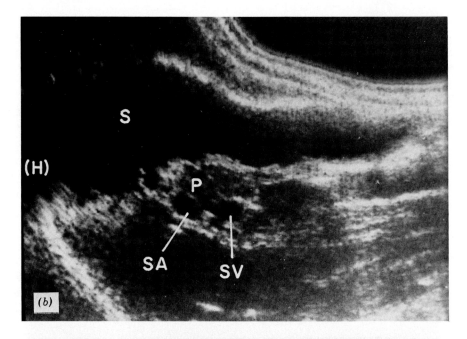

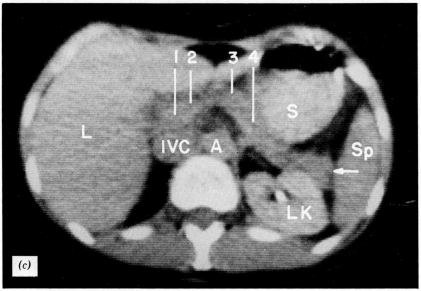

Figure 5-6 (*continued*)

to image the pancreas in that it displaces the stomach and lies immediately anterior to the pancreas (Fig. 5-1).[2] If the left lobe of the liver is not prominent, a frequently helpful maneuver is to elevate the patient's right side 45 degrees. This causes the liver to fall caudally, toward the left, and thus more over the pancreatic head. However, when the left lobe of the liver is small and the stomach and duodenum are gas-filled, ultrasound is frequently unable to visualize large parts of the gland even after elevation of the patient's right side. Bowel gas is usually lessened by scanning after a 4 to 6 hour fast, since the stomach is then either empty or filled with small amounts of secretions. When bowel gas persists, however, it may be displaced by the ingestion of fluid. The stomach is filled by having the patient drink water through a straw while lying left-side down to minimize ingestion of excessive amounts of air.[22] The patient is then repositioned right-side down so that the antrum and duodenum fill with water (Fig. 5-2b).[9] An additional view for the pancreatic head, permitting more complete imaging of the long axis of the common bile duct, is to scan at an oblique angle from the right shoulder toward the left hip, frequently with the right side of the patient slightly elevated (Figs. 5-2d and e).[23]

Neck and Body

The supine view is also commonly used in evaluating the pancreatic neck and body (Figs. 5-1, 5-3, and 5-4). These segments are anterior to the lumbar spine and, therefore, closer to the anterior abdominal wall. It has been found that gentle transducer pressure during scanning, particularly in thin patients, often displaces overlying gas-filled bowel, allowing more complete visualization.

Tail

The pancreatic tail is the most difficult region of the pancreas to evaluate completely. Gas in the stomach frequently causes the supine views to be inadequate, and, even when imaged, usually only the part of the tail slightly to the left of the spine is seen (Figs. 5-1 and 5-5). Prone ultrasound imaging through the left kidney infrequently allows better visualization of the normal pancreatic tail.[18,20] This view, however, is of greater value in the detection of tail enlargement (Fig. 5-7).[5,20] Care must be taken when performing prone scans that the transverse colon (in the region of the splenic flexure), small bowel loops (jejunum), and stomach are not mistaken for pancreatic tail masses (Fig. 5-7).[24]

Several techniques for imaging the tail of the pancreas have been proposed: (1) Supine scans with a water-filled stomach.[21] Water or any other ingested fluid may serve as both an anatomic landmark to the left upper quadrant and as an acoustic window to evaluate deeper structures.[25] While this view is frequently better for imaging the pancreatic head and body, it may be of value in imaging the tail in patients who cannot sit or stand.[25] (2) Erect or sitting-up scans without ingestion of water.[26] This technique may be of value in imaging more of the pancreas in any patient and is of particular value in patients who are not able to ingest fluids. Its advantages are that the gastric air rises to the fundus, the upper abdominal bowel falls toward the feet, the major abdominal veins become relatively distended, and the liver falls caudad proportionately more than does the pancreas, thereby serving as an acoustic window to image the pancreas. (3) Erect or sitting-up scans after ingestion of approximately 500 cc of water (Figs. 5-7a and b).[4,26,27] This combination gives better and more consistent pancreatic visualization than either maneuver alone. The previous success rates in routine supine imaging of the pancreatic head, body, and tail had been 77 to 90 percent, 70 to 90 percent, and 37 percent respectively.[4,18,19,28] In a study comparing the supine nonfluid-filled stomach technique with the erect fluid-filled stomach method, an increase from 49 to 84 percent was noted of adequate to excellent visualization for the head, from 52 to 92 percent for the body, and from 10 to 67 percent for the tail.[26] In addition, nonvisualization of any part of the pancreas decreased from 19 to 1 percent.[26] While these results are not outstanding for the head and body in which success rates of close to 90 percent had previously been reported, the erect water-filled stomach technique has significantly improved visualization of the pancreatic tail. In addition to permitting more consistent imaging of the tail, it also allows more complete detection of the pancreas extending the visualized area to the region of the left kidney and spleen (Figs. 5-7a and c). The use of real-time ultrasound has decreased the time of the water-filled examination to 5 to 10 minutes. Previous static images took 30 to 45 minutes, and a gastric motility inhibitor was frequently needed.[29]

Pancreatic Duct

In recent years, routine imaging of the main pancreatic duct, the duct of Wirsung, has been increasingly possible. This duct extends through the substance of the pancreas, starting at the tail, progressively enlarging as it courses to the head. The duct is imaged as an anechoic space surrounded by two

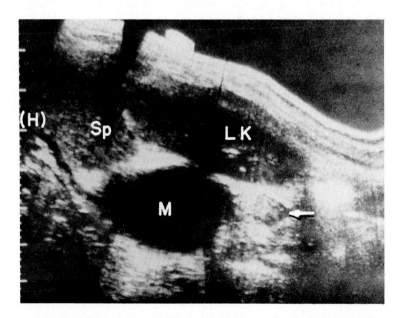

Figure 5-7 Pseudocyst in tail of the pancreas. Long-axis prone ultrasound scan performed through the left side of the back showing a pancreatic tail pseudocyst (M) between the spleen (Sp) and the left kidney (LK). Note a normally collapsed loop of small bowel (arrow). (H) = toward head of patient.

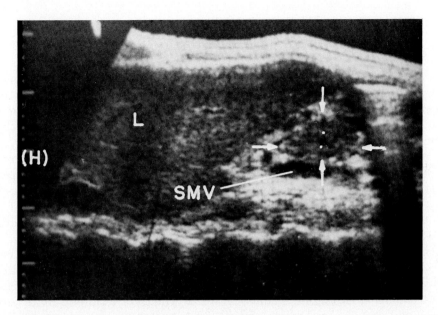

Figure 5-8 Normal pancreatic duct. Longitudinal scan 0.5 cm to the right of midline showing the pancreas (arrows) at the junction of the neck and body, immediately anterior to the superior mesenteric vein (SMV). The slightly prominent pancreatic duct (outlined by dots) can be identified in the midst of pancreatic tissue. L = liver; (H) = toward patient's head.

parallel hyperechoic lines resembling trolley tracks (Fig. 5-2b).[30,31,32] The maximum inner diameter, while not fully established, is considered normal if less than 2 mm and may be seen in approximately 82 to 84 percent of normal patients.[2,31,32] In the remaining 15 to 20 percent of nonvisualized normal pancreatic ducts, the use of intravenous secretin, causing physiologic distention, has led to duct identification in more than 80 percent.[31]

It is important to image the duct within the midst of the pancreatic tissue so that the more anteriorly situated collapsed stomach wall and the more posteriorly placed portal and splenic veins are not mistaken for the duct.[2,5] If a question arises as to whether the imaged structure is the duct or the collapsed stomach, fluid ingestion frequently resolves the problem.[4] Within the pancreatic body, the duct is usually parallel to the anterior abdominal wall and is, therefore, most reliably imaged within this segment (Fig. 5-8).[2,31,32] It is also felt that high-resolution real-time imaging allows more constant evaluation of the pancreatic duct, since it has been stated that static scans occasionally image only a single hyperechoic line for the pancreatic duct. While the resolution of both real-time and static images are similar, there has been an attempt to explain this discrepancy by suggesting that the pulsations of the adjacent aorta may blur the duct on the slower static scanners, thus causing a single line to be imaged.

ABNORMAL ULTRASOUND FINDINGS

Criteria

Abnormalities of the pancreas may be divided into processes causing diffuse enlargement, usually pancreatitis, and those creating focal distortion, most commonly neoplasms or sequelae of pancreatitis. Ultrasound can frequently detect these abnormalities by employing slight modifications of the same three criteria used to evaluate the normal pancreas, that is, echogenicity, size, and contour. Of these, echogenicity is the most consistent criterion since almost all pathologic processes distort pancreatic echo patterns; not all cause pancreatic enlargement and contour changes, however (Fig. 5-9a). Computed tomography is at times not as accurate as ultrasound, since it must rely predominantly on contour and size changes. Small lesions that do not distort the pancreatic outline are frequently missed (Fig. 5-9b).

In the ultrasound analysis of mass lesions (Table 5-2), the modified criteria are: (1) Ultrasound characteristics—cystic versus solid, overall echo pattern, sound absorption, and through-transmission. Sound absorption is inversely proportional to through-transmission so that when, for example, an ultrasonically solid mass lesion absorbs sound, the sound absorption is increased and through-transmission is decreased. (2) Size—normal or enlarged and, if enlarged, localized or diffuse. (3) Contour changes. (4) Additional features suggestive of a specific abnormality. It is important to remember that when an ultrasonically solid pancreatic mass is detected, accurate pathologic prediction is usually not possible (Tables 5-2 and 5-3). In one study, while hyperechoic solid masses were most likely malignant in 90 percent of cases, an additional 25 percent of inflammatory masses had similar ultrasound characteristics.[5] Therefore, pancreatic carcinoma, other primary peripancreatic malignancies, islet cell tumors, metastatic disease, focal pancreatitis, and lymphoma may be indistinguishable.[33]

Primary Adenocarcinoma

Primary adenocarcinoma of the pancreas is most commonly imaged as an ultrasonically solid, focally enlarged, lobulated abnormality with low-level echoes and increased sound absorption (Figs. 5-9 and 5-10).[5,11,19,33,34] Infrequently, primary pancreatic carcinoma may appear densely hyperechoic.[19] Since the majority of tumors have decreased echogenicity, it is on occasion difficult to separate an hypoechoic pancreatic mass from a pseudomass produced by overlying bowel gas and its distal reverberation, creating a false front and back wall.[19,33] When bowel gas is encountered, though, all the sound is reflected back to the transducer so that there is no through-transmission, while a solid pancreatic mass only absorbs some of the sound and therefore has through-transmission (Fig. 5-10).

Primary carcinoma most commonly occurs in the pancreatic head, where there is a high incidence of associated biliary obstruction and, occasionally, pancreatic duct obstruction as well (Fig. 5-11).[19,33] When a mass is imaged in the pancreatic head, therefore, both the common bile duct and pancreatic duct should be evaluated for dilatation.[11,33,35] Conversely, if the common bile duct

Table 5-2 Most Common Ultrasound Properties of Pancreatic Masses

Ultrasound characteristics	Pancreatic Carcinoma	Islet Cell Tumor	Metastatic Disease	Lymphoma	Cystadenoma Cystadeno-carcinoma	Pseudocyst	Abscess
Cyst or solid	Solid	Solid	Solid	Solid	Predominantly cystic with septations and irregular walls	Typically cystic	Complex, predominantly cystic
Echo pattern	Low-level echoes	Low-level echoes	Variable	Relatively hypoechoic	Relatively hypoechoic	Anechoic	Internal debris
Sound absorption	Increased	Increased	Increased	Some increase	Decreased	Decreased	Decreased
Through transmission	Decreased	Decreased	Decreased	Some decrease	Increased	Increased	Increased
Size							
Normal or enlarged	Enlarged	Enlarged	Enlarged	Enlarged	Enlarged	Enlarged	Enlarged
Localized or diffuse	Localized	Localized	Localized or diffuse	Localized or diffuse	Localized	Localized	Localized
Contour	Lobulated	Well circumscribed	Lumpy	Lumpy	Smooth or lobulated	Smooth	Smooth or irregular
Additional features	More likely to be in body and tail. Occasional cystic spaces within mass	Frequently displaces mesenteric vessel anteriorly	Frequently displaces mesenteric vessels anteriorly	More likely to be in body and tail	Occasionally may have thick walls, multiloculated or internal debris. May be seen in places distant from pancreas	Usually thick-walled. If bright areas within, may be gas

179

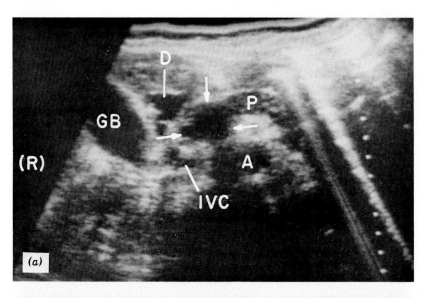

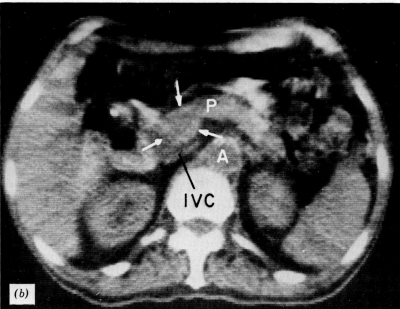

Figure 5-9 Primary adenocarcinoma of the pancreatic head. (*a*) Transverse ultrasound scan of the pancreas showing a hypoechoic solid mass in the pancreatic head (arrows) with only minimal rounding of the pancreatic contours and no gross enlargement. The right arrow denotes the normal-sized common bile duct in the posterolateral aspect of the pancreatic head. Note the normal pancreatic body (P) for comparison. GB = gallbladder; A = aorta; IVC = inferior vena cava; D = fluid-filled duodenal loop; (R) = toward right side of patient. (*b*) Transverse computed tomographic scan in the same patient and at the same level as Figure 8*a*. Note the normal-sized pancreatic head (arrows) with only minimal rounding and the adjacent normal pancreatic body (P) for comparison. IVC = inferior vena cava; A = aorta.

180

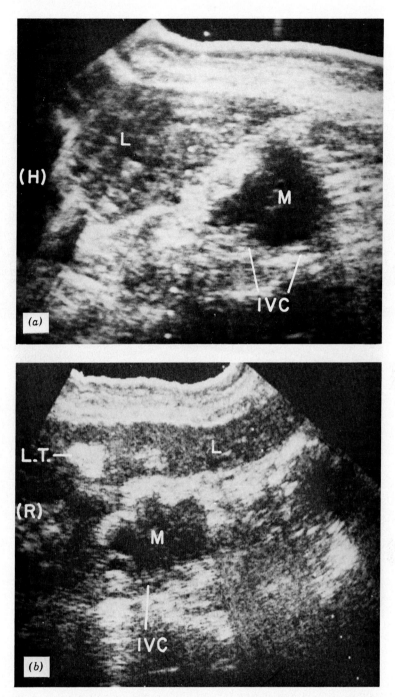

Figure 5-10 Primary adenocarcinoma of the pancreatic head. (*a*) Longitudinal ultrasound scan 2 cm to the right of the midline, showing a large lobulated hypoechoic solid mass (M) in the pancreatic head. Note the inferior vena cava (IVC) compressed posteriorly. L = liver; (H) = toward head of patient. (*b*) Transverse ultrasound scan of the pancreatic head in the same patient showing the same mass (M) compressing the inferior vena cava (IVC). L = liver; L.T. = ligamentum teres within the liver; (R) = toward right side of patient.

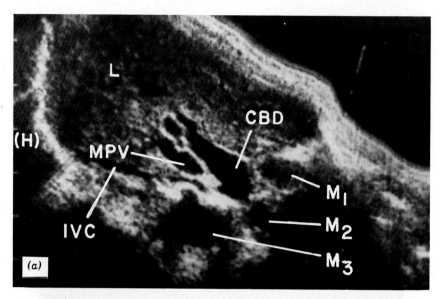

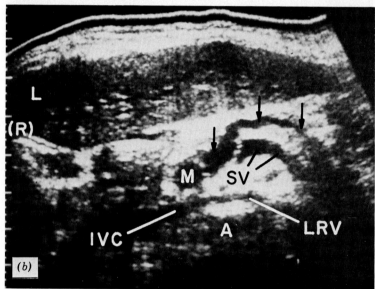

Figure 5-11 Dilated common bile duct and pancreatic duct secondary to primary adenocarcinoma of the pancreatic head. (*a*) Oblique long-axis ultrasound image of the pancreatic head, scanned from the right shoulder toward the left hip, showing a dilated common bile duct (CBD) tapering to a solid hypoechoic mass in the pancreatic head (M_2). Two similar hypoechoic masses (M_1 and M_3) represent retroperitoneal metastases. MPV = main portal vein; IVC = inferior vena cava; L = liver; (H) = toward head of patient. (*b*) Oblique ultrasound transverse image of the pancreas in another patient, scanned from the left shoulder toward the right hip, showing a dilated tortuous pancreatic duct (arrows) with slightly irregular walls extending to a solid hypoechoic mass (M) in the pancreatic head. Note the splenic vein (SV) posterior to the dilated duct and the mildly dilated hepatic bile ducts within the liver (L). IVC = inferior vena cava; A = aorta; LRV = left renal vein; (R) = toward right side of patient.

182

and/or pancreatic duct are dilated, a careful search for a pancreatic head mass should be undertaken. Even when a mass cannot be imaged, dilatation of either or both ductal systems still strongly implies abnormality within the head, not infrequently carcinoma. It is therefore important that scanning be performed in sequential intervals of 1 cm or less so that subtle abnormalities will not be missed.

When a pancreatic mass is imaged, raising the possibility of carcinoma, additional findings may lead to a definite diagnosis of malignancy. (1) Liver masses. Not infrequently, small multiple metastatic nodules are seen in the liver.[33] (2) Nodal masses. Lymphadenopathy is common, particularly in the liver hilum, para-aortic, and mesenteric areas (Fig. 5-11a). (3) Venous obstruction. If the adjacent splenic or portal vein cannot be imaged, this finding is suggestive of vascular occlusion, particularly if collateral vascular channels are detected.[11,33] However, since the nonvisualized venous structures may have been displaced or compressed instead, this finding is not foolproof (Fig. 5-12a). (4) Ascites. (5) Inferior vena cava compression. It has been observed that a pancreatic head malignancy markedly compresses the anterior surface of the inferior vena cava while a normal pancreas only slightly indents the anterior surface during maximum distension, and inflammatory pancreatic disease causes variable compression (Fig. 5-2a and 5-10).[34,36] This sign is not infallible either since (a) the inferior vena cava cannot be defined clearly in all normal patients and (b) the inferior vena cava is a very compressible vessel so that any

Table 5-3 Most Common Ultrasound Properties in Pancreatitis

	Acute Pancreatitis	*Chronic Pancreatitis*
Ultrasound characteristics		
Echo pattern	Uniformly hypoechoic	Variable, usually hyperechoic, coarsened pattern
Sound absorption	Decreased	Variable
Through transmission	Increased	Variable
Relative echogenicity to adjacent liver	Usually less than liver. May be equal to liver	Usually more than liver, may have echogenicity of adjacent retroperitoneal fat
Size		
Normal or enlarged	Enlarged	Normal or enlarged
Localized or diffuse	Diffuse	Usually diffuse but may be focal
Contour	Smooth	Irregular, may be lobulated
Additional features	Uncomplicated acute pancreatitis will return to normal on follow-up studies	May have normal ultrasound appearance. Occasionally may see bright discrete echoes of calcification. Dilated pancreatic duct

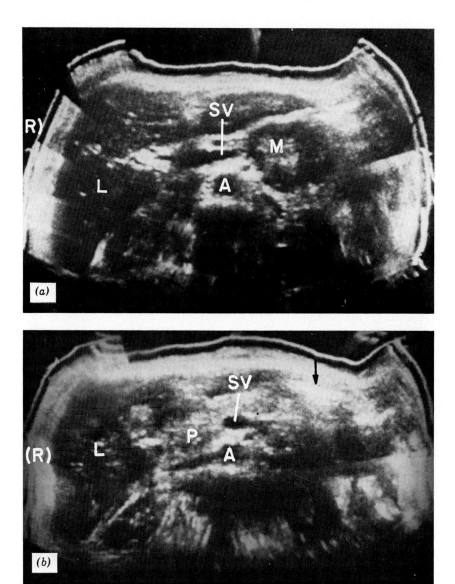

Figure 5-12 Islet cell tumor of the pancreatic tail. (*a*) Transverse ultrasound scan of the upper abdomen showing a well-circumscribed hypoechoic solid mass (M), with hyperechoic center, in the left upper quadrant. While the mass appears to be anterior and possibly compressing the splenic vein (SV), it could not be connected to the pancreas. At surgery, the mass was of pancreatic origin, anterior to the splenic vein, with compression rather than invasion of the vein. A = aorta; L = liver; (R) = toward right side of patient. (*b*) Transverse ultrasound scan in the same patient 1.5 cm caudad showing the pancreatic head and body (P). Note the bowel gas (arrow) obscuring the left upper quadrant. SV = splenic vein; A = aorta; L = liver; (R) = toward right side of patient.

184

pancreatic or parapancreatic enlargement, rather than malignancy alone, may cause marked compression.

Islet Cell Tumors

Islet cell tumors are rare, usually endocrinologically silent, and more common in the pancreatic body and tail where the greatest concentration of Langerhans' islets is located (Fig. 5-12).[37] They are well-circumscribed masses, frequently ultrasonically indistinguishable from pancreatic carcinoma but with occasional internal cystic areas (Table 5-2).[5,33,37] The only suggestion of malignancy, either ultrasonically or histologically, would be concomitant metastases.[37]

Metastatic Tumors and Lymphoma

Both metastatic disease and lymphoma may occupy the pancreatic bed, particularly in the region of the head and body where the main lymphatic chains are located.[19] If these masses are large, they may compress or displace the pancreas. When this occurs, the pancreas is frequently not appreciated, and the masses are mistaken for primary pancreatic carcinomas. To further add to the difficulty in differentiation, metastatic disease and infrequently lymphoma may have similar echo patterns to adenocarcinoma (Table 5-2). Usually, however, lymphoma is relatively anechoic and, when imaged as a rounded mass, may initially appear to be cystic until internal echoes are demonstrated at high power or gain settings. In the differentiation from primary carcinoma, metastatic disease and lymphoma are usually lumpier and more diffuse. In addition, while pancreatic carcinoma primarily occupies the area anterior to the splenic and portal veins, resulting in the posterior displacement of both structures, metastatic disease and lymphoma frequently occur posterior to these vessels, causing anterior displacement (Fig. 5-13).[5,33]

Cystadenomas and Cystadenocarcinomas

Pancreatic cystadenomas and cystadenocarcinomas are uncommon tumors, usually occurring in women between 30 and 60 years of age.[38,39] The majority are located in the pancreatic body and tail, are frequently clinically silent, and may therefore attain sizes of greater than 10 cm before becoming palpable.[38,39,40] The tumors are primarily cystic with septations, have thick walls, and are usually smooth or lobulated in contour (Table 5-2) (Fig. 5-14).[38] On occasion, hyperechoic soft tissue areas are imaged within the mass, felt to be caused by either calcification or the mucin-producing components of the tumor.[5,40] A definite diagnosis of calcification, however, can be made only if discrete shadowing is demonstrated posterior to the bright reflector. There are no specific criteria to separate a benign from a malignant tumor on either ultrasound or computed tomography so that, once the mass is detected, it must be considered potentially malignant.[40] The differential diagnosis of a cystadenoma or cystadenocarcinoma is usually either a complicated pseudocyst or less commonly an abscess (Fig. 5-15) (Table 5-2).[5,38,40] Rarely, solid tumors such as necrotic islet cell malignancies, mucinous adenocarcinomas, or solid anechoic lymphomatous masses may cause confusion.[5,38,40]

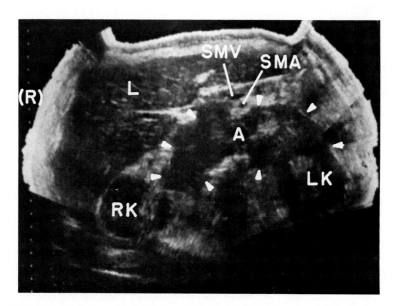

Figure 5-13 Metastases secondary to a primary bladder carcinoma. Transverse ultrasound scan in the region of the pancreatic head showing a bulky lobulated hypoechoic solid mass (arrowheads) surrounding the aorta (A) and displacing the superior mesenteric artery (SMA) and superior mesenteric vein (SMV) anteriorly. The normal pancreas was found at surgery to have been displaced anteriorly and superiorly. RK = right kidney; LK = left kidney; L = liver; (R) = toward right side of patient.

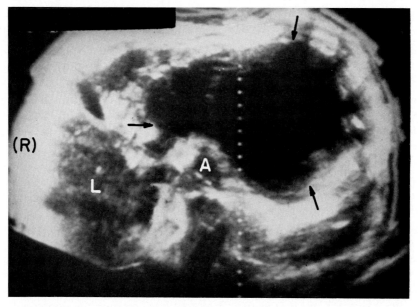

Figure 5-14 Mucinous cystadenocarcinoma of the pancreas. Transverse ultrasound image of the upper abdomen showing a large predominantly anechoic mass (arrows) in the left upper quadrant. The pancreatic tail and the splenic vein could not be imaged. The walls of the mass are irregular and thick, with internal septations.

186

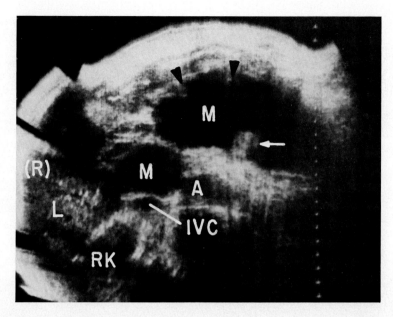

Figure 5-15 Complicated multiloculated pseudocyst. Transverse ultrasound scan of the upper abdomen through the area of the pancreas showing large anechoic masses (M) anterior to the aorta (A) and inferior vena cava (IVC). Note the thick septation (arrow) and wall irregularities (arrowheads) not dissimilar from those seen in pancreatic cystadenoma or cystadenocarcinoma. L = liver; (R) = toward patient's right side.

Difficulties in Imaging Pancreatic Masses

The left upper quadrant is a particularly difficult area to evaluate. Gas in the stomach and in the small and large bowel frequently obscures this region so that it is not uncommon for a mass to be either undetected or for its site of origin to be undetermined (Figs. 5-12*a* and 5-16*a*). In the evaulation for possible pancreatic origin, a mass should be analyzed for (*1*) its contiguity with the pancreatic head and body and (*2*) its relationship to the splenic vein. Only when a mass is directly anterior to the splenic vein and/or connected to the body of the pancreas can pancreatic origin be definitely diagnosed. If the mass compresses the splenic vein or displaces the pancreas, its site of origin becomes uncertain (Figs. 5-12 and 5-13). Computed tomography may aid in this evaluation since bowel gas does not obscure either the mass or adjacent normal structures (Fig. 5-16*b*), and it may be possible, on occasion, to opacify the splenic vein using high-dose intravenous contrast material.

The pancreatic duct is not infrequently dilated in pancreatic tumors, stones, and inflammation, on occasion up to 30 mm (Fig. 5-ll*b*).[30,31,35] When the duct is dilated, it can be traced from the pancreatic tail toward the head until a point of narrowing is found. While this is usually the site of pancreatic abnormality, with close correlation to endoscopic pancreatography, it is infrequent to image a discrete mass even in cases of carcinoma.[31] The irregularity or smoothness of the dilated ducts is also not of value in differentiating carcinoma from pancreatitis.[31]

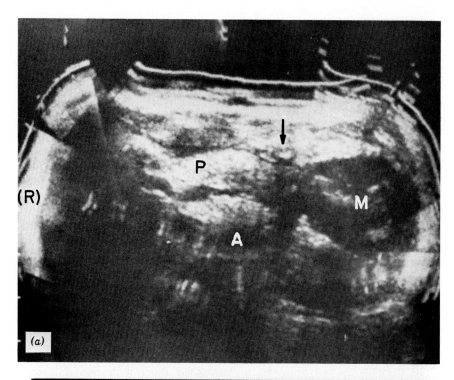

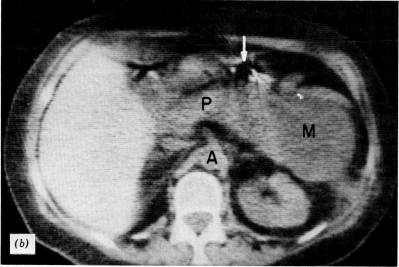

Figure 5-16 Infected pseudocyst (abscess) of the pancreatic tail. (*a*) Transverse ultrasound image of the upper abdomen showing a normal pancreatic head and body (P) and a separate left upper quadrant complex, irregularly hyperechoic mass (M). Note the interposed bowel gas (arrow) with shadowing. A = aorta; (R) = toward right side of patient. (*b*) Transverse computed tomographic image in the same patient and at the same level as part *a* showing the mass (M) connected to the pancreatic body (P). The interposed bowel gas (arrow) does not obscure the underlying pancreas. A = aorta.

188

Pancreatitis

In the analysis of diffuse pancreatic disease by ultrasound (Table 5-3), the criteria are modified as follows: (1) Ultrasound characteristics—echo pattern, sound absorption, through-transmission, and relative echogenicity compared to that of the adjacent liver. (2) Size—normal or enlarged and, if enlarged, localized or diffuse. (3) Contour changes. (4) Additional features that might lead to a specific diagnosis. While most diffuse diseases of the pancreas are related to pancreatitis, infrequently a large tumor may diffusely enlarge the pancreas or a small, strategically located tumor may obstruct the pancreatic duct causing distal diffuse pancreatitis. The combination of clinical history, laboratory data, and ultrasound findings may aid in making a definitive diagnosis of pancreatitis.

Acute Pancreatitis

The most common ultrasound findings in acute pancreatitis are diffusely decreased echogenicity, decreased sound absorption, and increased through-transmission (Table 5-3) (Figs. 5-17*a b*, and 5-18).[10,11,19] The echogenicity of the pancreas is usually decreased in relation to the adjacent liver, and the pancreas is uniformly enlarged in greater than 60 percent of cases, frequently with smooth contours.[10,11,19] The initial appearance commonly persists for days or weeks, usually reverting back to normal in uncomplicated cases.[10,11,19,41] Since concomitant paralytic ileus is not infrequently present, it is often difficult to evaluate the pancreas by ultrasound during the acute inflammatory phase.

There is a spectrum of severity in acute pancreatitis ranging from mild edema to fulminant pancreatic necrosis and hemorrhage (Figs. 5-17 and 5-19). Phlegmonous masses caused by the more severe pancreatic necrosis and hemorrhage occur in up to 18 percent of cases. These masses are usually confined to the region of the pancreatic bed, leading to diffuse enlargement, decreased echogenicity, decreased sound absorption, and increased through-transmission.[11,42,43] Computed tomography in these cases frequently shows extremely low attenuation numbers, consistent with fluid collections.[43] On occasion, however, phlegmons may cause only localized enlargement. In addition, the masses may infrequently demonstrate solid ultrasound characteristics of decreased echogenicity and increased sound absorption, with computed tomography demonstrating a mass in the solid CT number range. When this occurs, neither ultrasound nor computed tomography is able to differentiate inflammatory phlegmon from malignancy (Fig. 5-16).

Chronic Pancreatitis

The ultrasound properties in chronic pancreatitis are much more variable (Table 5-3). The echo pattern is usually increased and coarsened (Figs. 5-17*b* and *c*). On occasion, the echogenicity of the pancreas may even increase to approximate the hyperechoic properties of normal retroperitoneal fat and fibrous tissue so that the pancreas becomes difficult to separate from the surrounding retroperitoneum.[11] The pancreas is commonly diffusely enlarged (Fig. 5-17*c*). The pancreatic contours are usually irregular and lobulated.[10,44] Unfortunately, however, the pancreas may appear normal, even in cases of severe chronic relapsing pancreatitis.[10,13,45] In addition, a focal mass of chronic pancreatitis may be infrequently imaged, ultrasonically indistinguishable from a neoplasm.[10]

While many bright pancreatic echoes related to fibrosis and fatty infiltration are detected in chronic pancreatitis, these bright echoes may represent calcifications. The diagnosis of calcification can only be made by ultrasound if discrete distal shadowing is observed (Figs. 5-18 and 5-20a).[10,11,33] Since chronic pancreatitis has an additional high incidence of dilated pancreatic ducts associated with duct calculi, the calcifications may be within either the pancreatic substance or the ductal system.[31,33,46] To diagnose pancreatic duct calculi accurately, the parallel channels of the ducts must surround the bright reflectors.[46,47]

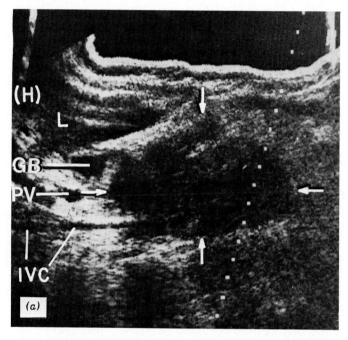

Figure 5-17 Pancreatitis: Progression from acute to chronic in same patient (a) Acute pancreatitis 2 days after initial symptoms. Longitudinal scan 2.5 cm to the right of the midline showing a hypoechoic mass (arrows) in the region of the pancreatic head. The echogenicity of the pancreas is considerably decreased when compared to the adjacent liver (L). Note the compression of the inferior vena cava (IVC) by the inflammation. Also note that the usually increased through-transmission is not present in this case. GB = contracted gallbladder. (b) Subacute pancreatitis 6 weeks after initial symptoms. Longitudinal scan 2.0 cm to the right of the midline showing a slightly smaller mass (arrows) in the pancreatic head with areas of decreased and increased echogenicity. Again note the anterior compression of the IVC by the mass. L = liver. (c) Chronic pancreatitis 5 months after initial symptoms. Longitudinal scan 2.0 cm to the right of the midline showing a much smaller mass (arrows and arrowheads) in the still prominent pancreatic head. The echo pattern is uniformly coarsened and bright, much more so than the adjacent liver (L). PV = portal vein; (H) = toward patient's head.

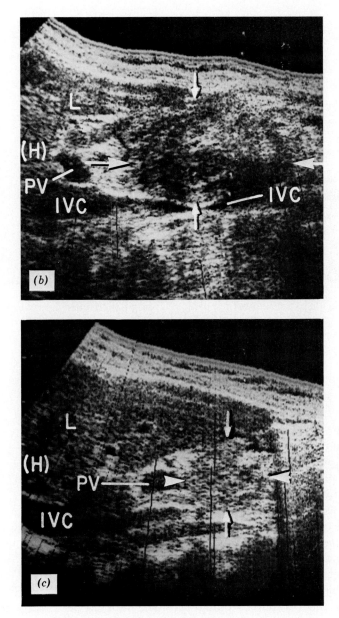

Figure 5-17 (*continued*)

Pseudocystic Disease

One of the most frequent complications in pancreatitis is pseudocyst formation. In acute pancreatitis pseudocysts occur in up to 18 percent, and in chronic pancreatitis they are found in up to 22 percent of cases (Table 5-2).[10,11] Uncomplicated pseudocysts are usually anechoic with smooth walls and good

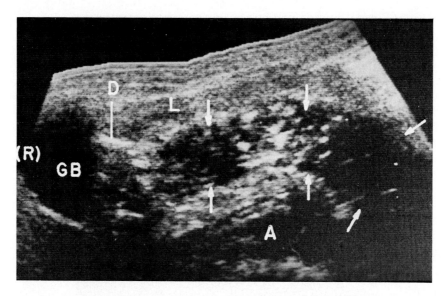

Figure 5-18 Acute exacerbation in chronic relapsing pancreatitis. Transverse ultrasound scan of the upper abdomen showing a diffusely enlarged pancreas (arrows). In the head and tail, the echo pattern is decreased with increased through-transmission, consistent with acute pancreatitis. In the body, there are bright echoes of calcification throughout the pancreatic parenchyma, consistent with chronic pancreatitis. No focal mass is seen. D = duodenum; GB = gallbladder; A = aorta; (R) = toward right side of patient.

sound transmission distally (Figs. 5-6, 5-20a, and 5-21a).[10,48,49] Infrequently, however, there may be internal debris, fluid-debris levels, uniform internal echoes, irregularities of the walls, septations, multiloculations, or bright curvilinear wall reflectors corresponding to calcification (Fig. 5-15).[10,48,49,50] When septations and irregularity of the wall occur, the differentiation from cystadenoma to cystadenocarcinoma may be difficult (Fig. 5-14). When a pseudocyst has internal echoes and irregular walls, there is difficulty in distinguishing it from an abscess (Fig. 5-16).[50] Usually, however, abscesses have more internal echoes and more wall irregularities than pseudocysts, and the detection of bright reflectors within the mass, representing gas, confirms the diagnosis of abscess (Table 5-2).[10,50] When gas or calcification are suggested, abdominal radiographs and computed tomography are valuable in making the specific diagnosis (Fig. 5-20b). On occasion, hematomas, loculated ascites, and fluid-filled loops of bowel may mimic pseudocysts.[48]

It has been shown that pseudocysts may mature rapidly, may be imaged as early as 6 days after an initial episode of acute pancreatitis, and may occasionally regress spontaneously without catastrophic consequences (Fig. 5-21).[50] In fact, there have been documented cases of the sudden asymptomatic disappearance of pseudocysts, presumably secondary to spontaneous drainage into the communicating pancreatic duct and then into the bowel. Pseudocysts are most commonly located in the peripancreatic region, frequently in the region of the

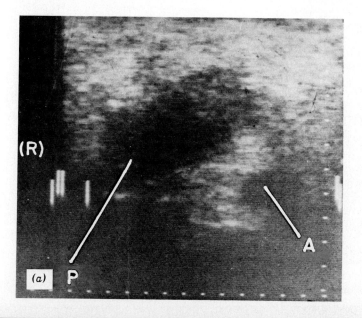

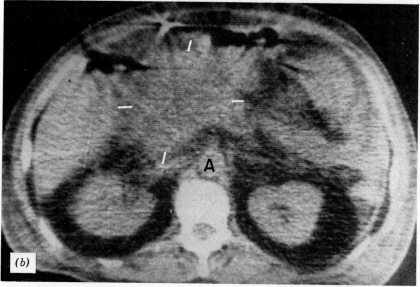

Figure 5-19 Phlegmonous pancreatitis. (*a*) Transverse ultrasound scan of the pancreatic head (P) showing a solid echo-poor irregular mass with decreased through-transmission. A = aorta; (R) = toward right side of patient. (*b*) Transverse computed tomography scan in the same patient and at the same level as part *a*. Note the solid mass (lines) in the pancreatic head. The number was elevated (+40 H), not near the usual water density of phlegmon. A = aorta.

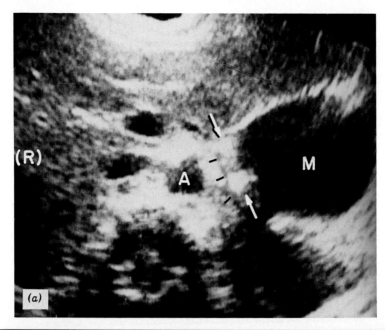

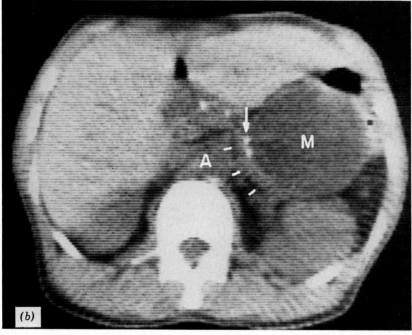

Figure 5-20 Chronic pancreatitis with uncomplicated pseudocyst in the lesser sac. (*a*) Transverse ultrasound image of the upper abdomen showing a small pancreatic tail (denoted by lines on its posterior aspect). There are multiple coarse discrete bright reflectors (arrows) and distal shadowing in the parenchyma of the pancreatic tail consistent with calcifications. In addition, there is a large left upper quadrant cystic mass (M), a pseudocyst, contiguous with the pancreatic tail. A = aorta; (R) = toward right side of patient. (*b*) Transverse computed tomographic image in the same patient and at the same level as part *a*. Again note the atrophic pancreatic tail (denoted posteriorly by lines), the calcifications (arrow), and the adjacent pseudocyst (M). A = aorta.

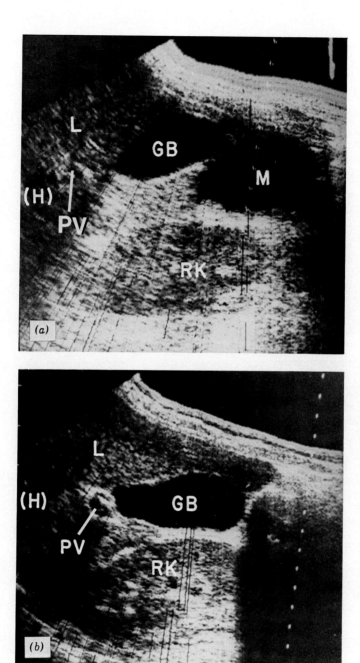

Figure 5-21 Asymptomatic pancreatic pseudocyst—sudden appearance and spontaneous regression. (*a*) Longitudinal scan 4 cm to the right of the midline in a patient 6 weeks after an acute episode of pancreatitis. The initial scan of acute pancreatitis had not shown a mass. Now, a cystic mass (M) is imaged anterior to the lower pole of the right kidney (RK), elevating the gallbladder (GB). (*b*) Longitudinal scan 4 cm to the right of the midline in same patient 8 weeks later. The gallbladder (GB) now lies directly anterior to the right kidney (RK), indicating resolution of the pseudocyst. L = liver; PV = right portal vein; (H) = toward patient's head.

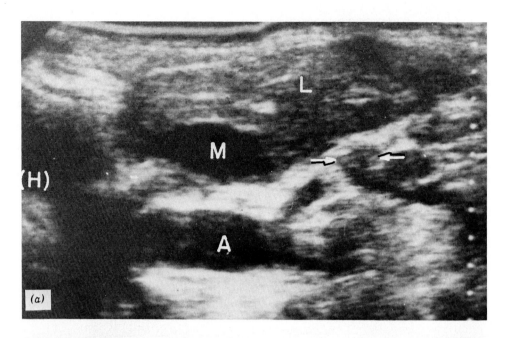

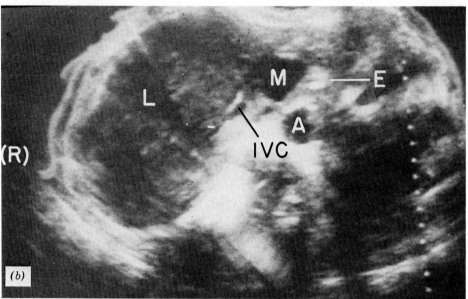

Figure 5-22 Upper retroperitoneal pseudocyst. (*a*) Longitudinal midline ultrasound scan showing a cystic mass (M) between the liver (L) and the abdominal aorta (A) near the diaphragm. Arrows = normal pancreatic tail; (H) = toward head of patient. (*b*) Transverse ultrasound scan in the same patient as part *a* showing the same cystic mass (M) displacing the esophagus (E) to the left. A = aorta; IVC = inferior vena cava; (R) = toward right side of patient.

lesser sac (Figs. 5-15 and 5-20).[11] On occasion, pseudocysts may dissect through the retroperitoneum anywhere from the mediastinum to the groin (Fig. 5-22), while rarely pseudocysts may replace the pancreatic core, occasionally with fluid-debris levels, leaving the normal overall pancreatic size intact.[10,11,42,51] It is suggested that at least one ultrasound examination of the pancreas be performed immediately after an acute episode of pancreatitis, allowing for a baseline evaluation of (1) pancreatic size and echo pattern, and (2) location and extent of possible pseudocyst or abscess formation. If a patient then shows clinical signs of worsening, another ultrasound examination can be performed and the results compared to the first.

COMPARISON OF DIFFERENT IMAGING MODALITIES

There have been a number of studies analyzing the relative efficacy of ultrasound, computed tomography, nuclear medicine, and barium studies in the detection of pancreatic disease (Table 5-4). To understand their value in the evaluation of the pancreas, certain statistical definitions are necessary:[52] (1) *Accuracy* is the ability to predict correctly whether or not disease is present. (2) A *true-positive rate* is the sensitivity in percent with the probability that the results of the test or procedure will be positive when the disease is present. (3) A true-negative rate is the specificity in percent with the probability that the results of the test or procedure will be negative when the disease is not present. (4) A false-positive rate is 100 minus specificity in percent and is the probability that the results of the test or procedure will be positive when the disease is not present. (5) A false-negative rate is 100 minus sensitivity in percent and is the probability that the results of the test or procedure will be negative when the disease is present.

The overall accuracy of barium studies for detecting pancreatic disease is 40 to 76 percent (Table 5-4).[4,53,54] This accuracy is increased with the use of hypotonic duodenography and in the presence of early acute pancreatitis.[53,54] However, the false-negative rate of 21 to 37 percent greatly decreases the value of these tests.[5,53]

Nuclear imaging of the pancreas has a high overall accuracy of 73 to 96 percent (Table 5-4).[53,55,56] However, the false-positive rate is also very high, between 30 and 75 percent, thus making the study far too non-specific for routine use.[45,54,55,56,57,58]

The two remaining noninvasive imaging modalities, ultrasound and computed tomography, have relatively high overall accuracy rates, approaching the mid-90s with much lower false-positive and false-negative rates than either barium or nuclear medicine examinations (Table 5-4).[5,7,8,14,19,44,45,53,57,59-62] While computed tomography and ultrasound are competing cross-sectional imaging modalities, they use different types of transmitted energies so that the images produced may be complementary. Nevertheless, when the pancreas is to be studied, three questions are always asked: (1) Which study should be performed first, ultrasound or computed tomography? (2) How reliable is the image produced, both in detecting abnormality and in ruling out disease? (3) After

Table 5-4   Overall Accuracy of Imaging Procedures in Detecting Pancreatic Abnormality[a]

Barium Studies 40 to 76%□	Nuclear Medicine (Selenomethionine SE 75) 73 to 96%*	Ultrasound 83 to 96%+	Computed Tomography 76 to 94%☉

Detection of Mass or Cancer (6 Series)	Range	Composite
Accuracy	80 to 98	89
True positive	81 to 94	88
False negative	6 to 19	12
False positive	1 to 19	10
True negative	78 to 99	90

Detection of Mass or Cancer (5 Series)	Range	Composite
Accuracy	78 to 90	85
True positive	84 to 90	87
False negative	10 to 16	13
False positive	8 to 35	16
True negative	65 to 92	84

[a] From 1975 to 1981.
KEY: □ = False negative = 21 to 37%; * = False positive = 30 to 75%; + = Part of pancreas termed nonvisualized due to bowel gas in up to 15 percent of cases. When possible, nonvisualized studies were excluded. In some studies, dilated common bile duct counted as positive for cancer; ☉ = No large studies performed on sub-10-second scanners. Pancreas termed indeterminate in up to 7 percent of cases. When possible, indeterminate studies excluded. In some studies, dilated common bile duct counted as positive for cancer.

the initial study, is any other test needed? In order to elucidate more fully the relative utility of ultrasound and computed tomography in the analysis of pancreatic disease, the advantages and disadvantages of each are discussed, comparative statistics are analyzed, and a flow chart for the workup of pancreatic diseases is proposed. Throughout this section, it is essential that two points be remembered: (1) Neither ultrasound nor computed tomography can consistently differentiate a malignant from a benign abnormality of the pancreas. (2) Neither ultrasound nor computed tomography can consistently evaluate masses less than 1 to 2 cm in size.

The advantages of ultrasound are (1) it is very accurate in imaging the pancreas in thin patients, even when there is a paucity of retroperitoneal fat, (2) it does not use ionizing radiation, (3) it is very accurate in analyzing biliary and, more recently, pancreatic duct obstruction, and (4) due to the rapid scan time of less than 1 second, particularly with real time, ultrasound can frequently image the pancreas despite respiratory or patient motion. The disadvantages of ultrasound are (1) the images are technically difficult to obtain and therefore are dependent on the skill of the person performing the scans[15] and (2) all or part of the pancreas is not visualized due to bowel gas and/or fat in up to 15 percent of patients.[5,19,56,60,63]

The advantages of computed tomography are (*1*) it is very accurate in imaging the pancreas in moderate to heavy patients, particularly in those where retroperitoneal fat surrounds the pancreas, (*2*) it allows complete cross-sectional imaging of the pancreas and the adjacent structures, (*3*) the pancreas can be imaged even when an abundance of overlying bowel gas is present,[5,43,54,64] and (*4*) images are technically easy to obtain. The disadvantages of computed tomography are (*1*) ionizing radiation is needed, (*2*) there is difficulty in imaging the pancreas in thin patients, and (*3*) respiratory and patient motion may significantly degrade the image.[54,62] Primarily due to motion degradation, pancreatic images have been judged to be nondiagnostic or indeterminate in up to 7 percent of patients studied.[7,59,62]

While both ultrasound and computed tomography are accurate in the detection of focal pancreatic masses, computed tomography appears to offer some additional value in staging carcinoma due to its ability to detect not only the mass but also malignant spread into surrounding tissues.[45] In the detection of uncomplicated pseudocysts, ultrasound has been found to be better in initial screening and follow-up, except for small pseudocysts of the pancreatic tail.[45,64,65] However, in complicated pseudocysts, computed tomography may be slightly more accurate.[65] In acute pancreatitis, computed tomography is usually of greater value than ultrasound since computed tomography can more consistently image the pancreas despite the frequently present paralytic ileus.[66] In addition, even when ultrasound is able to image the pancreas in acute pancreatitis, accurate evaluation of the degree of spread is frequently not possible, while computed tomography commonly detects peripancreatic extension into the lesser sac, the anterior and posterior pararenal spaces, and the flanks.[43,66,67,68] In chronic pancreatitis, both ultrasound and computed tomography are frequently inaccurate since the findings are commonly nonspecific. Computed tomography can diagnose chronic pancreatitis only when calcification, parenchymal pancreatic atrophy, and pancreatic duct dilatation are present (Fig. 5-17*b*).[64]

When ultrasound and computed tomography were analyzed statistically, three criteria were used: (*1*) Only studies performed since 1975 were included. While this is an arbitrary cut-off, it was hoped that after this date the most modern imaging equipment with the highest resolution was used for all published studies. (*2*) Only ultrasound studies examined on B-mode gray scale instrumentation were acceptable. (*3*) Only those computed tomography studies in which at least some of the examinations were performed on 20-second scanners were included. It is well known that slower computed tomography scanners have more artifacts than faster scanners. Studies performed solely on scanners with an examination time slower than 20 seconds were eliminated because of possible significant image degradation. Nevertheless, the supposition that the even faster sub-10-second scanners can further improve diagnostic accuracy has not as yet been demonstrated since no large studies of the pancreas have been performed on sub-10-second scanners. The lack of such data could be a potential shortcoming of this analysis. Nevertheless, when these criteria were used, the overall accuracy for ultrasound was 83 to 96 percent[5,14,19,44,53,60] and for computed tomography 76 to 94 percent (Table 5-4).[5,7,59,61,62]

In the more specific statistical analysis of accuracy in the detection of pancreatic mass or cancer (Table 5-4), four additional criteria were used: (1) At least 8 normals and 8 pancreatic carcinomas had to be included in each series. While these numbers were arbitrary, it was felt that a smaller series with fewer cases might not be accurate. (2) Whenever possible, ultrasound examinations were excluded when the pancreas was not visualized and computed tomography studies were excluded when termed "indeterminate." (3) Whenever possible, if a dilated common bile duct led to the diagnosis of pancreatic carcinoma, even without imaging of a mass, it was considered a correct diagnosis for both ultrasound and computed tomography. (4) The numbers of cases used to generate the true-positive, true-negative, false-positive, and false-negative rates had to be available for each series.

When these criteria were used, the detection rates of pancreatic mass or cancer could be analyzed in six series from five articles for ultrasound[5,14,28,53,56] and in five series from five articles for computed tomography[5,7,59,61,62] with wide statistical ranges encountered (Table 5-4). The major drawback in this analysis is the large variation in the number of patients analyzed in each series. If one computed tomographic series, for example, evaluated only 42 patients while another examined 145, detection of even two more cancers would be reflected by a much larger percentage of change in the smaller series. For this reason, it was decided to combine all of the series so that a composite statistical analysis could be obtained (Table 5-4). This allowed evaluation of 790 ultrasound examinations, 481 normals and 309 cancers, and 427 computed tomography patients, 273 normals and 154 cancers. The composite analysis revealed that ultrasound and computed tomography had similar true-positive values in the detection of cancer, 88 and 87 percent. Ultrasound was of greater value than computed tomography in ruling out disease (true-negative results), 90 to 84 percent, with fewer false-positive and false-negative results. While the difference between these results is not statistically significant, the value of ultrasound in pancreatic disease is apparent.

In the evaluation of pancreatitis, the consolidated statistics comparing ultrasound and computed tomography slightly favored computed tomography. The overall accuracy for computed tomography was 56 to 90 percent,[59,61,64,69,70] while for ultrasound the accuracy was 40 to 90 percent.[11,14,56,64,69] In acute pancreatitis, computed tomography was considerably superior to ultrasound both in imaging the pancreas regardless of the amount of bowel gas present and in evaluating peripancreatic spread.[66]

Three unresolved problems still persist in pancreatic evaluation. (1) Specific definitions for the normal and abnormal pancreas and for carcinoma and inflammation should be stated in each study. Some studies, while detecting abnormality, fail to give the criteria used in their evaluation.[28,59,72] (2) The best technique for optimum pancreatic imaging by ultrasound and computed tomography should be performed in every study. While most computed tomographic studies have routinely used oral contrast, intravenous contrast, and intravenous or intramuscular glucagon to obtain adequate pancreatic images in up to 98 percent of cases,[5,71] few ultrasound studies routinely use a water-filled stomach, erect pancreatic scanning, or a combination of the two. In our analysis, the only study employing these techniques reported a visualization rate of 98 percent,[28] while the others failed to image the pancreas in up to 15 percent of cases.[5,14,53,56] Some additional series, also not using these techniques, have reported nonvisualization rates as high as 46 percent.[71,72] (3) What is the optimum statistical approach to evaluate ultrasound and computed tomography in pancreatic mass detection? Recently, it has been proposed that the use of receiver operating characteristic (ROC) curves may be more valid than the use of true-positive, true-negative, false-positive and false-negative rates.[73] In a recent study evaluating ultrasound and computed tomography in pancreatic disease, five categories ranging from definitely normal to definitely abnormal were obtained.[72] While this study did not state definitions for pancreatic disease, that is, normal, carcinoma, and inflammation, it did find that computed tomography was more sensitive, .87 to .69, and more specific, .90 to .82, than ultrasound in detecting abnormality.[72] It is important that these problems be addressed before further analyses are performed.

Nevertheless, a flow chart is proposed for the work-up of pancreatic diseases (Table 5-5). Since the composite statistical analysis has shown ultrasound to be equal to computed tomography in mass evaluation and better in determining normalcy (Table 5-4), ultrasound should be the primary imaging modality (Table 5-5). The flow chart may then be divided into three sections: normal, abnormal, and nonvisualized. Obviously, if ultrasound cannot image any part of the pancreas, computed tomography should be performed. However, if a normal or an abnormal pancreas is imaged, the remainder of the work-up depends on (a) the degree of clinical suspicion that pancreatic disease could be present and (b) whether that suspicion points toward malignancy or toward pancreatitis. The only pancreatic lesion that should not be included in this flow chart would be an islet cell tumor. Its small size and frequent hypervascularity makes angiography the initial procedure of choice.

When the ultrasound examination is normal and there is a low degree of clinical suspicion, there would usually be no need for further work-up. If, however, there is a high clinical suspicion of malignancy, computed tomography and perhaps additional tests would be indicated, even after a normal ultrasound study (Table 5-5). If, instead, a diagnosis of pancreatitis is clinically suspected with a normal ultrasound study, it would remain a clinical judgment as to whether further work-up was needed. As an alternative, it might be appropriate, in such a situation, to perform follow-up ultrasound examinations at predetermined intervals.

When an abnormal pancreas is imaged by ultrasound, the clinical suspicion would again modify the decision concerning further evaluation (Table 5-5). With a suspicion of malignancy, when subtle pancreatic irregularities are detected by ultrasound, computed tomography and perhaps other tests would be indicated. For a well-defined mass, biopsy or surgery would be the appropriate next step. If there is dilatation of the common bile duct without a well-defined mass, however, a percutaneous or transhepatic cholangiogram would be the recommended next procedure even when the intrahepatic ducts are not grossly distended.

When an abnormal pancreas is imaged and there is clinical suspicion of pancreatitis, the remainder of the work-up would depend on the severity of the clinical symptoms. If the ultrasound findings are consistent with the clinical findings, it would be possible to follow the pancreas with ultrasound exami-

Table 5-5 Flow Chart: Suggested Work-Up of Pancreas

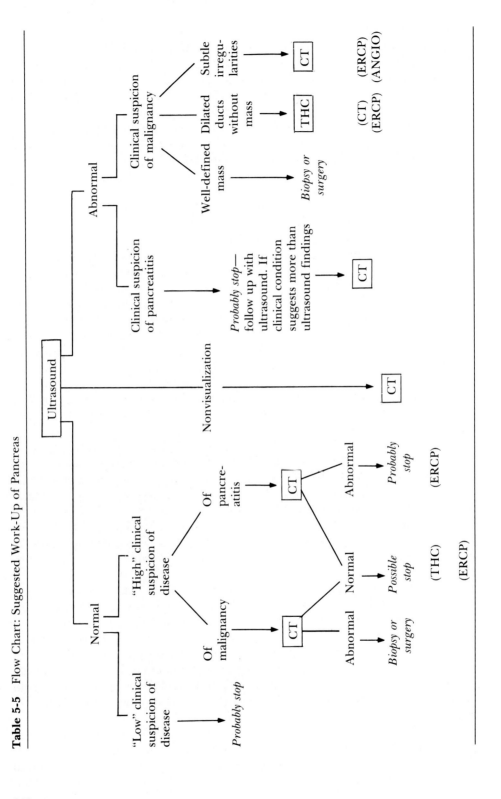

202

nations at suitable intervals as the clinical course dictated. If, however, the patient's clinical condition is more severe than is suggested by the ultrasound findings, computed tomography would be indicated to evaluate for peripancreatic spread and possible gas-containing abscesses.

At present, no imaging modality is optimal for the pancreas. In the correct hands, ultrasound is extremely valuable in the detection of both a normal and an abnormal pancreas. Computed tomography is also an important test and, when these are used together, occasionally more information is gained than when either test is used alone.

In the evaluation of the pancreas, the future of ultrasound and computed tomography will depend, at least partially, on the ability of these studies to predict whether an abnormality is malignant or inflammatory. For computed tomography, recent work in a small series with a sub-5-second scanner and high intravenous bolus of contrast has shown that accurate prediction can be made between pancreatitis and cancer.[74] Dynamic computed tomography scanning has been shown to be of value in differentiating liver lesions and perhaps may be of value in the pancreas.[75] For ultrasound, the avenues for future improvement may lie with tissue characterization and with Doppler evaluation of detected lesions.[76,77] Finally, the detection of subtle pancreatic duct dilatation, even when no mass is imaged, may allow the earlier detection of pancreatic lesions.

REFERENCES

1. Gray H: The pancreas, in Goss CM (ed): *Gray's Anatomy*, ed. 28. Philadelphia, Lea & Febiger, 1966, pp 1,257–1,261.

2. Weinstein BJ, Weinstein DP: Sonographic anatomy of the pancreas. *Semins Ultrasound* 1(3):156–165, 1980.

3. Sample WF: Techniques for improved delineation of normal anatomy of the upper abdomen and high retroperitoneum with gray scale ultrasound. *Radiology* 124:197–202, 1977.

4. Weill F, Schraub A, Eisenscher A, Bourgoin A: Ultrasonography of the normal pancreas. *Radiology* 123:417–423, 1977.

5. Katz RJ, Behan M, Herbstman C, et al: Sonography and CT of the pancreas. *Semin Ultrasound* 1(3):209–227, 1980.

6. Ghorashi B, Rector WR: Gray scale sonographic anatomy of the pancreas. *J. Clin Ultrasound* 5(1):25–29, 1977.

7. Sheedy PF, Stephens, DH, Hattery RR, MacCarty RL: Computed tomography in the evaluation of patients with suspected carcinoma of the pancreas. *Radiology* 124:731–737, 1977.

8. Lee JKT, Stanley RJ, Melson GL, Sagel SS: Pancreatic imaging by ultrasound and computed tomography. *Rad Clin North Am* 16(1):105–117, 1979.

9. Taylor KJW, Pollock D, Crade M: Pancreatic ultrasonography: Techniques, artifacts, and clinical results, in Moss AA, Goldbert HI (eds): *Computed Tomography, Ultrasound and X-ray: An Integrated Approach.* San Francisco, University of California Press, 1980, pp 81–87.

10. Sarti DA, King W: The ultrasonic findings in inflammatory pancreatic disease. *Semin Ultrasound* 1(3):178–191, 1980.

11. Johnson ML, Mack LA: Ultrasonic evaluation of the pancreas. *Gastrointest Radiol* 3:257–266, 1978.

12. Marks WM, Filly RA, Callen PW: Ultrasonic evaluation of normal pancreatic echogenicity and its relationship to fat deposition. *Radiology* 137:475–479, 1980.

13. Doust BD, Pearce JD: Gray-scale ultrasonic properties of the normal and inflamed pancreas. *Radiology* 120:653–657, 1976.

14. Lawson TL: Sensitivity of pancreatic ultrasonography in the detection of pancreatic disease. *Radiology* 128:733–736, 1978.

15. Shaff MI, Walker WJ: Ultrasound in pancreatic disease. *Appl Radiol/Ultrasound* 88–96, 1980.

16. Filly RA, London SS: The normal pancreas: Acoustic characteristics and frequency of imaging. *J Clin Ultrasound* 121–124, 1979.

17. deGraaff CS, Taylor KJW, Simonds BD, Rosenfield AJ: Gray-scale echography of the pancreas. *Radiology* 129:157–161, 1978.

18. Haber K, Freimanis AK, Asher WM: Demonstration and dimensional analysis of the normal pancreas with gray-scale echography. *AJR* 126:624–628, 1976.

19. Arger PH, Mulhern CB, Bonavita JA: An analysis of pancreatic sonography in suspected pancreatic disease. *J Clin Ultrasound* 7:91–97, 1979.

20. Goldstein HM, Katragadda CS: Prone view ultrasonography for pancreatic tail neoplasms. *AJR* 131:231–234, 1978.

21. Coleman BG, Arger PA, Rosenberg HK, Mulhern CB, Ortega W, Stanffer D: Gray-scale sonographic assessments of pancreatitis in children. *Radiology* 146:145–150, 1983.

22. Crade M, Taylor KJW, Rosenfield AT: Water distention of the gut in the evaluation of the pancreas by ultrasound. *AJR* 131:348–349, 1978.

23. Behan M, Kazam E: Sonography of the common bile duct: Value of the right anterior oblique view. *AJR* 130:701–709, 1978.

24. Berger M, Smith EH, Bartrum RJ, et al: False-positive diagnosis of pancreatic tail lesions caused by colon. *J Clin Ultrasound* 5:343–345, 1977.

25. Warren PS, Garrett WJ, Phil D, Kossoff G: The liquid-filled stomach: An ultrasonic window to the upper abdomen. *J Clin Ultrasound* 6(5):295–382, 1978.

26. MacMahon H, Bowie JD, Beezhold C: Erect scanning of pancreas using a gastric window. *AJR* 132:587–591, 1979.

27. Jacobson P, Crade M, Taylor KJW: The upright position while giving water for the evaluation of the pancreas. *J Clin Ultrasound* 6:353–354, 1978.

28. Taylor KJW, Buchin PJ, Viscomi GN, Rosenfield AT: Ultrasonographic scanning of the pancreas. *Radiology* 138:211–213, 1981.

29. Bowie JD, MacMahon H: Improved techniques in pancreatic sonography. *Semin Ultrasound* 1(3):170–177, 1980.

30. Weinstein DP, Weinstein BJ: Ultrasonic demonstration of the pancreatic duct: An analysis of 41 cases. *Radiology* 130:729–734, 1979.

31. Ohto M, Saotome N, Saisho H, et al: Real-time sonography of the pancreatic duct: Application to percutaneous pancreatic ductography. *AJR* 134:647–652, 1980.

32. Parulekar SG: Ultrasonic evaluation of the pancreatic duct. *J Clin Ultrasound* 8:457–463, 1980.

33. Weinstein DP, Weinstein BJ: Pancreas, in Goldberg BB (ed): *Ultrasound in Cancer.* New York, Churchill Livingstone, 1981.

34. Wright CH, Maklad F, Rosenthal SJ: Grey-scale ultrasonic characteristics of carcinoma of the pancreas. *Br J Radiol* 52:281–288, 1979.

35. Gosink BB, Leopold GR: The dilated pancreatic duct: Ultrasonic evaluation. *Radiology* 126:475–478, 1978.

36. Walls WJ, Templeton AW: The ultrasonic demonstration of inferior vena caval compression: A guide to pancreatic head enlargement with emphasis on neoplasm. *Radiology* 123:165–167, 1977.

37. Raghavendra BN, Glickstein ML: Sonography of islet cell tumor of the pancreas: Report of two cases. *J Clin Ultrasound* 9:331–333, 1981.

38. Wolson AH, Walls WJ: Ultrasonic characteristics of cystadenoma of the pancreas. *Radiology* 119:203–205, 1976.

39. Hodgkinson DJ, ReMine WH, Weiland LH: Pancreatic cystadenoma: A clinicopathologic study of 45 cases. *Arch Surg* 113:512–519, 1978.

40. Carroll B, Sample WF: Pancreatic cystadenocarcinoma: CT body scan and gray scale ultrasound appearance. *AJR* 131:339–341, 1978.

41. Slovis TL, VonBerg VJ, Mikelic V: Sonography in the diagnosis and management of pancreatic pseudocysts and effusions in childhood. *Radiology* 135:153–155, 1980.

42. Burrell M, Gold JA, Simeone J, et al: Liquefactive necrosis of the pancreas. *Radiology* 135:157–160, 1980.

43. Mendez G, Isikoff MB, Hill MC: CT of acute pancreatitis: Interim assessment. *AJR* 135:463–469, 1980.

44. Lees WR, Vallon AG, Denyer ME, et al: Prospective study of ultrasonography in chronic pancreatic disease. Br *Med J* 1:162–164, 1979.

45. Simeone JF, Wittenberg J, Ferrucci JT: Modern concepts of imaging of the pancreas, in Margulis AR (ed): *Progress in Clinical Radiology*. New York, Lippincott, 1980.

46. Weinstein BJ, Weinstein DP, Brodmerkel GJ: Ultrasonography of pancreatic lithiasis. *Radiology* 134:185–189, 1980.

47. Isikoff MB, Hill MC: Ultrasonic demonstration of intraductal pancreatic calculi: A report of two cases. *J Clin Ultrasound* 8:449–452, 1980.

48. Miller CE, Cooperberg PL, Cohen MM: Pitfalls in the ultrasonographic diagnosis of the pancreatic pseudocyst. *J Can Assoc Radiol* 29:239–242, 1978.

49. Laing FC, Gooding GAW, Brown T, Leopold GE: Atypical pseudocysts in the pancreas: An ultrasonographic evaluation. *J Clin Ultrasound* 7:27–33, 1979.

50. Sarti DA: Rapid development and spontaneous regression of pancreatic pseudocysts documented by ultrasound. *Radiology* 125:789–793, 1977.

51. Gooding GAW: Pseudocyst of the pancreas with mediastinal extension: An ultrasonographic demonstration. *J Clin Ultrasound* 5(2):121–123, 1976.

52. Griner PF, Mayewski RJ, Mushlin AI, Greenland P: Selection and interpretation of diagnostic tests and procedures: Principles and applications. *Ann Intern Med* 94(4/2):553–600, 1981.

53. Walls WJ, Gonzalez G, Martin NL, Templeton AW: B-scan ultrasound evaluation of the pancreas: Advantages and accuracy compared to other diagnostic techniques. *Radiology* 114:127–134, 1975.

54. Partain CL, Staab EV, McCartney WH: Multiple Imaging Modalities for the study of pancreatic disease. *Semin Nucl Med* 9(1):36–42, 1979.

55. Barkin J, Vining D, Miale A, et al: Computerized tomography, diagnostic ultrasound, and radionuclide scanning. *JAMA* 238(19):2,040–2,042, 1977.

56. Berger LA, Agnew JE, Chudleigh PM, Screening for pancreatic disease: A comparison of grey-scale ultrasonography and isotope scanning. *Lancet*, 633–635, March, 1979.

57. DiMagno EP, Malagelada JR, Taylor WF, Go VLW: A prospective comparison of

current diagnostic tests for pancreatic cancer. *New Engl J Med* 297(14):737–742, 1977.

58. Braganza JM, Fawcitt RA, Forbes WSC, et al: A clinical evaluation of isotope scanning, ultrasonography, and computed tomography in pancreatic disease. *Clin Radiol* 29:639–646, 1978.

59. Moss AA, Federle M, Shapiro HA, et al: The combined use of computed tomography and endoscopic retrograde cholangiopancreatography in the assessment of suspected pancreatic neoplasm: A blind clinical evaluation. *Radiology* 134:159–163, 1980.

60. Mackie CR, Cooper MJ, Lewis MH, Moossa AR: Nonoperative differentiation between pancreatic cancer and chronic pancreatitis. *Ann Surg* 189(4):480–487, 1979.

61. Haaga JR, Alfidi RJ, Havrilla TR, et al: Definitive role of CT scanning of the pancreas. *Radiology* 124:723–730, 1977.

62. Stanley RJ, Sagel SS, Levitt RG: Computed tomographic evaluation of the pancreas. *Radiology* 124:715–722, 1977.

63. Cotton PB, Lees WR, Vallon AG, et al: Gray-scale ultrasonography and endoscopic pancreatography in pancreatic diagnosis. *Radiology* 134:453–459, 1980.

64. Ferrucci JT, Wittenberg J, Black EB, et al: Computed body tomography in chronic pancreatitis. *Radiology* 130:175–182, 1979.

65. Kressel HY, Margulis AR, Gooding GW, et al: CT scanning and ultrasound in the evaluation of pancreatic pseudocysts: A preliminary comparison. *Radiology* 126:153–157, 1978.

66. Silverstein W, Isikoff MB, Hill MC, Barkin J: Diagnostic imaging of acute pancreatitis: Prospective study using CT and sonography. *AJR* 137:497–502, 1981.

67. Siegelman SS, Copeland BE, Saba GP, et al: CT of fluid collections associated with pancreatitis. *AJR* 134:1,121–1,132, 1980.

68. Dembner AG, Jaffe CC, Simeone J, Walsh J: A new computed tomographic sign of pancreatitis. *AJR* 133:477–479, 1979.

69. Foley WD, Stewart ET, Lawson TL, et al: Computed tomography, ultrasonography, and endoscopic retrograde cholangiopancreatography in the diagnosis of pancreatic disease: A comparative study. *Gastrointest Radiol* 5:29–35, 1980.

70. Fawcitt RA, Forbes WSC, Isherwood I, et al: Computed tomography in pancreatic disease. *Br J Radiol* 51:1–4, 1978.

71. Kamin PD, Bernardino ME, Wallace S, Jing B-S: Comparison of ultrasound and computed tomography in the detection of pancreatic malignancy. *Cancer* 46:2,410–2,412, 1980.

72. Hessel SJ, Siegelman SS, McNeil BJ, et al: A prospective evaluation of computed tomography and ultrasound of the pancreas. *Radiology* 143:129–133, 1982.

73. Hanley JA, McNeil BJ: The meaning and use of the area under a receiver operating characteristic (ROC) curve. *Radiology* 143:29–36, 1982.

74. Marchal G, Baert AL, Wilms G: Intravenous pancreaticography in computed tomography. *J Comput Assist Tomogr* 3(6):727–732, 1979.

75. Araki T, Itai Y, Furui S, Tasaka A: Dynamic CT densitometry of hepatic tumors. *AJR* 135:1,037–1,043, 1980.

76. Rosenfield AT, Taylor KJW, Jaffe CC: Clinical applications of ultrasound tissue characterization. *Radiol Clinics North Am* 18(1), 1980.

77. White DN, Cledgett PR: Breast carcinoma detection by ultrasonic doppler signals. *Ultrasound Med Biol* 4:329–335, 1978.

6

Reticuloendothelial System

Kenneth J. W. Taylor

INTRODUCTION

The *reticuloendothelial system* is a collective term for anatomically widespread tissue that exhibits phagocytosis. Cells of this system can be identified by their uptake of intravenously injected particles or dyes such as Indian ink or trypan blue. Cells of the reticuloendothelial system, varying in number and morphology, exist in the following anatomic sites:

1. In connective tissues, in which they are called *histiocytes* and in the brain where they are called microglia
2. In blood, where they are represented by large mononuclear cells
3. In the spleen, liver, thymus, bone marrow, medulla of the suprarenal gland, and the anterior lobe of the hypophysis
4. In the lymph nodes and lymphoid aggregates throughout the body, such as the tonsils

Due to the ability of these cells to ingest particles actively, they are involved in the immediate body defense against microorganisms and also with the establishment of a specific immune response. Two categories of cells are involved in the immune response:

1. Cells engaged in trapping, processing, and accomplishing the recognition of a foreign antigen
2. Immunologically competent cells, both for the cell-mediated and humoral antibody responses

These two types of cells represent the receptor and effector limbs of the immunologic response respectively.

In fetal life, the reticuloendothelial system of the spleen, liver, and bone marrow are important sites of hematopoiesis, and this function is retained postnatally in the bone marrow. In certain disease states associated with increased erythropoiesis, the cells of the liver and spleen may regain their hematopoietic function.

The lymph vessels comprise a network of minute capillaries that are blind-ending, but are capable of absorbing lymph that has filtered out of the blood capillaries. Because of this function, obstruction of these vessels results in the accumulation of free tissue fluid, producing edema, ascites, or an effusion, depending on the anatomic site. These small lymphatic plexuses form vessels of 1 to 2 mm in diameter that accompany the superficial veins and deep arteries. These channels are interrupted by lymph nodes. Lymph nodes are bean-shaped lymphoid masses; most lymph nodes are 2 to 3 mm in size, but they may be as large as 2 cm in length. They act as mechanical filters for the lymph returning from the tissues to the bloodstream, while the immunologically competent cells that are contained within the lymph nodes can initiate the response to microorganisms or other foreign protein.

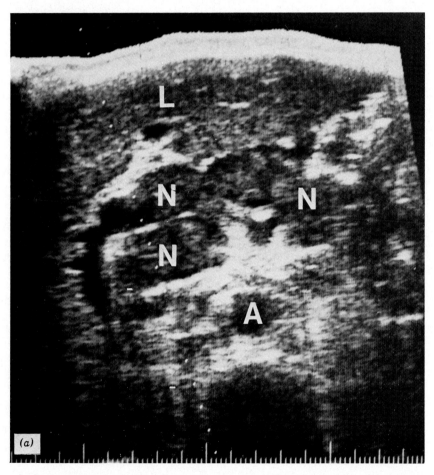

Figure 6-1 (*a*) Transverse scan through the upper abdomen showing the liver (L) anteriorly. Anterior to the aorta (A) a homogeneous lobulated mass is seen (N). These appearances are consistent with marked upper para-aortic lymphadenopathy in a patient with lymphoma. (*b*) Longitudinal scan through the upper abdomen showing liver (L) and aorta (A) posteriorly. Again the lobulated lymph node mass (N) is seen.

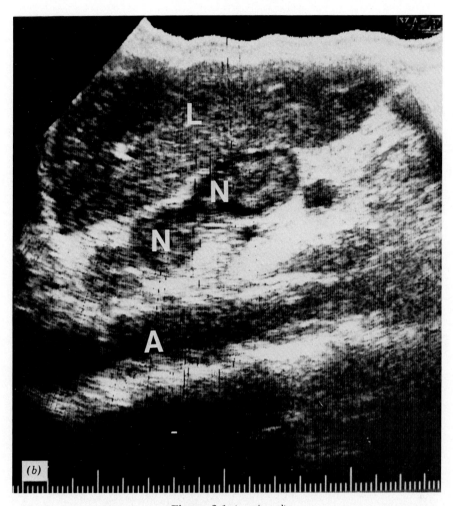

Figure 6-1 (*continued*)

The spleen is the largest lymphoid organ in the body and measures some 11 × 7 × 3 cm with an average weight of 150 g. The spleen is surrounded by a glistening capsule except at the hilum, which is in the center of its inferior surface and is the site at which branches of the splenic artery and splenic veins enter and leave the spleen respectively.

The splenic artery is a branch of the celiac artery, and both of these vessels are well seen on transverse ultrasonograms. The splenic artery travels along the superior or posterior border of the pancreas and usually divides into several branches before entering the splenic hilum. The artery is accompanied by the splenic vein, which is joined by the inferior and superior mesenteric veins to form the portal vein behind the neck of the pancreas.

The spleen contains aggregates of lymphoid tissue known as malpighian corpuscles, which have a structure similar to the follicles in the lymph nodes. Lymphoid tissue comprising the splenic cords alternate with splenic sinuses, which are long irregular channels lined by endothelial cells. Highly phagocytic cells are present within the spleen, and these can entrap abnormal particles or effete red cells.

As a part of the reticuloendothelial system, the spleen is important in the immunologic response of the body. However, the spleen is not essential to life, although there is considerable evidence of an increased susceptibility to infection in children who have had a splenectomy. In view of this tendency, a conservative approach is usually taken toward splenic rupture unless catastrophic blood loss occurs.

Attempts to image the reticuloendothelial system in the normal state by ultrasonography are limited largely to the display of the spleen, although normal lymph nodes can now be visualized with high-resolution small parts scanners. In other anatomic sites, such as the thyroid and gut, lymphoid

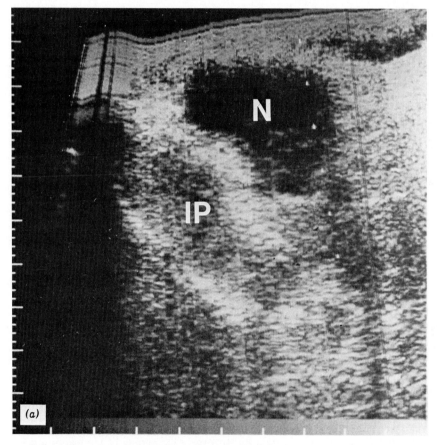

Figure 6-2 (*a*) Transverse scan through right iliac fossa. The iliopsoas (IP) muscle is seen posteriorly. There is a lobulated homogeneous mass of nodes (N) that was lymphadenopathy due to Hodgkin's disease. (*b*) Transverse scan of the pelvis with a distended bladder. Highly homogeneous masses are seen in the superficial tissues due to inguinal lymphadenopathy.

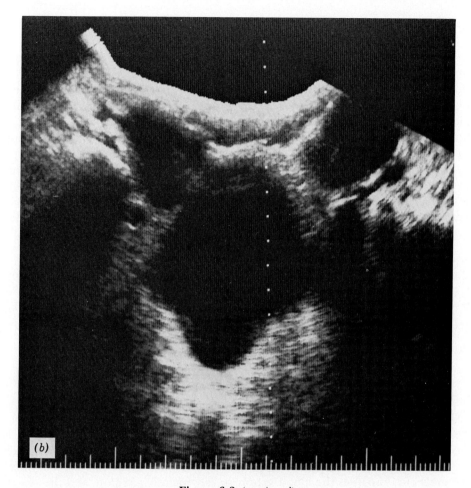

(b)

Figure 6-2 *(continued)*

aggregations are normally present only in microscopic amounts, although abnormal proliferation resulting in gross lymphoid masses that are apparent on ultrasound examination may occur. In addition, enlargement of the abdominal and pelvic lymph nodes may be diagnosed reliably by ultrasound scanning.

In addition to the ability to display an abnormal lymphoid mass, whether nodal or extranodal, ultrasonic examination frequently discloses secondary effects produced by the pressure of such masses on adjacent viscera. For example, para-aortic lymphadenopathy may produce varying degrees of hydronephrosis, and this condition is easily detected by ultrasound scanning. More rarely, upper abdominal para-aortic lymphadenopathy may produce pathologic distension of the biliary tree, and these secondary effects may allow the examiner to infer the presence of abnormalities even when the primary cause of the pathology is obscured by gas in the intestine.

ABDOMINAL AND PELVIC LYMPHADENOPATHY

Lymphangiography is a highly effective means of imaging the para-aortic lymph nodes, and by serial studies subsequent to opacification, neoplastic activity in nodes may be assessed.[1] Gallium citrate[67] (^{67}Ga) is also used widely to demonstrate tumor activity in nodes too high to be opacified by bipedal lymphangiography,[2] and it is effective for detecting small foci of melanoma and a limited number of other tumor types.[3] The combination of an ultrasound image to reveal enlarged nodes and a ^{67}Ga uptake study to demonstrate neoplastic activity within them may be an effective and practical alternative to lymphangiography. Lymphangiography does require special expertise that is not always available, and ultrasound examination with or without a complementary ^{67}Ga study provides a meaningful alternative to lymphangiography, especially under one of five conditions:

1. When operator expertise in lymphography is not available
2. Where previous lymphographic examinations and/or obesity render lymphography difficult or impossible, despite operator expertise
3. In the demonstration of high para-aortic lymphadenopathy not opacified by lymphography
4. In patients with severe allergies to iodine in whom contrast media may produce morbidity or even mortality
5. When necessary to demonstrate nodes such as the mesenteric lymph nodes which are outside the para-aortic chain

In searching for abdominal and pelvic lymphadenopathy, it is important to recall that the lymphatic channels accompany the blood vessels. Thus, it is essential for the ultrasonologist to be aware of the lymphatic drainage of each organ. For example, despite the superficial position of the testes, the lymphatic drainage accompanies the blood supply to the epigastric region, and the search for lymphadenopathy from testicular tumors should be directed to the high pre-aortic region.

The development of body computerized tomography (BCT) has provided yet another technique for demonstrating abnormal retroperitoneal masses. In the obese patient, CT may be dramatically better than ultrasound since fat provides a superb contrast medium for the retroperitoneal space. In addition, confusion with gut can be averted by the use of oral contrast medium. However, not infrequently, patients with advanced malignancy have no retroperitoneal fat and may be frankly cachectic. In such thin patients, the ultrasound image may be superior to the CT image. It should be noted that both ultrasound and CT produce an anatomic image and do not allow differentiation between malignant enlargement of lymph nodes and hyperplasia. Ga[67] uptake denotes functional activity, but again cannot differentiate between malignant and inflammatory processes.

Technique

Real-time ultrasound scanners, now widely commercially available, greatly increase the speed with which the abdomen and pelvis can be surveyed. With the current generation of manually operated static ultrasound scanners, the longitudinal midline scan is first performed (sagittal plane). With modern gray scale equipment, this scan can be carried out in a single linear sweep down the anterior surface of the abdomen, using paraffin oil or an aqueous gel as a coupling agent. The scanning arm is then moved one centimeter to the right and the procedure repeated. The scan can be initiated by a simple sector scan through the liver substance using previously established techniques[4] and then continued as a linear scan down the abdomen. The mechanical arm is then moved another centimeter toward the right and the procedure repeated. In this way, a series of paramedian scans are obtained to the right and left of the median plane. Lymphadenopathy is apparent as a lobulated mass that is acoustically highly homogeneous, that is, relatively echo-free or producing very weak internal echoes.[5]

These sagittal scans are augmented by serial transverse scans, commencing at the xiphisternum. Although the best resolution of the upper abdominal

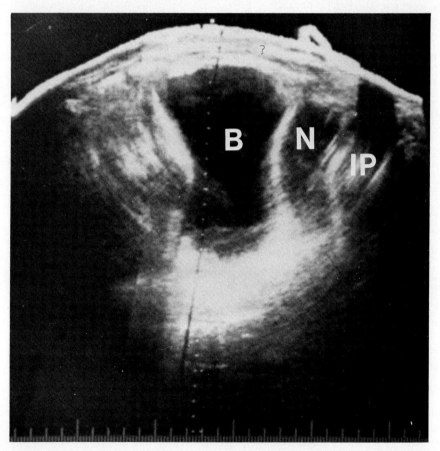

Figure 6-3 Transverse scan through the pelvis showing a distended bladder (B). Note that the walls of the bladder are convex medially due to a mass of homogeneous tissue (N) lying on the sidewalls of the pelvis. The iliopsoas (IP) muscle is seen more laterally.

vasculature is obtained by limited sector scans, in the demonstration of lymph-adenopathy it may be advantageous to compound, to some extent, on transverse scanning. Upper para-aortic lymphadenopathy is again apparent as a lobulated highly homogenous mass in the pre-aortic and para-aortic position (Fig. 6-1). A lymph node mass often surrounds the aorta. Mesenteric lymphadenopathy has the same lobulated and homogeneous characteristics, although the mass tends to be located more to the left of the midline. Pelvic lymphadenopathy presents a similar appearance in relation to the iliac vessels (Fig. 6-2) and may form masses that encroach on the pelvic cavity (Fig. 6-3).

In a significant number of patients, air in the gut prevents visualization of the retroperitoneal areas. This disadvantage is particularly apparent in patients who have been hospitalized for a long period of time with consequent immo-bilization. Gut preparation can be carried out on these patients, initially by oral

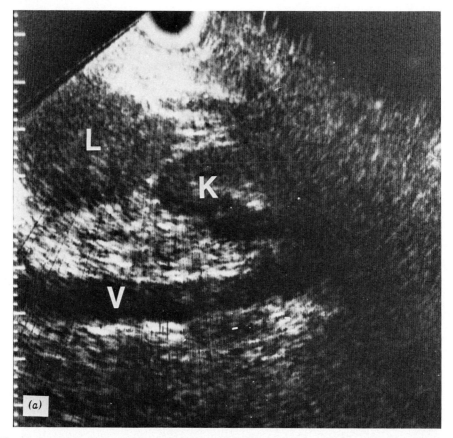

Figure 6-4 (a) Left decubitus approach to the normal upper retroperitoneum. A coronal section shows the liver (L), the right kidney (K), and the inferior vena cava (V). (b) Right decubitus approach to the normal upper retroperitoneum. A coronal scan shows the spleen (S), the left kidney (K), and the aorta (A). (c) Decubitus scan showing the spleen (S) and left kidney (K). Medial to the spleen, there are small lobulated masses consistent with lymphadenopathy.

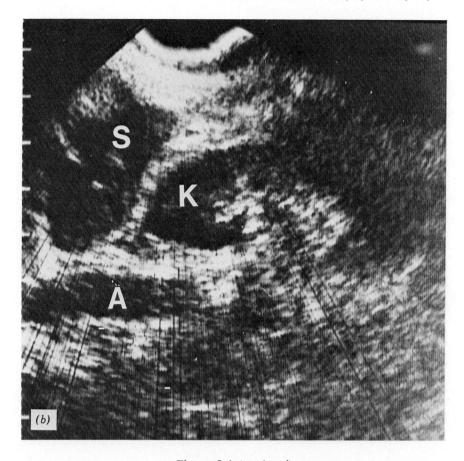

Figure 6-4 (*continued*)

cathartics, but, if necessary, enemas can be administered. When an anterior approach is impossible, decubitus positions can be effective using the liver and spleen as acoustic windows to the para-aortic region (Fig. 6-4).

Large retroperitoneal masses tend to displace air-containing gut and render the retroperitoneal area more amenable to ultrasonic visualization. Despite all attempts at gut preparation, there remain a minority of patients, possibly 10 percent, in whom the retroperitoneal area cannot be displayed adequately by ultrasound and in whom CT is necessary. In such patients, para-aortic lymphadenopathy should be suspected if the disease has produced a partial ureteric obstruction with consequent hydroureter and some degree of hydronephrosis. Both kidneys can be scanned satisfactorily by simple sector scans from the posterolateral aspects of the trunk, using previously established techniques.[6] These techniques allow a minimal degree of hydronephrosis to be reliably identified.

Rather infrequently, the presence of upper para-aortic lymphadenopathy may cause some obstruction of the bile ducts and result in dilatation of the intrahepatic and even extrahepatic parts of the biliary tree. Thus, whenever

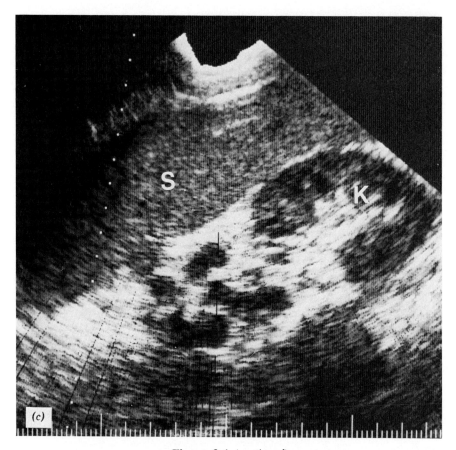

Figure 6-4 (*continued*)

dilated bile ducts are noted, determined efforts must be made to delineate the anatomic site and the cause of the obstruction and to exclude the presence of either a nodal or extranodal lymphomatous mass. Retrocaval lymph node masses may displace the inferior vena cava (Fig. 6-5) or compress the lumen resulting in peripheral edema.

RETROPERITONEAL EXTRANODAL LYMPHOID MASSES

Like pancreatic neoplasms in a similar anatomic situation, retroperitoneal lymphoid masses were very difficult to diagnose before the advent of ultrasound and computerized tomography. Either of these techniques can now be used depending on the facilities available and the bodily configuration of the patient. Such extranodal masses are found particularly in the non-Hodgkin's lymphomas, and, as with para-aortic lymphadenopathy, it is important to search for secondary signs of pressure in terms of hydronephrosis or biliary obstruction.

Lymphomatous masses tend to be highly homogeneous tumors in that they display low reflectivity. Extranodal lymphoid masses tend to be much more irregular in shape than lymphadenopathy and do not display the lobulated pattern that is characteristic of enlarged lymph nodes.

Lymphoma is highly sensitive to radiation therapy. Ultrasound and computerized tomography can be used for therapy planning to attack the tumor while sparing the kidneys as much as possible. For radiation therapy planning purposes, the complete tomogram produced by CT is much more satisfactory than the ultrasound image.

Diagnostic aspiration and biopsy procedures can be carried out under ultrasound or CT guidance. This simple procedure may save the patient unnecessary surgery, and histology is essential before implementation of rational therapy. (These techniques are detailed in Chapter 12.) The use of a 22-gauge

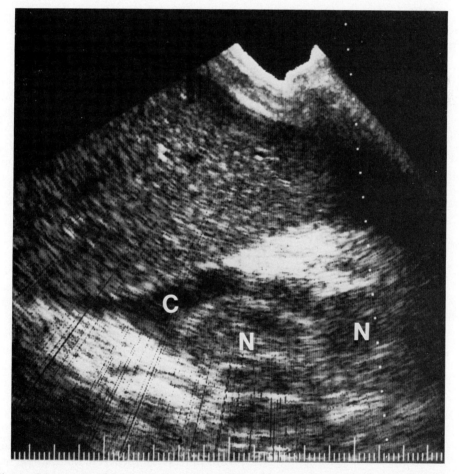

Figure 6-5 Longitudinal scan through the liver with the inferior vena cava posteriorly. The cava (C) is bowed anteriorly by enlarged lymph nodes (N). This mass must be differentiated from an adrenal mass that lies in the same anatomic position.

needle appears to allow biopsy in close proximity to the gut without hazard.[7] Even perforation of the gut appears to be without sequelae. Some authors prefer CT for guiding biopsy, since a scan with the needle in position allows the examiner to ensure that the needle is correctly sited.[8] However, in my view, it is more important to know that a diagnosis has been attained than to have a scan that demonstrates the position of the needle. Thus, in practice, we biopsy the mass and obtain an immediate preliminary reading from a cytologist. If we have failed to obtain an adequate cytologic specimen, more passes are made until adequate material has been obtained. The major advantage of ultrasound techniques for biopsy of these masses is the availability of instrumentation. A biopsy tends to be a lengthy procedure, especially when it is necessary to wait for the cytologic results. It is most advantageous, therefore, to use machines that are inexpensive and readily available in considerable numbers. However, patients are best served by a flexible approach; biopsy under CT guidance should be employed for those patients who are poorly visualized by ultrasound.

ULTRASOUND OF THE SPLEEN

Ultrasound examination of the spleen discloses its size and position even when under the cover of the rib cage and thus not clinically palpable. Apart from disclosing the normal spleen, ultrasound also demonstrates both focal disease and diffuse splenomegaly.

To a large extent, spleen scintigraphy is redundant after ultrasound scanning of the spleen. The size, shape, and position of the organ may be inferred from either examination and the presence of focal defects identified. Ultrasound is more specific in that it allows further differentiation of masses between those that are cystic and those that are solid.

Scanning Techniques

The normal spleen is under the cover of the lower left ribs, and thus techniques to image it by ultrasound must employ the lower left intercostal spaces.[9] The patient lies in the right (side down) decubitus position with the left arm extended above the head. This extension opens up the lower left intercostal spaces, and access can be exaggerated if necessary by placing a pillow under the patient's right side. The spleen can then be examined either obliquely or longitudinally in the coronal plane. The examiner identifies the plane of the tenth and eleventh intercostal spaces and aligns the gantry with this plane. A transducer with a small face (13 mm in diameter) at a frequency of 3.5 or 5 MHz allows optimal penetration of the space. The transducer can then be swept through a wide angle (approaching 180 degrees) to image the entire spleen along its longitudinal axis. (Fig. 6-6a). If the spleen is found to be higher or lower, adjacent intercostal spaces can be used up to the level of the left hemidiaphragm.

A scan in the coronal plane is also extremely valuable for imaging the spleen, left adrenal, left subphrenic space, or the left hemidiaphragm (Fig. 6-6b). The gantry of the scanning arm is arranged in the coronal plane (midaxillary) of the patient with the scanning arm toward the patient's feet. Again, a transducer

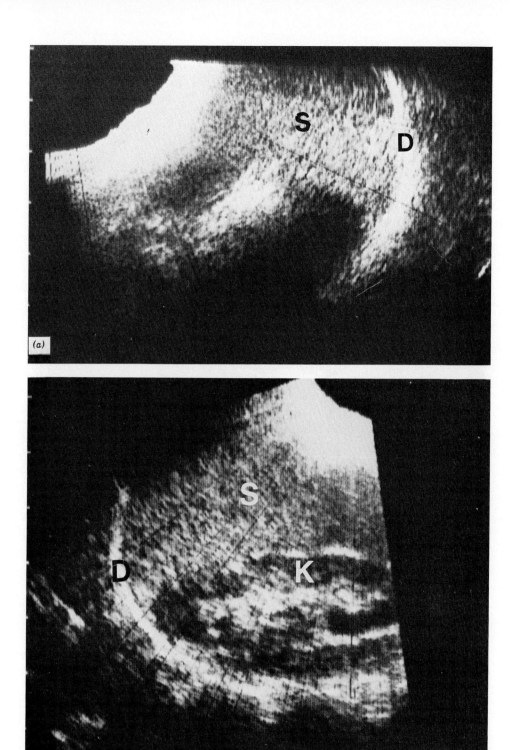

Figure 6-6 (*a*) Oblique scan showing normal spleen (S). The left hemidiaphragm (D) is seen limiting the spleen superiorly and posteriorly. (*b*) Coronal scan of the spleen performed with the patient in the right decubitus position. The spleen (S) is limited above by the left hemidiaphragm (D) and posteriorly by the left kidney (K).

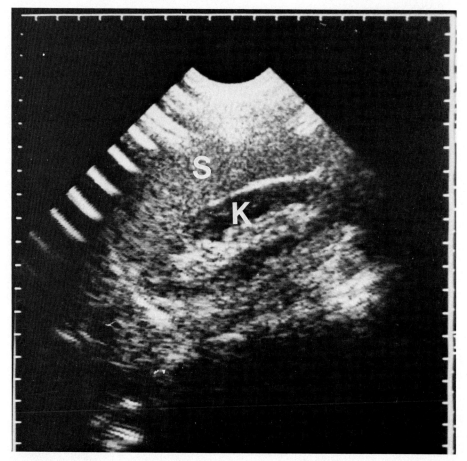

Figure 6-7 Real-time (mechanical sector) scan in the coronal plane showing the spleen (S) and the left kidney (K).

with a small contact face is placed in the tenth or eleventh interspace in the midaxillary line and is moved through a wide sector approaching 180 degrees. This displays the left hemidiaphragm, spleen, the region of the adrenal gland, and the upper pole of the left kidney (Fig. 6-6). Using these two techniques, the spleen can be imaged in every patient, and, in addition, the spleen provides an acoustic window to the left subphrenic space, left adrenal gland, and upper pole of the left kidney, all notoriously difficult areas for ultrasound examination unless the decubitus position is adopted.

The same scanning planes are used with a real-time device that can provide very adequate scans of the spleen (Fig. 6-7). The major difficulties that may be encountered with a real-time device are the limited field of view obtainable with some of the sector scanners or the presence of shadowing from the ribs that occurs with some of the linear array scanners and other scanners that require a large surface area of contact. Rotating or rocking sector scanners with wide angles of view are, however, entirely suitable for rapid scanning of the left upper quadrant.

Ultrasound Scanning of Splenic Pathology

Congenital Disorders

Aplasia of the spleen is a rare disorder that is usually associated with other congenital anomalies. A more common finding is hypoplasia. (Fig. 6-8). Accessory spleens are extremely common and are discovered in 20 to 30 percent of all postmortem examinations.[10] They are usually found in the region of the tail of the pancreas and may simulate a tumor on ultrasound scanning. Under these circumstances, liver scintigraphy is particularly beneficial since uptake of colloid indicates that the mass has phagocytic activity and, therefore, is an accessory spleen. Even after splenectomy, hypertrophy of the accessory spleen or splenic remnant may lead to a recurrence of the spleen, and this regenerated tissue has been termed the *born again spleen*.[11]

Abnormalities in the position of the spleen may occur, especially in young, usually multiparous women.[12] A wandering spleen may occur during pregnancy,

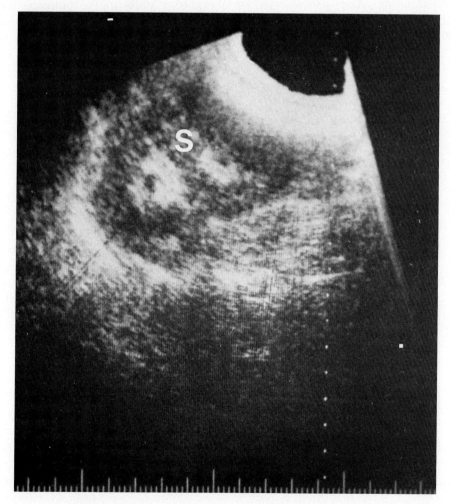

Figure 6-8 Coronal scan shows hypoplastic spleen (S).

and movement of the spleen is permitted by the presence of a long pedicle. Thus, a homogeneous mass may be found in the pelvis or in any other position in the abdominal or pelvic cavity.[13] Although the characteristic splenic texture may suggest the diagnosis by ultrasound, in my opinion, specific uptake of technetium-99m-labelled colloid allows a more specific diagnosis.

Splenic Cysts

Martin classified splenic cysts into primary, or true, cysts of the spleen and secondary, or pseudocysts, of the spleen occurring after trauma. (Table 6-1).[14]

Parasitic cysts are the most common cysts of the spleen worldwide. However, in the United States, nonparasitic cysts are more common, and 10 percent of these are epidermoid. The remaining 90 percent comprise dermoids, lymphangiomas, cavernous hemangiomas, and congenital cysts.[15] Multiple congenital epidermoid cysts are shown in Figure 6-9. True cysts by definition have an epithelial lining in contrast to secondary cysts or pseudocysts that have no true cellular lining. Also, psuedocysts are about four times more common than primary cysts (Fig. 6-10). Typically, they are associated with trauma occurring most frequently in childhood whether the trauma is recalled or not. About 70

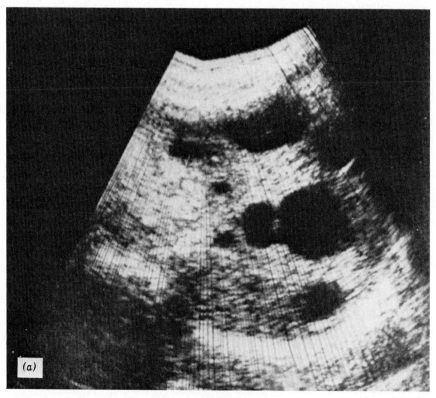

Figure 6-9 (*a*) Splenic scan demonstrating multiple cysts that proved to be epidermoid in origin. (This figure is shown by courtesy of the editors, *Journal of Clinical Ultrasound.*) (*b*) Surgical specimen of the spleen shown in part *a*.

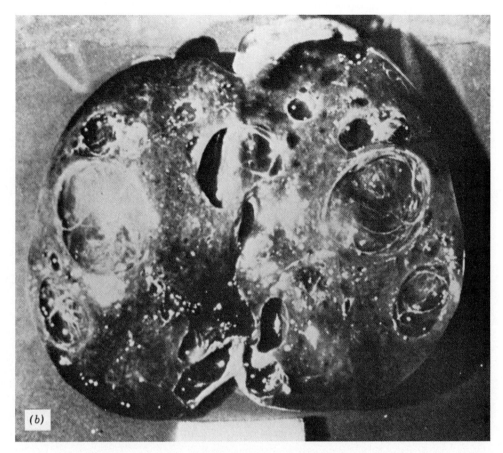

(b)

Figure 6-9 (*continued*)

percent of the patients are asymptomatic.[16] Symptoms are most commonly due to progressive distension.

Ultrasound allows an immediate assessment and definitive diagnosis of an intrasplenic cystic mass.[17,18,19] This finding may preclude the need for other radiologic studies. Calcification may be seen in the cyst wall in about 10 percent of cases, especially with echinoccocal or secondary posttraumatic cysts.[20] The left hemidiaphragm may be elevated on a chest radiograph.[4] An intravenous

Table 6-1   Classification of Splenic Cysts

Primary (True cysts)
  Parasitic
  Nonparasitic
   Congenital
   Neoplastic
Secondary (Pseudocysts or posttraumatic cysts)

urogram usually demonstrates downward displacement of the left kidney, and the stomach is usually displaced medially. CT can demonstrate the same findings as ultrasound, but, in this situation, it is virtually entirely repetitive and is seldom if ever necessary to make the diagnosis. If there is any doubt as to the relation of the spleen to the mass, liver/spleen scintigraphy[21] is a highly specific means of identifying splenic tissue, and further invasive studies such as angiography or splenoportography are then unnecessary.[22]

Splenic Rupture

Rupture of the spleen may occur due to direct trauma to the spleen or spontaneously because of abnormality of the spleen. The spleen may be unduly friable because of involvement by an infective or neoplastic process, most commonly malaria[23] and infectious mononucleosis.[24] A list of the diseases associated with spontaneous splenic rupture is shown in Table 6-2.[25] Figure 6-11 shows free fluid around the right lobe of the liver of a 20-year-old man with infectious mononucleosis who was in shock. Despite a normal liver/spleen scan, the presence of free fluid around the liver raised the possibility of a hemoperitoneum. Investigation disclosed a falling hematocrit, and a presumptive diagnosis of a ruptured spleen was made. Under ultrasound visualization, 40 ml of virtually pure blood were aspirated. The patient was treated with bed rest and intravenous fluids.

This case illustrates a conservative approach to splenic rupture, and, indeed, the diagnosis was never surgically proven. However, the clinical state of the patient and the diagnostic tap of the hemoperitoneum allowed successful diagnosis and conservative treatment.

Splenic trauma is common in children, and any blow to the left lower ribs, whether causing rib fracture or not, may cause subsequent splenic rupture. In

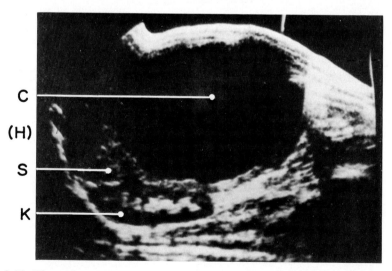

Figure 6-10 Ultrasonogram through left upper quadrant mass in an 11-year-old boy. Hugh cystic cavity (C) is seen lying superficially with a compressed spleen (S) and left kidney (K) posteriorly.

Table 6-2 Causes of Spontaneous Splenic Rupture

Infectious Diseases	Hematologic Disorders	Miscellaneous
Malaria	Hodgkin's disease	Tumors
Infectious mononucleosis	Leukemia	Malignant melanoma
Viral hepatitis	Sarcoma	Gastric cancer
Actinomycosis	Multiple myeloma	Sarcoidosis
Infectious endocarditis	Amyloidosis	Primary cyst
Typhoid fever	Polycythemia vera	Pregnancy
Influenza	Hemophilia	Gaucher's disease
Typhus	Myeloid metaplasia	Systemic lupus
Tularemia	Congenital hemolytic anemia	Splenic infarct
Echinococcosis	Felty's syndrome	Splenic vein thrombosis
Paratyphus		Portal vein thrombosis
Pneumonia		Gastric ulcer
Relapsing fever		Pancreatitis
Blastomycosis		Crohn's disease
Chicken pox		

young adults, motor vehicle accidents are a most frequent cause of splenic rupture.

During the past 30 years, there has been a gradual move toward a more conservative approach in the management of patients with splenic rupture. Splenic rupture used to be treated by splenectomy, but more recently, the late sequelae of splenectomy have led many surgeons to reexamine the desirability of this procedure.

King and Schumacker[26] noted fatal sepsis in children after splenectomy, and a later review by Singer showed a death rate from sepsis some 60 times greater in asplenic children than in normal ones.[27] Postsplenectomy sepsis follows a rapidly progressive infective course, usually with meningitis or pneumonia. Although it may occur at any time after splenectomy and at any age, it is more common in infants and within the first 1 or 2 years after surgery.[28] It is now accepted practice that, where possible, splenic rupture be treated by surgical repair of the spleen (splenorrhaphy) and hemostasis.[29] In many children, splenic rupture not leading to exsanguination may be treated conservatively by bed rest and transfusion.

Postsplenectomy syndrome in adults is limited to a few case reports, and the significance is unknown.[30,31] One interesting study demonstrated significantly increased mortality from both pneumonia and ischemic heart disease in a long-term follow-up of normal adults who were splenectomized for trauma during World War II.[32]

Since it is no longer considered necessary to explore every patient with possible splenic rupture, a reliable noninvasive diagnostic method becomes more important. For these purposes, ultrasound and/or splenic scintigraphy are valuable. After splenectomy, the operative site may fill with hematoma and

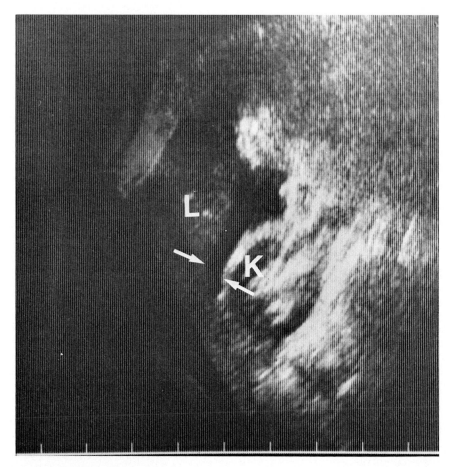

Figure 6-11 Limited transverse scan through right lower intercostal space shows liver (L) and right kidney (K). A small amount of fluid is seen in the hepatorenal angle (arrow), and guided aspiration demonstrated pure blood in a patient with a ruptured spleen.

produce a "pseudo-spleen" (Fig. 6-12). In the longer period, hypertrophy of accessory spleens may produce a "born again spleen."[11]

Splenic Abscess

A solitary abscess of the spleen is uncommon. Chulay and Lankarani (1976)[33] reported only 10 cases in nearly 100,000 admissions to the Cleveland Metropolitan Hospital over a 10-year period. However, bacterial endocarditis due to intravenous narcotic abuse has increased in prevalence in recent years, and hemorrhagic infarcts of the spleen are common. Some of these may progress to abscess formation.[34] However, unless gas bubbles appear, we are unable by ultrasound alone to differentiate between a hematoma and a splenic abscess (Fig. 6-13). It is probable that infected hematomas are frequently successfully treated medically by the long-term antibiotic therapy regime necessary for the treatment of endocarditis.

Air contained within a cystic lesion must raise the strong possibility of abscess formation by a gas-producing organism. This may make ultrasound recognition of the abscess extremely difficult. In the presence of gas, diagnosis by CT may be much easier,[35] as in the following patient.

A 68-year-old woman was admitted with fevers to 107° F and a history of prior treatment of adenocarcinoma of the cervix.[5] A recurrent tumor was found in the upper vagina, and an enlarged spleen was noted. Ultrasound examination (Fig. 6-14*a*) revealed a central area of low-amplitude echoes with a focus of high-level echoes suggesting the presence of gas. An abdominal CT (Fig. 6-14*b*) demonstrated a gas-containing, low-density lesion in the center of the spleen. Gallium 67 scan showed increased activity in the region of the splenic hilum. At surgery, a gastric mass was found that had produced a fistula

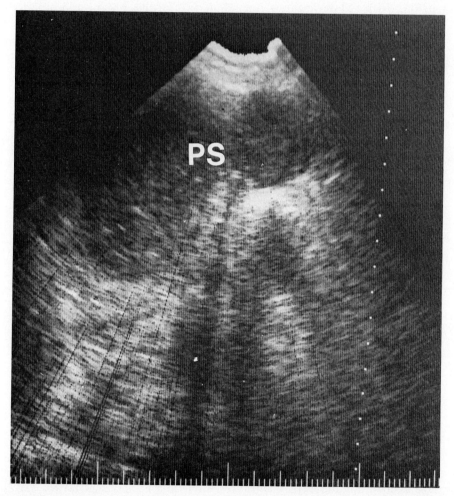

Figure 6-12 Oblique scans through the left upper quadrant in a patient following splenectomy. An echogenic area (PS) simulates the appearance of the spleen. This was due to a postoperative hematoma.

into the splenic hilum, and a gas-containing abscess had formed. The gas content of the lesion is very obvious on the CT scan but could easily be misinterpreted as air in adjacent gut on ultrasound. In the presence of recurrent tumor, the uptake of ^{67}Ga is nonspecific.

Almost invariably, there is a predisposing cause for a splenic abscess. Sengupta and Mukhergi (1975)[36] found that 70 percent of splenic abscesses were due to hematogeneous spread from an infective focus elsewhere, 10 percent were due to local sepsis, as, for example, from a carcinoma of the colon, and 15 percent followed trauma to the spleen.

Splenic Infarcts

Infarcts of the spleen are common in association with bacterial endocarditis. As stated above, there may be irregular fluid-filled areas indistinguishable from an abscess, but resolving without further symptoms or signs on medical therapy alone (Fig. 6-13). These infarcts may show progressive organization, and the

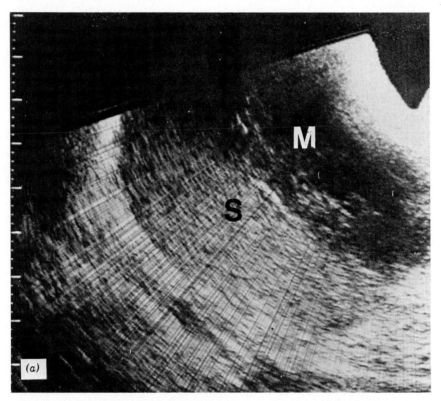

Figure 6-13 (*a*) Splenic scan showing a homogeneous mass (M) with compressed splenic tissue (S) more posteriorly. These approaches were seen in a patient with documented bacterial endocarditis and were assumed to be due to a hemorrhagic infarct. (*b*) The same patient as shown in part *a* 8 months later. There has been organization of the abnormal area (M), which appears to be walled off from an otherwise normal spleen (S).

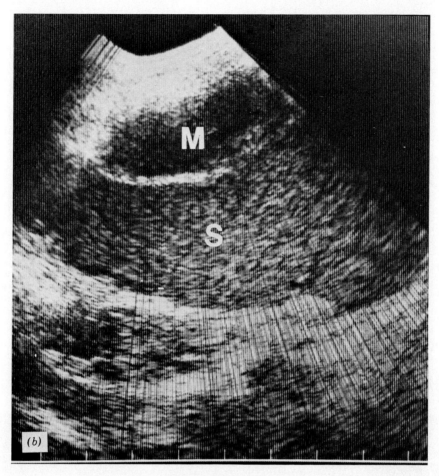

Figure 6-13 (*continued*)

irregular cystic area may progress to an echogenic focus, typically wedge-shaped with the base to the capsule of the spleen (Fig. 6-15).

Histoplasmosis

Histoplasmosis is caused by *Histoplasma capsulatum*, which has a worldwide distribution. The disease is contracted by inhalation of fungal spores that develop in yeast. The original lung lesion is similar to a tuberculous reaction. Occasionally, systemic dissemination of the lung lesion occurs, generally without clinical change, yielding calcified lesions in the liver, spleen, lymph nodes, brain, and other viscera. Thus, patients with histoplasmosis of the spleen have splenomegaly with high-level foci throughout the organ, often with some shadowing (Fig. 6-16).

Focal Tumor of the Spleen

Although the spleen is very frequently diffusely involved with tumor in both lymphoma and leukemia, the presence of splenomegaly is a poor indicator of

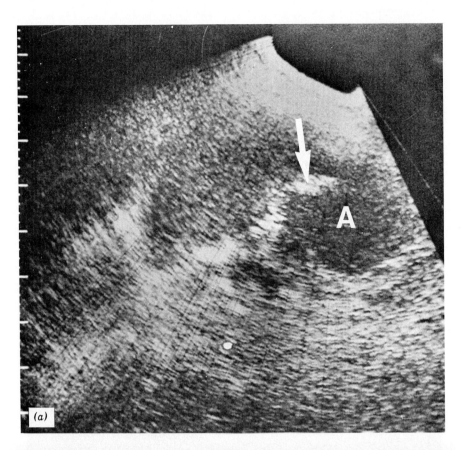

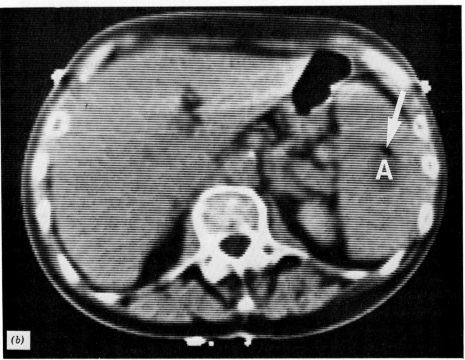

230

Figure 6-14 (*a*) Gas-containing splenic abscess (A). Notice the high-level echoes (arrow) due to the presence of contained air. (This figure is shown by courtesy of the *Yale Journal of Medicine and Biology*.) (*b*) CT scan of the same patient as that shown in part *a*. A small amount of air (arrow) is shown within a small abscess cavity (A) within the spleen.

←———————————————————————————————————

involvement.[37] Focal deposits do occur, although rather rarely, but particularly in lymphoma and melanoma, and are usually less echogenic than the surrounding normal splenic parenchyma in my experience (Fig. 6-17).[38,39] Such homogeneous deposits may be confused with an abscess.[40] On two occasions, I have seen an echogenic focus that proved to be due to leukemic infiltration. On two further occasions, an echogenic focal defect of the spleen has proved to be a rare metastatic deposit from a primary carcinoma in the colon (Fig. 6-18). Echogenic deposits from melanoma[33] and ovarian cancer[41] have been described.

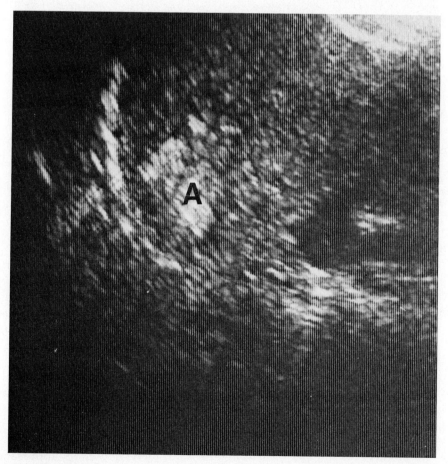

Figure 6-15 Splenic scan shows echogenic area (A) in a patient after documented bacterial endocarditis. Appearances are consistent with a splenic infarct.

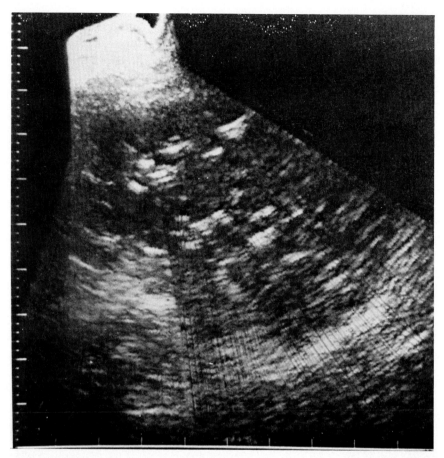

Figure 6-16 Splenic scan showing multiple small echogenic areas throughout. The plain film also demonstrated calcifications. Appearances are consistent with past histoplasmosis.

Diffuse Splenomegaly

The longitudinal axis of the spleen can easily be measured by ultrasound techniques and is usually 11 cm or less, and 12 cm is certainly abnormal in my experience. If multiple serial sections are taken through the organ, the volume may be computed.[42,43] The addition of gray scale technique not only allows more reliable detection of focal disease but also allows some differential diagnosis on the cause of splenomegaly by the tissue texture revealed.

Taylor and Milan[44] first noted some association between the echogenicity of the splenic parenchyma and pathology, although this relationship is not absolute. Nevertheless, an enlarged spleen of low echogenicity tends to be found in a malignant involvement, whereas inflammatory causes of splenomegaly tend to have a high echogenicity (Fig. 6-19). Of course, exceptions exist.[45] It must be stressed that these observations relate only to patients when they are seen initially. Aggressive therapy of neoplastic spleens may result in an appearance identical to that of many inflammatory or congestive causes of splenomegaly. For a true comparison, the scans must be performed at constant gain and TGC settings and at the same frequency. Computerized A-scan analysis of the amplitude of echoes performed at constant gain and TGC settings and at the same frequency confirmed the finding that low echogenicity tends to be associated with malignancy and high echogenicity with an inflammatory process in splenomegaly.[43] This relation has also been confirmed by other authors.[41]

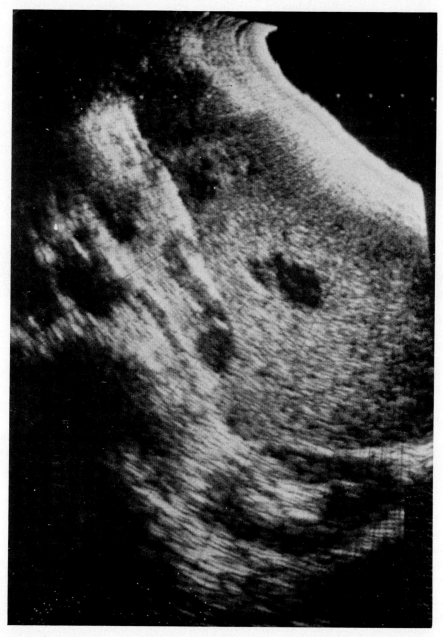

Figure 6-17 Splenic scan showing an enlarged organ with several well-marked defects. Appearances were due to splenic infiltration with local lymphoma.

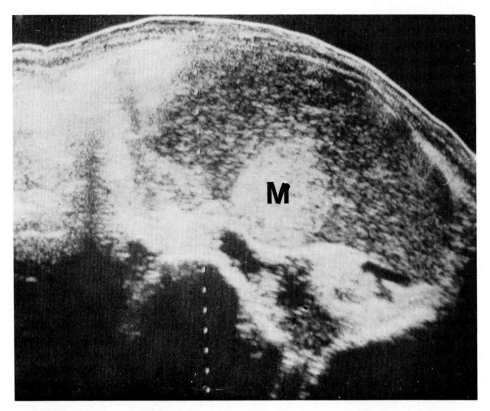

Figure 6-18 A well defined echogenic mass (M) is seen within the spleen. This was due to a metastasis from a carcinoma of the colon.

Mittelstaedt and Partain reported that the normal echogenicity of the spleen was similar to that of the liver, but this was also noted in a number of patients with splenomegaly who had pathologic conditions associated with erythropoiesis, increased reticuloendothelial activity, or congestion.[41]

Examination of the spleen is also useful in the assessment of portal hypertension secondary to cirrhosis of the liver, or more rarely, congenital hepatic fibrosis. Indeed, portal hypertension is the most common cause of splenomegaly in the United States. In portal hypertension, progressive obliteration of the portal venous channels by fibrosis within the liver leads to reduction of blood flow and eventually to a reversal of flow in the portal vein. This back pressure produces congestive splenomegaly. Thus, in any patient with cirrhosis of the liver, the spleen should also be scanned to search for possible evidence of portal hypertension. In addition, the portal vein may be enlarged and tortuous, although this is variable. Recently, a patent left umbilical vein has been observed

→

Figure 6-19 (*a*) Scans of the left upper quadrant show an echogenic spleen (S) surrounded by a subphrenic abscess (A). Above the left hemidiaphragm there is a large left pleural effusion (E). At surgery, a phlegmon of the spleen was found surrounded by a subphrenic abscess. (*b*) Splenomegaly in a patient with chronic lymphocytic leukemia on long-term chemotherapy. The echogenicity is markedly less than that seen in part *a*.

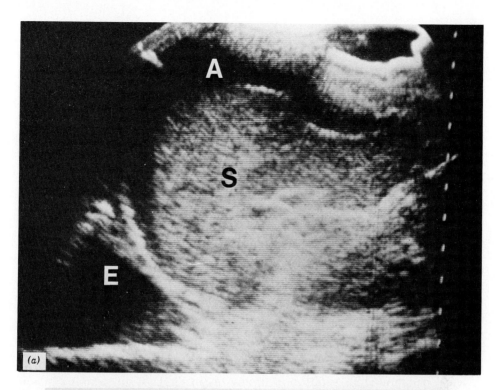

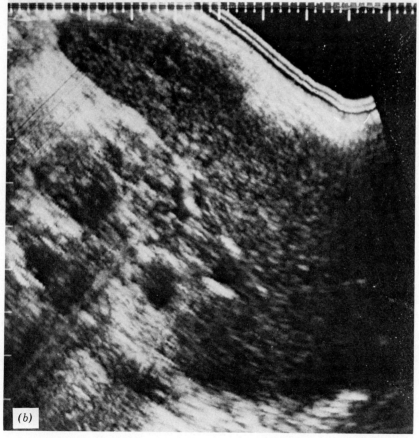

as a sign of portal hypertension and is claimed to be entirely specific.[46,47,48] However, similar anastomotic channels can open after superior vena caval compression, so this sign may not be as specific as was originally considered. In addition, the majority of patients with portal hypertension do not have evidence of a patent umbilical vein. In the longer term, the availability of pulsed Doppler devices should permit routine determination of the direction of flow and measurement of the absolute flow in the portal vein.

OTHER SITES OF RETICULOENDOTHELIAL PROLIFERATION

Abnormal reticuloendothelial proliferation may occur in many sites other than the retroperitoneal area in various neoplastic conditions. It is important to note that this abnormal lymphoid tissue in any anatomic site tends to have the same ultrasonic characteristics, which consist of low attenuation and low echo amplitude in the untreated state. Lymphomatous infiltration of the liver is common in an advanced state of disease, and this gives rise to well-delineated areas of very low echo amplitude (Fig. 6-20a). Subsequent chemotherapy may alter this pattern greatly and lead to disappearance of the lesion (Fig. 6-20b). Similar homogeneous masses occur in lymphomatous infiltration of the kidneys.

Thus, lymphomatous infiltration in any organ tends to give tumors of low attenuation and low echo amplitude. Enlargement of the thymus gland, as in thymoma, is seen as a low echo-producing area anterior to the heart, while mediastinal nodes show a typical lobulated low echo-producing area, but are much better visualized by CT. Neoplastic proliferation of the lymphoid tissue in the thyroid produces acoustically highly homogeneous tumors, as do lymphomas arising in the retroorbital site.

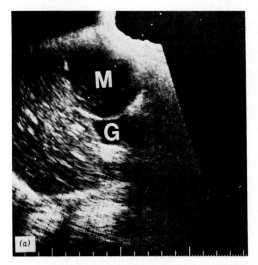 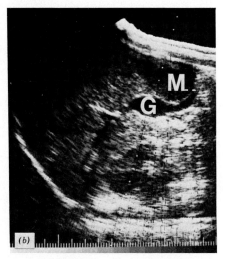

Figure 6-20 (a) The liver is shown in a young patient with Burkitt's lymphoma. A large focal mass (M) is seen compressing the lumen of the gallbladder (G). (b) Same patient as in part a showing marked diminution in the size of the mass (M) after therapy.

In conclusion, the reticuloendothelial system is a diffuse anatomic entity of which only the spleen can be imaged adequately by current ultrasonic techniques in the normal patient. In disease states, abnormal lymphoid masses may be visualized by ultrasound in many different sites, including the retroperitoneum and enlarged para-aortic and mesenteric nodes.

REFERENCES

1. Castellino RA, Billingham M, Dorfman RF: Lymphographic accuracy in Hodgkin's disease and malignant lymphoma: The note on the "reactive" lymph node as a cause of most false-positive lymphograms. *Invest Radiol* 9:155–165, 174.

2. King DJ, Dawson AA, McDonald AM: Gallium scanning in lymphoma. *Clin Radiol* 31:729–732, 1980.

3. Hoffer PB: Status of [67]gallium tumor detection. *J Nuc Med* 21:394–398, 1980.

4. Taylor KJW, Hill CR: Scanning techniques in gray scale ultrasonography. *Br J Radiol* 48:918–920, 1975.

5. Freimanis AK, Asher WM: Development of diagnostic criteria in echographic study of abdominal lesions. *AJR* 108:747–755, 1970.

6. Chulay JD, Lankarani MR: Splenic abscess: Report of 10 cases and review of the literature. *Am J Med* 61:513–522, 1976.

7. Holm HH, Als O, Gammelgaard J: Percutaneous aspiration and biopsy procedure under ultrasound visualization, in Taylor KJW (ed): *Clinics in Diagnostic Ultrasound: Diagnostic Ultrasound in Gastrointestinal Disease.* 1979, Vol 1, p 137.

8. Wittenberg J, Ferrucci JT: Radiographically guided needle biopsy of abdominal neoplasms: Who, how, where, why. *J Clin Gastroenterol* 1:273–284, 1979.

9. Moulton D, Taylor KJW, Simonds BD, Rosenfield AT: New ultrasonic scanning techniques to display the left upper quadrant, in White D, Lyons EA (eds): *Ultrasound in Medicine.* New York, Plenum Press, 1977, Vol 4, pp 619–622.

10. Robbins SL: *Pathologic Basis of Disease.* Philadelphia, W.B. Saunders Co, 1974, p 769.

11. Pearson HA, Johnston D, Smith K: The born-again spleen: Return of splenic function after splenectomy for trauma. *New Engl J Med* 298:1,389–1,392, 1978.

12. Miller EI: Wandering spleen in pregnancy: Case report. *J Clin Ultrasound* 3:281–282, 1975.

13. Gordon, DH, Burrell MI, Levin DC, et al: Wandering spleen: The radiological and clinical spectrum. *Radiology* 125:39–46, 1977.

14. Martin JW: Congenital splenic cysts. *Am J Surg* 96:302–308, 1958.

15. Sirinek KR, Evans WE: Nonparasitic splenic cysts. *Am J Surg* 126:8–13, 1973.

16. Blank E, Campbell JR: Epidermoid cysts of the spleen. *Pediatrics* 51:75–84, 1973.

17. Kaufman RA, Silver TM, Wesley JR: Preoperative diagnosis of splenic cysts in children by gray scale ultrasonography. *J Pediatr Surg* 14:450–454, 1979.

18. Bhimji SD, Cooperberg PL, Naiman S, et al.: Ultrasound diagnosis of splenic cysts. *Radiology* 122:787–789, 1977.

19. Dembner AG, Taylor KJW: Gray scale sonographic diagnosis: Multiple congenital splenic cysts. *J Clin Ultrasound* 6:143–214, 1978.

20. Fowler RH: Cystic tumors of the spleen. *Int Abst Surg* 70:213–223, 1940.

21. Pearson HA, Touloukian RJ, Spencer RP: The binary spleen: A radioisotope scan sign of splenic pseudocyst. *J Pediatr* 77:215–220, 1970.

22. Sloan CE, Bramis J, Janowitz HD, et al: Epidermoid cyst of the spleen: Case report and discussion. *Mt Sinai J Med* 43:372–376, 1976.

23. Ellison EH: Spontaneous rupture of the diseased spleen. *Arch Surg* 59:298–299, 1949.

24. Rutkow IM: Rupture of the spleen in infectious mononucleosis: A clinical review. *Arch Surg* 113:718–720, 1978.

25. Nichols TW, Wright SM, Pyeatte JC, et al: Spontaneous rupture of the spleen. *Am J Gastroenterol* 75:226–228, 1981.

26. King H, Schumacker HB: Susceptibility to infection after splenectomy performed in infancy. *Ann Surg* 136:239–242, 1952.

27. Singer DG: Post-splenectomy sepsis. *Perspect Pediatr Pathol* 1:285–311. 1973.

28. Eraklis AJ, Filler RM: Splenectomy in childhood: A review of 1413 cases. *J Pediatr Surg* 7:382–388, 1972.

29. Giuliano AE, Lim RC: Is splenic salvage safe in the traumatized patient. *Arch Surg* 116:651–656, 1981.

30. Grinblat J, Gilboa Y: Overwhelming pneumococcal sepsis 25 years after splenectomy. *Am J Med Sci* 270:523–524, 1975.

31. Karatsas NB: Fatal pneumococcal septicema after splenectomy. *Br Med J* 2:1,500–1,501, 1966.

32. Robinette CD, Fraumeni JF: Splenectomy and subsequent mortality in veterans in the 1939–1945 war. *Lancet* 2:127–129, 1977.

33. Murphy JF, Bernadino ME: The sonographic findings of splenic metastases. *J Clin Ultrasound* 7:195–197, 1979.

34. Dubbins PA: Ultrasound in the diagnosis of splenic abscess. *Br J Radiol* 53:488–489, 1980.

35. Somer FG, Gonazlez R, Taylor, KJW: Computed tomography and ultrasound findings of a gas-containing abscess. *Yale J Med Biol* 53:161–163, 1980.

36. Sangupta D, Mukherjie B: Amebic abscess of the spleen. *J Indian Med Assoc* 64:45–47, 1975.

37. Carroll BA, Ta HN: The ultrasonic appearance of extranodal abdominal lymphoma. *Radiology* 136:419–425, 1980.

38. Glees JP, Taylor KJW, Gazet JC, et al: Accuracy of gray scale ultrasonography of liver and spleen in Hodgkin's disease and other lymphomas compared with isotope scans. *Clin Radiol* 28:223–238, 1977.

39. deGraaf CS, Taylor KJW, Jacobson P: Gray scale echography of the spleen: Follow-up in 67 patients. *Ultrasound Med Biol* 5:13–21, 1979.

40. Cunningham JJ: Ultrasonic findings in isolated lymphoma of the spleen simulating splenic abscess. *J Clin Ultrasound* 6:377–414, 1978.

41. Mittelstaedt CA, Partain CL: Ultrasonic-pathologic classification of splenic abnormalities: Gray-scale patterns. *Radiology* 134:697–705, 1980.

42. Kardel T, Holm HH, Rasmussen SN, Mortensen T: Ultrasonic determination of liver and spleen volume. *Scand J Clin Lab Invest* 27:123–128, 1971.

43. Koga T: Correlation between cross-sectional area of the spleen by ultrasonic tomography and actual volume of the removed spleen. *J Clin Ultrasound* 7:119–120, 1979.

44. Taylor, KJW, Milan J: Differential diagnosis of chronic splenomegaly by gray-scale ultrasonography: Clinical observations and digital A-scan analysis. *Br J Radiol* 49:519–525, 1976.

45. Siler J, Hunter TB, Weiss J, Haber K: Increased echogenicity of the spleen in benign and malignant disease. *Am J Radiol* 134:1,011–1,014, 1980.

46. Funston MR, Goudre E, Richter IA, et al: Ultrasound diagnosis of the recanalised umbilical vein in portal hypertension. *J Clin Ultrasound* 8:244–246, 1980.

47. Schabel SI, Rittenberg GM, Javid LH, et al: The "bull's-eye" falciform ligament: A sonographic finding of portal hypertension. *Radiology* 136:157–159, 1980.

48. Glazer GM, Laing FC, Brown TW, et al: Sonographic demonstration of portal hypertension: The patent umbilical vein. *Radiology* 136:161–163, 1980.

7

Intraabdominal Fluid Collections

Paul A. Dubbins
Alfred B. Kurtz

INTRODUCTION

The detection and characterization of intraabdominal fluid collections remain challenging diagnostic problems. The demonstration of ascites in a patient with chronic liver disease denotes a degree of liver decompensation perhaps not detectable by clinical means, while the demonstration of intraperitoneal fluid in a patient with malignant disease alters staging and subsequent management. The detection and localization of hematomas, seromas, and lymphoceles allows a more rational approach to the management of abdominal fluid collections including those associated with surgery. Prompt and accurate diagnosis of intraabdominal pus, however, probably remains the most significant and important challenge to the efficacy of the various abdominal imaging techniques. Several authors attest to the seriousness of the problem of intraabdominal abscess,[1-3] and the mortality associated with even treated abdominal abscess remains high at about 30 percent.[1] The morbidity, too, of intraabdominal abscess is common, varied, and disabling.[4-6]

The ability of ultrasound to demonstrate fluid within the abdomen and thus differentiate a cyst from a solid mass has resulted in the use of this modality for the diagnosis of the various intraabdominal fluids.[3,7-12] To a large degree, the demonstration of fluid by ultrasound is a nonspecific finding in that there is no absolute method of differentiation among various types of fluid. Certain echo patterns, however, are seen more commonly with particular fluid collections, and knowledge of these patterns may allow a specific diagnosis in the correct clinical setting.

This chapter discusses the role of ultrasound in the diagnosis of fluid collections within the abdomen. In particular, the use of ultrasound to localize fluid collections is considered and, where possible, specific echo patterns are described. It is not proposed to consider in detail the nature or appearance of fluid collections within solid organs as these have been described in the relevant chapters. Similarly, pancreatic pseudocyst is considered in the chapter on ultrasound of the pancreas and is, therefore, not discussed here.

GENERAL ANATOMY OF THE ABDOMEN[13]

The Abdominal Musculature

There are three pairs of broad, flat muscles that form the major part of the anterolateral abdominal wall (from exterior inward: the external oblique, the internal oblique, and the transversus abdominis muscle) and a strap-like muscle, the rectus abdominis, situated on each side of the midline (Fig. 7–1). The aponeuroses of the anterolateral muscles meet at the anterior midline where the intertwining of the tendon fibers form the linea alba. In addition, the strap-like rectus abdominis muscle is ensheathed by the decussation of these aponeuroses close to the midline.

The muscles contributing to the posterior abdominal wall are the quadratus lumborum, extending from the iliac crest to the transverse processes of the lumbar vertebrae, and the iliopsoas muscle. The iliopsoas is made up of the psoas major, arising from the lumbar vertebral bodies and transverse process, and the iliacus arising from the inner surface of the wing of the ilium, joining together in the pelvis to insert into the upper part of the femur.

The cephalad muscular boundary of the abdominal cavity is formed by the diaphragm. Caudad, the muscles of the pelvic floor and the bladder provide the inferior boundary.

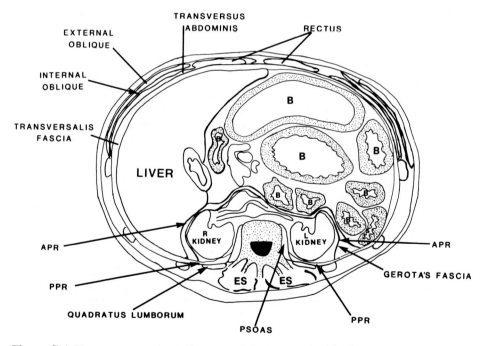

Figure 7-1 Transverse section of upper abdomen at the level of the second lumbar vertebral body, demonstrating the peritoneal and retroperitoneal spaces. APR = anterior pararenal space; PPR = posterior pararenal space; B = bowel loops; ES = erector spinae muscle. The muscles of the abdominal wall are demonstrated.

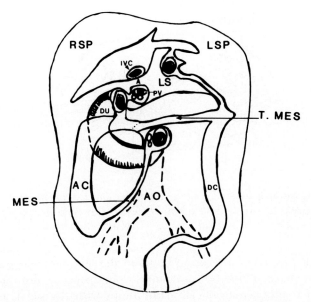

Figure 7-2 The peritoneal attachments of the posterior abdominal wall. RSP = right subphrenic space; LSP = left subphrenic space; IVC = inferior vena cava; LS = the lesser sac; A = the aditus to the lesser sac; PV = the portal vein; DU = the duodenum; T.MES = the attachment for the transverse mesocolon; AC = the ascending colon; DC = the descending colon; MES = the root of the mesentery; AO = the aorta. The attachment of the various peritoneal reflections determines the routes of spread and compartmentalization of intraabdominal fluid.

The Peritoneal Cavity

The peritoneal cavity is a blind sac reduced to slit-like proportions through the continuity of its parietal and visceral layers. It is, by definition, empty except for a film of fluid. However, those structures that are projected into the cavity by a mesentery and can only be reached through the peritoneal cavity are described as being intraperitoneal; these structures include the stomach and small bowel, the transverse colon, the liver, and the spleen. Those structures that have no mesentery are considered retroperitoneal and include the ascending and descending colon, the pancreas, the duodenum, and the kidneys.

The peritoneal reflections and mesenteric attachments determine the routes of spread of intraperitoneal fluid, serving as boundaries for compartmentalization (Fig. 7-2).[14] The transverse mesocolon, the mesentery of the transverse colon, contributes the major barrier dividing the abdominal cavity into supra- and inframesocolic compartments. The root of the small bowel mesentery further divides the lower compartment into two unequal inframesocolic spaces. Communication between supra- and inframesocolic spaces occurs via the paracolic gutters. The right paracolic gutter is continuous with the right subhepatic space; its posterior extension, the hepatorenal fossa (Morrison's pouch) (Fig. 7-3); and the right subphrenic space. The falciform ligament separates the right and left subphrenic and subhepatic spaces. The phrenicocolic ligament fixes the splenic flexure of the colon to the left diaphragm, thus

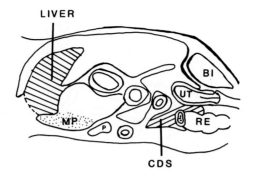

Figure 7-3 Longitudinal section in the midline demonstrating the potential peritoneal spaces and the areas in which fluid tends to collect. MP = Morrison's pouch; CDS = cul-de-sac; UT = uterus; Bl = bladder; RE = rectum; P = pancreas.

partially obstructing communication between the left paracolic gutter and the left perisplenic space. While both inframesocolic spaces communicate with the pelvis, the left is more anatomically continuous with the pelvic cavity than is the right. In general, intraperitoneal spread occurs more commonly on the right than on the left side. It is important to remember, though, that while the above routes of spread are most common, the reflections and attachments are not always complete, so that abnormalities may occasionally extend into unexpected areas.

The lesser omentum is an area between the lesser curvature of the stomach and proximal duodenum and the visceral surface of the liver. There is a potential space between the lesser omentum, stomach, duodenum, and the peritoneal surface covering the pancreas that is referred to as the *omental bursa* or *lesser sac* (Fig. 7-2). The major entrance to this sac is via the small epiploic foramen in the right upper quadrant within the free edge of the hepatoduodenal ligament. Although a possible site of fluid collection, spread of fluid from without rarely occurs via the small epiploic foramen, and fluid primarily collects in the lesser sac due to direct involvement either by a penetrating gastric ulcer or, more commonly, a pancreatic pseudocyst. Occasionally, fluid collections in the lesser sac may result from gastric or gallbladder surgery.

In the pelvis, the peritoneum is reflected over the fundus of the bladder, the anterior and posterior surface of the uterus in women, and over the superior portion of the rectum (Fig. 7-3). In men there is a single potential space for fluid collection, while in women there are two: the anterior cul-de-sac between the bladder and uterus and the posterior cul-de-sac (pouch of Douglas) between the uterus and the rectum. When the patient is supine, the most dependent portions of the abdomen are the pelvis, the hepatorenal recesses, and the paracolic gutters. While fluid may spread through the peritoneum via the described pathways, it commonly gravitates to these particular sites (Fig. 7-3).

Retroperitoneum

Lying on the muscles of the posterior abdominal wall and covered only on their anterior surface by the parietal peritoneum are the retroperitoneal structures:

the duodenum, the abdominal vessels, the pancreas, the kidneys and adrenal glands. Fluid may track in any direction in the retroperitoneum and may extend across the midline. The single most effective boundary to the spread of fluid in the retroperitoneum is the renal (Gerota's) fascia, a loose condensation of connective tissue that surrounds the kidney and adrenal gland and separates the perirenal from the pararenal spaces. This fascia effectively prevents the ingress and egress of fluid from the perirenal space. However, while the density of connective tissue is sufficiently loose to allow fluid within the perirenal space to expand this area, even from diaphragm to pelvic brim, it usually prevents fluid from crossing the midline.

Thus, the extraperitoneal region has been described as being clearly demarcated into three spaces:[15,16] (a) The anterior pararenal space, lying between the posterior parietal peritoneum and the anterior renal fascia and containing the pancreas and the retroperitoneal parts of the alimentary tract. (b) The perirenal space lying within the confines of the anterior and posterior renal fascia. (c) The posterior pararenal space lying between the posterior renal fascia and the transversalis fascia and containing no organs. Computed tomography is capable of demonstrating the three distinct anatomically defined extraperitoneal compartments,[17] but ultrasound can only infer the position of a fluid collection by the relative displacement of retroperitoneal organs.

TECHNIQUE

While the general principles of ultrasound technique have been described in previous chapters, when a fluid collection is suspected, the examination of the abdomen requires meticulous attention to technique but with a flexible approach. Although the examination may be performed with static B-mode equipment, the need for multiple scan planes and various patient positions means that high-resolution real-time equipment is ideally suited for the purpose. Not only can the patient be more quickly and more adequately examined in the ultrasound facility, but the mobility of the real-time units also allows examination of the seriously ill patient without the need for transportation to the ultrasound department.

Patient preparation is kept to a minimum. Although an overnight fast is desirable to reduce the amount of abdominal bowel gas, many examinations are performed as a matter of some urgency and thus must be done without preparation. However, many of the patients are already on a very restricted diet, which tends to reduce the problem of bowel gas. Scanning following recent surgery, nevertheless, is complicated by the presence of the recent wound, surgical dressings, and drainage tubes. Examination in these situations requires inventiveness on the part of the examiner, using oblique scan planes, angling the transducer toward the area of interest from a remote skin surface, and making various changes in patient position. It is important to remove as many of the dressings as is possible without compromising the sterility of any open wound. Using real time, particularly a sector scanner, allows the necessary versatile approach in such a patient.

Sufficient power or gain should be used to ensure that there is penetration of the sound beam to the retroperitoneum, so as not to confuse relatively echo-poor masses, such as lymphoma, with collections of fluid. However, it is also important to maintain any adjacent structures known to be fluid-containing, such as the bladder or the gallbladder, as echo-free.[18] This requires appropriate adjustment of the time-compensated gain curve and proper selection of the transducer to ensure that the zone of maximum focus is within the area of interest. Then, whenever an abnormality appears cystic at low to moderate power or gain settings, the power or gain should be increased, while still maintaining no echoes within a known echo-free structure, to determine if the mass is truly cystic or if it has low-level echoes (Fig. 7.4).

Since fluid tends to collect in certain predetermined sites, the examination of the abdomen by ultrasound is directed toward these specific sites, unless there are features that localize the fluid collection more accurately before the performance of the examination. The attention of the ultrasonographer is, therefore, concentrated on the right subphrenic and subhepatic spaces, the left perihepatic and perisplenic spaces, the paracolic gutters, and the pelvis. When examining the right subhepatic and subphrenic spaces, the patient is examined in the supine, prone, and left lateral decubitus positions. Similarly, the prone and the right lateral decubitus positions are used for examination of the perisplenic space.[18] It is frequently necessary to use the intercostal spaces to visualize both right and left upper quadrants. The paracolic gutters are probably best examined from an anterior and lateral approach while the patient is lying supine. Both supine and oblique positions are used in the examination of the pelvis, using the filled or partially filled urinary bladder as an acoustic window to the pelvic structures. Those parts of the peritoneum occupied by small bowel are exceedingly difficult to visualize by ultrasound, and it is fortunate that it is uncommon for fluid collections to occur in these locations.[19]

A similar flexible attitude is required in the examination of the retroperitoneum. The high retroperitoneum is usually examined with the patient supine, although further information can be obtained with the patient erect, both before and after filling the stomach with fluid to provide an acoustic window. The right peri- and pararenal spaces may be examined in the supine, decubitus, and prone positions; the left peri- and pararenal spaces may be examined in the decubitus and prone position.

The use of varied positions for the examination of the abdomen serves to define not only the best approach for accurate delineation of the fluid collection, but also to establish whether the fluid collection is free, contained in bowel, or loculated. Performing the examination in more than one position also helps minimize artifact-related errors.

In those patients with suspected abdominal abscesses and particularly those with open abdominal wounds, care must be taken to avoid contamination of the machine and personnel, with resultant cross-infection. It is therefore suggested that whenever possible patients with suspected abscesses should be scanned at the end of an examination session so that adequate cleansing of the equipment can be performed without disrupting workload. Both the transducer and the machine controls should be cleaned with an appropriate disinfectant after these studies, and the operator's hands should be thoroughly washed. In certain circumstances, a "dirty" and "clean" operator are required to avoid contamination of the equipment.

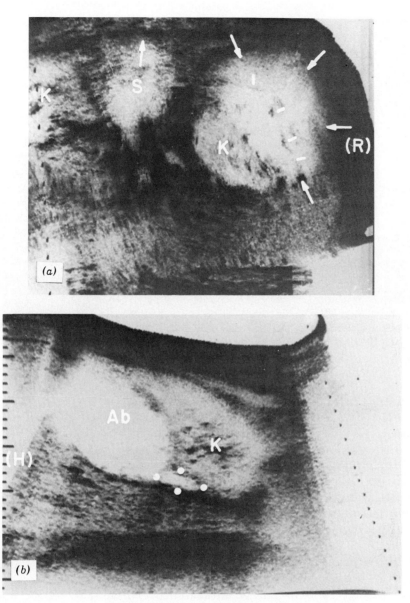

Figure 7-4 Right renal abscess. (*a*) Prone transverse scan of the right renal area demonstrating a subcapsular collection of pus that distorts the renal outline and stretches the renal capsule (short lines). In addition, there is a perirenal collection (arrows) that displaces the kidney anteriorly and medially. It is interesting to note that the perirenal collection contains more echoes than the subcapsular collection, and yet both were abscesses. (*b*) Longitudinal prone scan at low-power settings showing a subcapsular echo-free abscess (Ab). Note the small perirenal component, denoted by dots. (*c*) Longitudinal scan of part *b* at higher power settings demonstrating the echogenic content of the subcapsular abscess (Ab). (H) = toward patient's head; (R) = toward patient's right side.

247

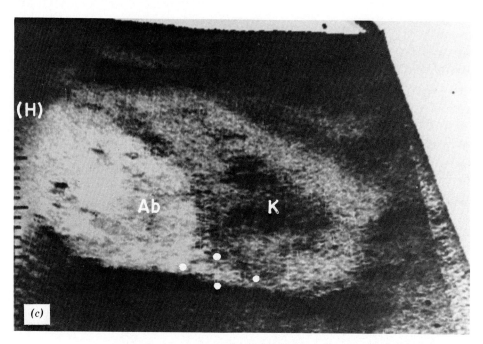

Figure 7-4 (*continued*)

DETERMINATION OF SITE OF FLUID COLLECTION

Although the ideal endpoint of any imaging procedure is the exact diagnosis of a lesion, simple detection and localization of a fluid collection provides important information. Determination of the site and volume of a fluid collection helps in the choice of appropriate treatment, be it "wait and see," percutaneous drainage, or surgical intervention.

Fluid may collect subcutaneously, within the muscles, between the muscle layers, or between muscles and peritoneal surfaces (Fig. 7-5). The fluid may be intraperitoneal or extraperitoneal, generalized or loculated. If related to a solid viscus, recognition of the location of the thin, brightly echogenic capsule of that organ becomes important in determining whether the fluid is located in an extracapsular, subcapsular, or intraparenchymal site (Fig. 7-4. See also Fig. 7-16).

DIFFERENTIATION AMONG TYPES OF FLUID

The typical echo characteristics of a fluid collection have been described as an anechoic space, sharply marginated with a clearly defined back wall and good through transmission of sound (Fig. 7-6).[18,20] Similarly, it has been suggested that different types of fluid can be distinguished on the basis of their shape, margination, and the echo characteristics of the fluid itself.[21,22] However, the nature and echo characteristics of abdominal fluid are extremely varied so that

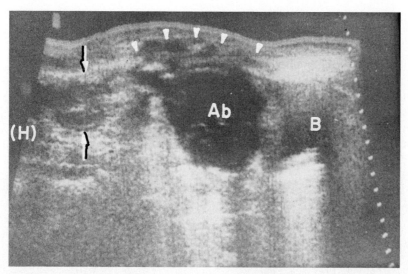

Figure 7-5 Pelvic abscess. Coronal scan in left lateral decubitus position showing a well-defined, hypoechoic collection (Ab) just cephalad to the bladder (B) representing a postoperative abscess. The arrows outline the "target" appearance of adjacent thickened bowel wall, and the arrowheads indicate extension of the abscess into the tissue planes of the anterior abdominal wall. (H) = toward patient's head.

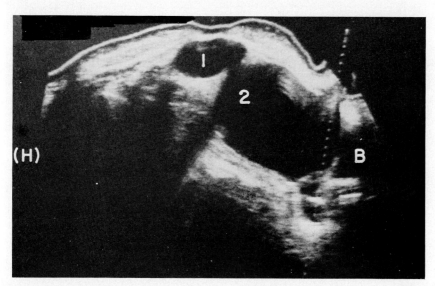

Figure 7-6 Longitudinal scan in a patient with loculated bilomas (1 and 2) in the lower abdomen and pelvis demonstrating the typical ultrasound appearance of a cystic fluid collection, a well-defined anechoic space except for anterior reverberation artifact, a clearly defined back wall and posterior acoustic accentuation. B = bladder; (H) = toward patient's head. (From Zegel HG et al: Ultrasonic characteristics of bilomas. *Clin Ultrasound* 9:21–24, 1981)

collections of blood, pus, urine, lymph, transudate, bile, etc. may have similar echo patterns, shape, and contour.[20,23]

The typical abscess is described as an ellipsoidal structure, with finely irregular walls containing either no echoes or weakly echoing material evenly dispersed through the cavity (Fig. 7-4b and c). Some abscesses, however, have a surrounding halo of increased echoes, whereas others are surrounded by a ring of tissue that is almost anechoic. In 20 percent of cases, abscess walls tend to lack the sharpness of the walls of such fluid-containing organs as the urinary bladder and such fluid collections as lymphoceles, hematomas, and urinomas (Figs. 7-

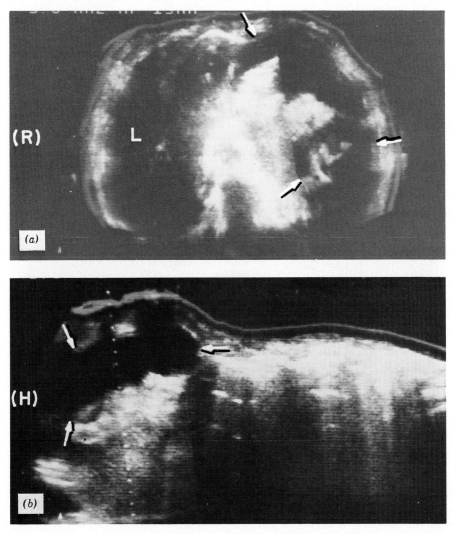

Figure 7-7 Abscess in left upper quadrant. (a) The transverse, and (b) the longitudinal sections of the left upper quadrant demonstrating areas (arrows) that are completely anechoic and others that contain coarse echogenic debris. Note the indistinctness of the boundaries. (H) = toward patient's head; (R) = toward patient's right side.

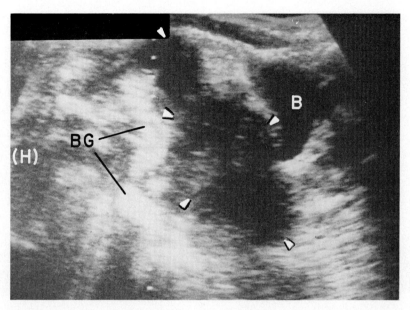

Figure 7-8 Pelvic (appendiceal) abscess. Longitudinal scan to the right of midline, demonstrating an irregular anechoic area (arrowheads) with indistinct boundaries just cephalad to the bladder (B). The brightly echogenic areas posterior and cephalad to the abscess collection represent bowel gas (BG), but could on occasion be mistaken for areas of gas within an abscess. (H) = toward patient's head.

5, 7-7, and 7-8).[20] Occasionally, fluid-fluid levels or bright reflectors may be identified, presumably as a result of the settling of debris or gas respectively (Fig. 7-9).[20,24]

The appearance of hematomas is dependent on the age of the lesion and the nature of the clotting process. It has been demonstrated in vitro that fresh, unclotted or homogeneously clotted blood has no internal echoes. With fragmentation of the clot, internal echoes are demonstrated.[25] Doust et al. stated that if hematomas are examined within 24 hours of their occurrence, they will be anechoic, presumably due either to absence of clot formation or because clot fragmentation has not yet occurred.[22] By contrast, Fleischer claimed that echoes occur much earlier in the natural history of a hematoma and may be demonstrated within a few hours of occurrence.[26]

In all probability the speed of clotting depends on many factors, including the patient's coagulation status, the site of the hematoma, and its relationship to other organs. After 24 hours, hematomas tend to adopt an ellipsoidal shape, usually demonstrating either a coarsely echogenic mass or one containing brightly echo-producing debris, presumably the consequence of aggregates of blood clot (Figs. 7-10, 7-11a and b). This appearance remains largely unchanged for about 30 days, after which the echogenic contents gradually decrease, becoming a chronic seroma (cystic-type collection) (Figs. 7-11c and d).[27] Alternatively, the hematoma may become organized and subsequently may even partly calcify at this stage yielding a solid-type pattern.

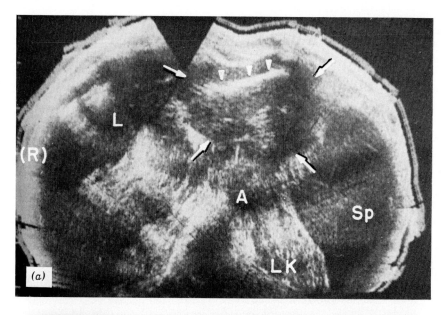

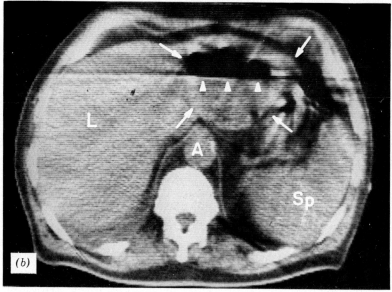

Figure 7-9 Hepatic abscess. (*a*) The transverse ultrasound section of the upper abdomen, and (*b*) the CT scan at the same level in a patient with an abscess in the left lobe of the liver (arrows). The arrowheads point to gas within the abscess, demonstrated on ultrasound as a hyperechoic band and on CT as an area of low attenuation. L = liver; A = aorta; SP = spleen; LK = left kidney. (From Kurtz AB et al: Ultrasound and computed tomography of the liver. *CRC Crit Rev Diagn Imaging* in press)

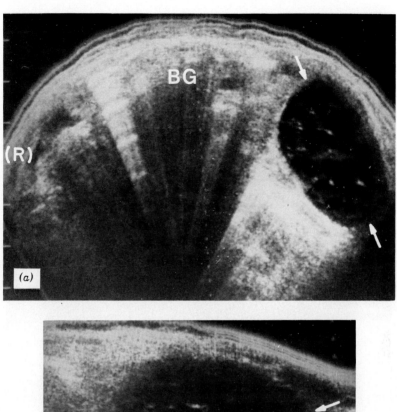

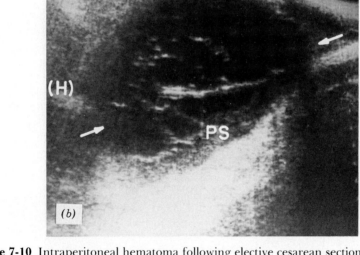

Figure 7-10 Intraperitoneal hematoma following elective cesarean section 3 days earlier (*a*) The transverse scan 10 cm below the xyphoid, and (*b*) the longitudinal scan approximately 7 cm to the left of midline. A well-defined mass, indicated by the arrows, is demonstrated in the left side of the abdomen anterior to the psoas muscle (PS). There are multiple coarse echoes and septations within the mass, presumably representing aggregates of blood clot. In the central abdomen, the "dirty" shadowing of bowel gas (BG) is demonstrated. (R) = toward patient's right side; (H) = toward patient's head.

253

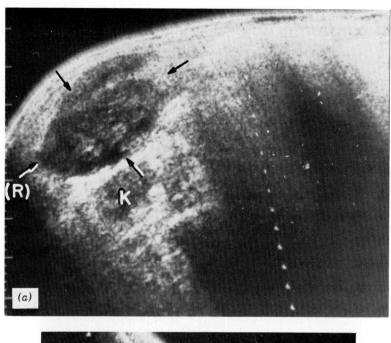

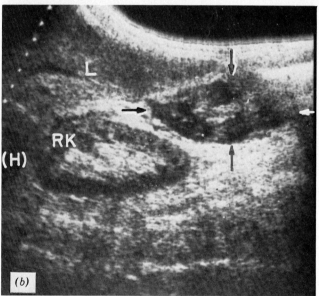

Figure 7-11 Intraabdominal hematoma. (*a*) The transverse, and (*b*) the longitudinal ultrasound images of a hematoma (arrows) 36 hours after an attempted right renal biopsy. Note the coarse hyperechoic debris due to clot aggregates. (*c*) The transverse and (*d*) the longitudinal ultrasound images in the same patient at 5 days, now demonstrating an enlarged, totally anechoic hematoma (arrows). While this is an unusual time course for the progression of a hematoma's echo characteristics, the change from echogenic to echo-free is typical. RK = right kidney; L = liver; (R) = toward patient's right side; (H) = toward patient's head.

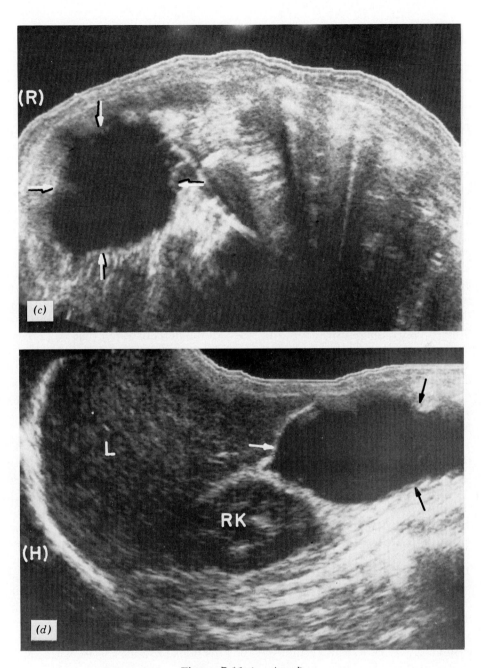

Figure 7-11 (*continued*)

Lymphoceles, which arise when a lymphatic trunk is severed or occluded, usually contain no echogenic debris, but are commonly loculated by one or more septa (Fig. 7-12). Urinomas are usually anechoic without septa or debris although we have encountered a case where fine septations were prominent (Fig. 7-13).

Classification of fluid collections into specific etiologies on the basis of echo pattern is not, however, without its disadvantages. In Doust's series, 30 percent of the abscesses were described as atypical, containing either coarse echoes, large amounts of debris, or septa.[21] Moreover, 25 percent of those considered as typical abscesses were totally anechoic and, therefore, could not be distinguished from cysts, bilomas, urinomas, etc. clearly on the basis of echo characteristics (Fig. 7-6).[18] Furthermore, one of the important complications of a hematoma and infrequently of a lymphocele is the development of infection with subsequent conversion into an abscess (Fig. 7-12a), which is unfortunately often not accompanied by any change in echo characteristics.

The appearance of gas-containing abscesses has been described.[28,29] As might be expected, when abscesses contain either small microbubbles or larger collections of gas, hyperechoic areas appear within the masses, with or without distal acoustic shadowing (Fig. 7-9). Plain film findings in 82 patients with right upper quadrant abscesses from the Mayo Clinic demonstrated that 70 percent had radiographically demonstrable gas within the abscesses.[1] From this study, an examiner could expect to demonstrate hyperechoic masses on ultrasound in the majority of right upper quadrant abscesses. While the Mayo Clinic series may represent an unusual selection of patients, it is also possible that our apparently low detection rate of gas-containing abscesses may be related to misinterpretation of the echoes as adjacent bowel gas.

More recently, in vitro work has demonstrated that many different types of fluid are anechoic, but the amount of sound through transmission varies with the nature of the fluid.[30] For example, packed red cells, hemolysate, whole blood, and serum were shown to be entirely anechoic, but the through transmission of serum and hemolysate was much more marked than whole blood, and more marked still than packed red cells. However, at present, methods of measuring sound through transmission in vivo are largely subjective.

Clearly, the echo patterns of fluid collections are not always characteristic. Therefore, the diagnosis of intraabdominal fluid collections cannot depend solely on the shape and echo characteristics of the fluid. Rather, the diagnosis must rely on careful attention to clinical history, physical examination, (including that available to the ultrasonographer at the time of the examination), as well as observation of the site, shape, margination, and echo characteristics of the lesion (Fig. 7-14). Rarely, certain specific infections produce specific ultrasound characteristics. Hydatid disease, more properly considered an infestation, usually demonstrates a characteristic pattern of multiple cysts of varying size that may be arranged in a spoke-wheel or a more disordered "soap bubble" pattern (Fig. 7-15).[31] Similarly, certain clinical presentations are characteristic, and, in these situations, ultrasound serves to confirm the diagnosis, to localize and determine the extent of the lesion, and to determine whether the fluid is free or loculated.

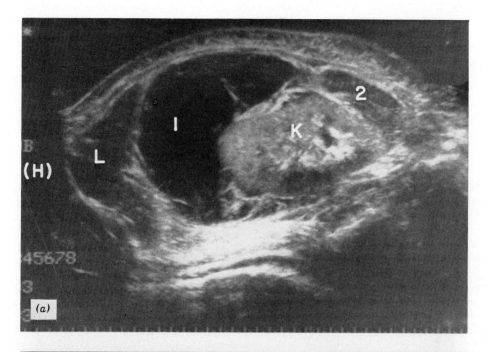

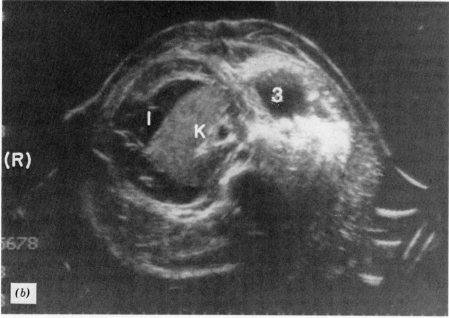

Figure 7-12 Lymphoceles following renal transplantation. (*a*) The longitudinal scan of the right lower quadrant, and (*b*) the transverse scan of the pelviabdominal region. A multiloculated fluid-containing area (labeled 1, 2 and 3) is seen to surround the transplanted kidney (K). Collections 1 and 3 are typically anechoic, whereas 2 is hyperechoic. At aspiration, collection 2 was an infected lymphocele. (H) = toward patient's head; (R) toward patient's right side.

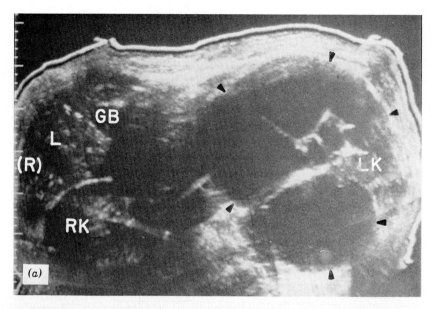

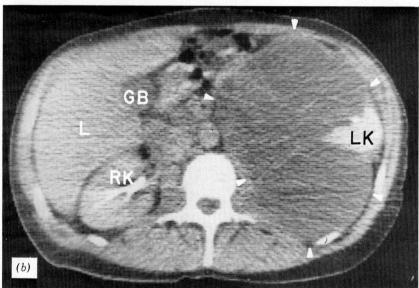

Figure 7-13 Urinoma surrounding left kidney secondary to obstruction. (*a*) The ultrasound transverse section of the upper abdomen, and (*b*) the CT section at the same level, showing a large septated cystic mass in the left side of the abdomen in a patient with acute obstructive uropathy. The presence of septations demonstrated both on ultrasound and CT are unusual for a urinoma. LK = left kidney; RK = right kidney; GB = gall bladder; L = liver; (R) = toward patient's right side.

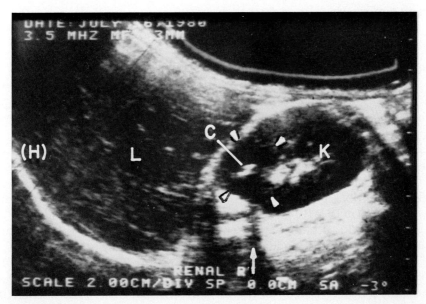

Figure 7-14 Tuberculous renal abscess. Longitudinal scan 5 cm to the right of midline showing a relatively anechoic space (arrowheads) at the upper pole of the right kidney (K) that demonstrates good through-transmission of sound. Within this anechoic space is a brightly hyperechoic area (C) representing calcium with distal acoustic shadow (arrows). L = liver; (H) = toward patient's head.

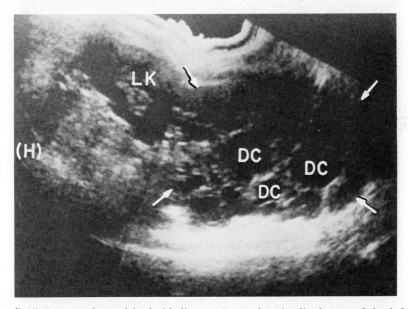

Figure 7-15 Retroperitoneal hydatid disease. Prone longitudinal scan of the left lower quadrant demonstrating a "soap bubble" pattern of multiple daughter cysts (DC) creating a larger multicystic mass (arrows) of hydatid disease just inferior to the left kidney (LK). (From Dr. Ruth Shilo, Municipal Hospital Ichilov, Tel Aviv, Israel.)

LOCULATED FLUID

Right Subphrenic Collection

Right subphrenic abscesses may be purely subphrenic or may be subphrenic and subhepatic, subphrenic and intrahepatic, or a combination of all three (Fig. 7-16). There are often localizing clinical signs as well as plain radiographic findings of an elevated right hemidiaphragm, pleural effusion, or extraintestinal gas in the right upper quadrant.[1,2,15,32–35] In addition, it is not infrequent for the diaphragm to be "fixed" by the inflammation and, therefore, not move on ultrasound examination despite deep inspiration and expiration. Careful attention must be paid to locating the strong curvilinear echo of the diaphragm and the rather less thick but also strong linear echo of the liver capsule in order to differentiate pleural effusion from subphrenic abscess and to identify the subcapsular or intrahepatic component (Figs. 7-16 and 7-17). For this purpose, the longitudinal scan is mandatory to identify clearly the relationship of the fluid collection to the diaphragm (Fig. 7-16).[36,37] If the abscess is purely subphrenic, it may be crescentic as it lies between the diaphragm and the dome of the liver. However, if the liver capsule is breached and there is an intrahepatic component, then the margins become much more ragged and less well defined. Certain organisms may, in fact, breach the diaphragm, thus producing an empyema and/or lung abscess (e.g. amebic abscess).

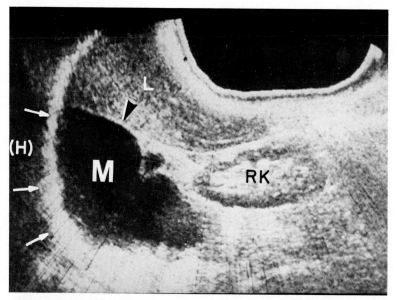

Figure 7-16 Right subphrenic abscess. Longitudinal scan to the right of midline demonstrating a space-occupying mass immediately inferior to the thick echo of the diaphragm (arrows) and posterior to the liver (L). Arrowhead denotes the thin hyperechoic liver capsule. The mass (M) is predominantly anechoic, but there is some hyperechoic debris in the dependent portion. Note that this abscess appears to be tracking posterior to the right kidney (RK). (H) = toward patient's head.

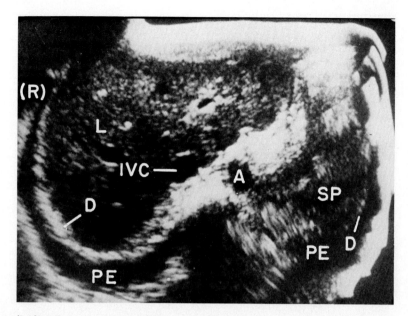

Figure 7-17 Bilateral pleural effusions. Transverse scan of the upper abdomen demonstrating pleural effusions (PE). The diaphragms (D) are identified as thick, curvilinear echoes, but the liver capsule cannot be separately identified. The pleural effusion extends to the spine and posterior to the crus of the diaphragm, thus allowing differentiation from ascites. Nevertheless, the diaphragms are more easily recognized on longitudinal scans. IVC = inferior vena cava; L = liver; SP = spleen; A = aorta; (R) = toward patient's right side.

Subhepatic abscesses may occur either in isolation or in association with subphrenic abscesses. Here the abscess is more commonly ellipsoid and displaces adjacent organs. It must be differentiated from a distended gallbladder, which may result from a prolonged fast.[38] This is most significant in the postoperative patient who has often been subjected to prolonged parenteral fluid therapy.

Left Perisplenic Fluid Collection

The left upper quadrant is more difficult to examine with ultrasound, though an adequate view of the left subphrenic region can usually be achieved with the patient in the right lateral decubitus position, scanning in the intercostal spaces (Fig. 7-18). Since sound may be attenuated either generally or focally by the ribs, care must be taken to ensure that a hypoechoic spleen, or a relatively hypoechoic area within the spleen, caused by rib artifact is not confused with an abscess or other fluid collection. Following splenectomy, the stomach frequently is displaced into the splenic bed[39] and, in cases of suspected subphrenic fluid collection following splenectomy, care must be taken to identify the stomach by scanning the patient in various positions and by administrating fluid by mouth so as not to confuse the stomach with a subphrenic collection. Examination with real time during the swallowing of fluid is of particular value. The typical pattern of many small bright echoes derived from gas microbubbles

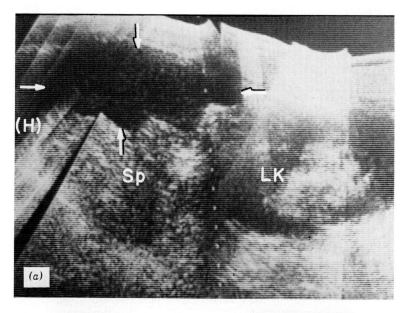

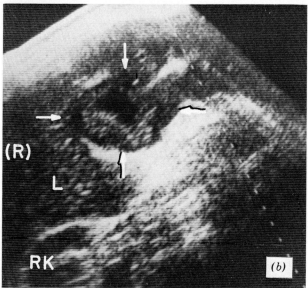

Figure 7-18 Left subphrenic abscess and intrahepatic abscess in a drug addict. (*a*) Coronal scan of the left upper quadrant demonstrating an irregular, relatively anechoic area (arrows) lateral to the spleen (Sp) and cephalad to the left kidney (LK). (*b*) Transverse scan of the liver (L) in the same patient demonstrating an additional intrahepatic solid mass with necrotic center (arrows). RK = right kidney; (R) = toward patient's right side; (H) = toward patient's head. (From Dr. Carl Rubin, Frankford Hospital, Philadelphia, Pennsylvania.)

262

as the fluid enters the stomach in turbulent fashion clearly separates the stomach from an abnormal collection.[40,41]

Fluid Collections in the MidAbdomen

Fluid collections in the paracolic gutters, peripheral in location, are usually more easily identified than those in the central abdomen. These paracolic collections may be loculated or free, intraperitoneal, or extraperitoneal (Fig. 7-10), and abscesses derived from large bowel are usually situated in the anterior pararenal space. In the central abdomen, the mixed ultrasound appearance of large and small bowel makes the diagnosis of an abdominal fluid collection most difficult. Bowel filled with gas may mimic a gas-containing abscess, while bowel filled with fluid may look like an uncomplicated abscess (Fig. 7-8). In these situations, real time is invaluable to assess the changing position, shape, and contents of bowel loops with peristalsis. Unfortunately, a paralytic ileus, not infrequently associated with the postoperative state and particularly with inflammatory lesions in close proximity to the bowel, for example, pancreatitis, may result in one or more stationary fluid-filled loops of bowel. Since there is no peristalsis in this situation, examination with real time does not solve the problem. Occasionally, a follow-up study after 24 hours demonstrates a change in appearances and allows differentiation of bowel, but, if not, other investigations including contrast radiography and computed tomography may be necessary.

Fluid Collections in the Pelvis

Pelvic abscesses may result from the spread of infection from elsewhere into this anatomic sump, from inflammatory processes involving the large and small bowel locally and, in women, from primary disease of the reproductive tract.[42] The ultrasound appearances of pelvic abscesses are similar to those of abscesses elsewhere (Figs. 7-5 and 7-8), but not infrequently demonstrate septations and multiple loculations. The echographic features are not specific, and in particular, it is difficult to differentiate pelvic abscesses from endometriosis and ectopic pregnancy. It may also be difficult to differentiate pelvic abscesses from hemorrhagic ovarian cysts as well as from ovarian cystadenomas and cystadenocarcinomas, unless normal ovaries can be separately identified. In these situations, the importance of clinical history, physical findings, and the results of other laboratory investigations such as the pregnancy test become of paramount importance.

Fluid Collections in the Renal Bed

The anatomy of the retroperitoneum has been described above. Fluid collections deriving from paraspinal musculature and the vertebrae may involve the posterior pararenal space and those from bowel the anterior pararenal space. Fluid collections of renal origin are usually confined to the perirenal space, but may also involve both the posterior and anterior pararenal spaces. However, Gerota's fascia provides an effective boundary to fluid communication between peri- and pararenal spaces so that both spaces are rarely jointly involved (Fig.

7-4). Ultrasound is not capable of resolving the tissue planes between these compartments, and CT is required if such resolution is deemed necessary.[17] However, certain inferences may be made about the location of the fluid by its relationship to the kidney and the nature of renal displacement. Thus, posterior pararenal collections tend to displace the kidney anteriorly; anterior pararenal collections produce renal compression and posterior displacement; perirenal collections tend to occupy more than one surface of the kidney (Fig. 7-4). Fluid collections may be of various origins so that, while abscesses occur as a result of primary renal infections, urinomas and lymphoceles may occur as a result of obstruction of ureter and lymphatics respectively, and hematoma as the result of trauma (Figs. 7-12, 7-13, and 7-14).

Transplanted Kidney

Fluid collections are a common complication of renal transplantation (Figs. 7-12 and 7-19). In a recent series, 51 percent of transplant recipients had abnormal fluid collections, and, of these, 18 patients required surgery.[43] The predominant fluid collections associated with renal transplantation are lymphoceles and abscesses, although urinomas and hematomas also occur. In the patient following renal transplantation, symptomatology may be confusing, at least in part due to immune suppression. It may, therefore, be important to diagnose the nature of the fluid in the absence of an appropriate history. It is clear from the foregoing discussion that no echo pattern is, in and of itself, specific for any fluid type. While septations are more common in lymphoceles and hematomas, they may also be seen in abscesses and, rarely, in urinomas (Figs. 7-10, 7-12, and 7-13). Since almost all the fluid collections in the series reported by Silver et al. contained echoes and since fluid-fluid levels were demonstrated even in urinomas, of greatest value in determining the type of abnormality imaged was the characteristic time course of these abnormalities.[43] Urinomas tended to occur earlier (mean 13 days), lymphoceles at an intermediate stage (mean 23 days), while abscesses and hematomas appeared progressively later (mean 39 and 53.5 days, respectively). However, since there is overlap, the exact diagnosis can only be achieved by percutaneous diagnostic aspiration of the fluid. This is generally a simple procedure in the transplanted kidney, since the renal transplant and the fluid collection are both superficially placed.

Ultrasound is invaluable in the evaluation of the renal transplant. Not only can the presence of fluid be detected, but also abnormalities of renal parenchyma can be shown. Early hydronephrosis can also be demonstrated, either as a complication of an obstructing fluid collection or secondary to ureteric anastomotic stenosis.

Fluid Collections Involving Muscles

Both hematomas and infections affecting muscles result initially in the generalized enlargement of the muscle. Subsequently, fluid-filled areas may develop due to either ischemic necrosis or focal abscess formation. The most commonly affected muscles are the iliopsoas and the rectus abdominis. Rectus sheath hematomas may be consequent on direct trauma, unaccustomed exercise, severe

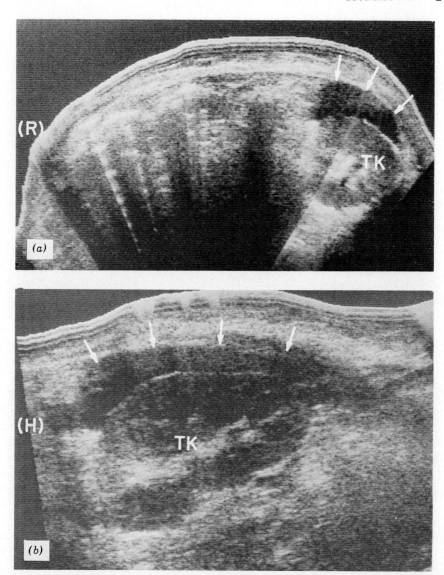

Figure 7-19 Transplanted kidney with anterior hematoma. (*a*) The transverse and (*b*) the longitudinal scan of the transplanted kidney (TK). There is an elliptical fluid collection anterior and lateral with internal echoes, outlined by arrows, found to be a hematoma on aspiration. (H) = toward patient's head; (R) = toward patient's right side.

coughing, stretching due to pregnancy, tumor, or bleeding diathesis.[44,45] Clinically, hernias and tumors, etc. have been confused with the diagnosis of rectus sheath hematomas, but, with ultrasound, it is generally not difficult to detect the asymmetric enlargement of one rectus sheath (Fig. 7-20). Enlargement of one or both psoas muscles may be the result of either infection or hemorrhage. In the past, psoas abscesses were primarily derived from infections of the spine,

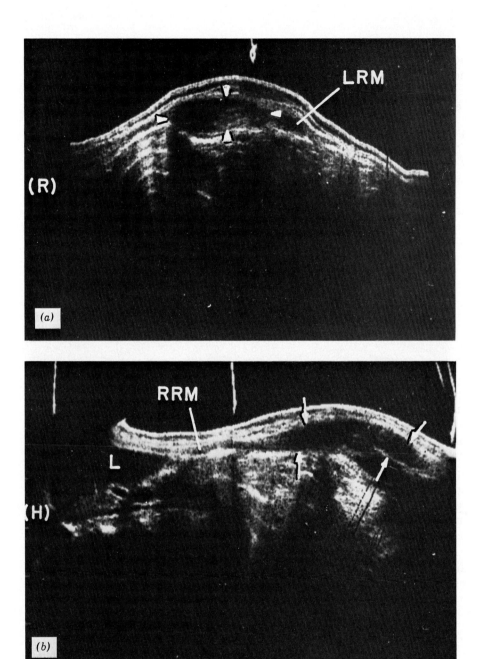

Figure 7-20 Rectus sheath hematoma, secondary to excessive exertion. (*a*) A transverse scan of the midabdomen, and (*b*) a longitudinal scan 2 cm to the right of the midline in a patient with a diffuse enlargement (arrows) of the distal aspect of the right rectus muscle (RRM). Note the normal left rectus muscle (LRM). (H) = toward patient's head; (R) = toward patient's right side.

266

but now are more commonly associated with focal infections, for example in the pararenal space.[46] Hematomas of the iliopsoas or iliacus muscles may be the result of direct trauma or derived from a bleeding diathesis.

Hemorrhage Associated with a Bleeding Diathesis

Spontaneous hemorrhage may occur within a muscle,[47,48] within the retroperitoneum,[48] within the mesentery,[49] or within the bowel wall.[50] The diagnosis of intraabdominal hemorrhage is vital to ensure the proper management of the patient. It is important, for instance, to differentiate a psoas or iliacus muscle hematoma from a hemarthrosis of the hip or knee joint, both of which may have similar symptomology (Fig. 7-21). Management of a hemarthrosis requires much earlier mobilization of the patient than does a muscle hematoma. In all cases of intraabdominal hemorrhage, achieving a prompt diagnosis allows early administration of the appropriate clotting factors.

Hemorrhage Associated with Abdominal Trauma

Blunt or penetrating injury to the abdomen may cause damage to a solid viscus, to the spine, the retroperitoneum, the bowel, the vessels, or the pelvic viscera. In the evaluation of penetrating injuries, iatrogenic trauma should be considered, and, in this connection, the radiologist is acutely aware of the complications of such percutaneous procedures as translumbar aortography. The extent of injury in all cases of trauma is difficult to diagnose clinically, and, although conventional and contrast radiography, radionuclide scanning, and angiography have played, and continue to play, a role in management, the newer sectional imaging modalities provide further information not previously available. Several workers have stressed the advantage of computed tomography because of superior anatomic detail and the ability to image all intraabdominal organs simultaneously.[51,52] However, ultrasound has also been found to be useful in the diagnosis of renal trauma, including renal fracture and associated hematomas,[53] mesenteric hemorrhage,[54] high retroperitoneal trauma including pancreatic hematomas,[55] and splenic or perisplenic trauma (Fig. 7-22).[56,57]

The choice of imaging modality depends on many factors, including availability of instrumentation and local expertise. Perhaps the most important factor, however, is the clinical impression. Penetrating injuries are correctly managed by immediate laparotomy because of the impending risk of bowel perforation or vascular damage. Similarly, situations where the trauma has resulted in severe blood loss and where the patient is admitted to the hospital in shock demand immediate intervention. Real-time ultrasound evaluation in the emergency room or in the operating room immediately before surgery may help in planning the operative approach.

Both ultrasound and CT probably find most use in the examination of blunt trauma. Here the extent of injury may be assessed, the size and location of associated fluid collection may be determined, and complications such as hydronephrosis, biliary obstruction and pancreatitis may be detected early (Fig. 7-23). Follow-up examination by either ultrasound or computed tomography provides assurance of adequate and complete resolution of the effects of trauma if no intervention is contemplated.

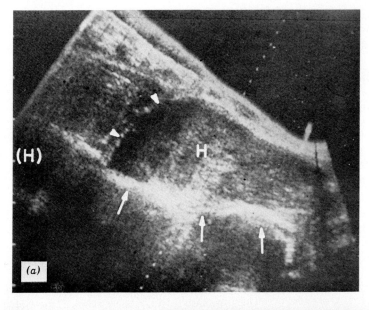

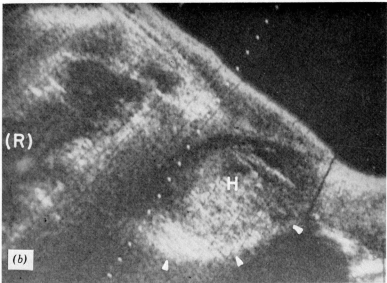

Figure 7-21 Left iliacus muscle hematoma in a patient with hemophilia. (*a*) A longitudinal and (*b*) a transverse scan of left lower quadrant showing diffuse hyperechoic enlargement of the iliacus muscle bounded cephalad by its insertion into the iliac crest (arrowheads) and posteriorly by the iliac bone (arrows). The appearance of the hematoma (H) is indistinguishable from muscle enlargement and echogenicity when secondary to an abscess or tumor. (H) = toward patient's head; (R) = toward patient's right side.

268

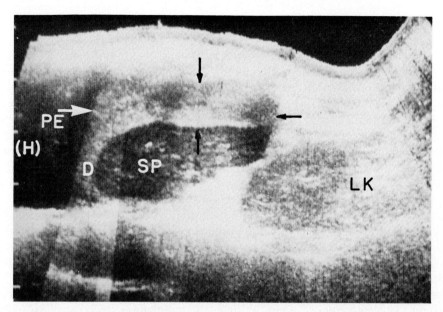

Figure 7-22 Perisplenic hematoma, secondary to bleed following partial gastrectomy. Coronal scan of the left upper quadrant demonstrating a large ellipsoidal hyperechoic fluid collection (arrows) lateral to the spleen (SP), inferior to the diaphragm (D), and cephalad to the left kidney (LK). There is a coincident left pleural effusion (PE). (H) = toward patient' head.

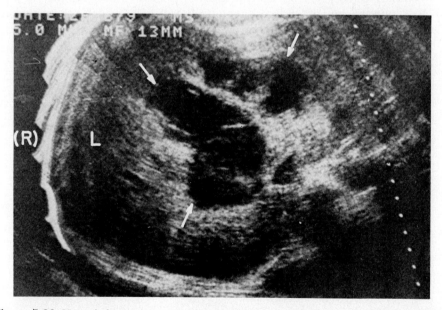

Figure 7-23 Hepatic hematoma. Transverse scan of the liver in a patient following blunt abdominal trauma. The relatively hypoechoic collections are irregularly angulated in shape (arrows) hepatic lacerations. L = liver; (R) = toward patient's right side. (From Kurtz AB et al: Ultrasound and computed tomography of the liver. *CRC Crit Rev Diagn Imaging* in press.)

FREE INTRAPERITONEAL FLUID

The detection of ascites and its differentiation from other forms of intraabdominal fluid collections is usually not difficult.[58,59] Typically, ascites is anechoic is freely mobile within the peritoneal cavity, does not displace adjacent organs but rather insinuates itself between them, and allows bowel loops to float freely when they contain gas or to sink when they contain fluid (Fig. 7-24).[60] Ascitic fluid usually collects in the most dependent portions of the abdominal cavity. When the patient is lying supine, these will, of course, be the pelvis, hepatorenal fossa, and paracolic gutters. Experimentally, very small amounts of fluid (less than 100 cc) can be detected by ultrasound.[61] In vivo, when the person is prone in the hand/knee position, fluid collects against the anterior abdominal wall, and detection of small amounts of fluid is facilitated. When very small amounts of peritoneal fluid are present, fluid collections will occasionally not be seen in the typical positions. Instead, the fluid collects in a thin film around solid intraperitoneal structures such as the liver, presumably secondary to a capillary form of flow such as a meniscus (Fig. 7-25). When ascites is consequent on hypoalbuminemia, it may be reflected by thickening of the gallbladder wall[62] with an associated halo of ascitic fluid in the gallbladder bed (Fig. 7-26). With larger amounts of fluid, the ascites tends to gravitate toward the flanks and pelvis, and the bowel tends to aggregate in the middle of the abdomen (Figs. 7-27 and 7-28a). This is in contradistinction to certain very large, predominantly cystic tumors that occupy a large part of the abdomen, which may be confused with clinically tense ascites. When a mass is present, however, the bowel is displaced upward and laterally so that no bowel loops can be demonstrated floating within the fluid-containing mass (Figs. 7-28b, 7-29, and 7-30).[63]

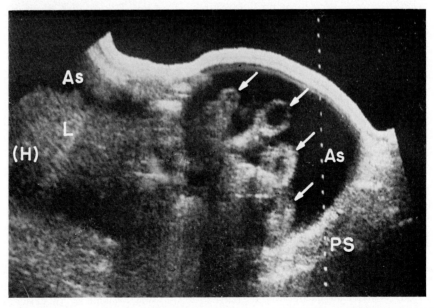

Figure 7-24 Transudative ascites. Longitudinal scan to the right of midline in a patient with ascites (As), within which bowel loops (arrows) float freely in the pelvis anterior to the psoas muscle (PS). L = liver; (H) = toward patient's head.

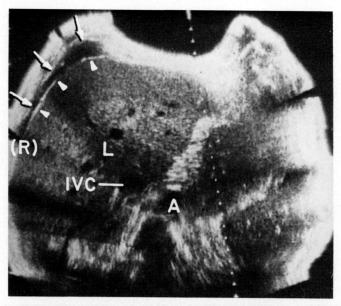

Figure 7-25 Transudative ascites. Transverse scan of the upper abdomen in a patient with chronic liver disease and consequent ascites. There is a small collection of fluid between the anterior abdominal wall (arrows) and the liver capsule (arrowheads). This fluid was initially in this single location without fluid in the flanks or in Morrison's pouch. It was not loculated, as the patient later developed widespread, freely communicating ascites. L = liver; IVC = inferior vena cava; A = aorta; (R) = toward right side of patient.

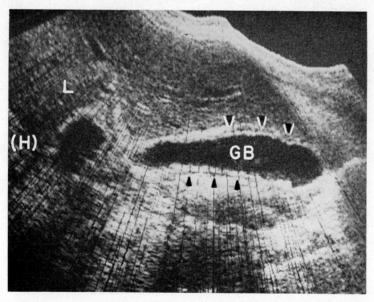

Figure 7-26 Ascites. Longitudinal scan of the gallbladder (GB) in a patient with early ascites showing a small amount of fluid in the gallbladder bed (arrowheads). This ultrasound picture is difficult to differentiate from acute cholecystitis. L = liver; (H) = toward patient's head.

271

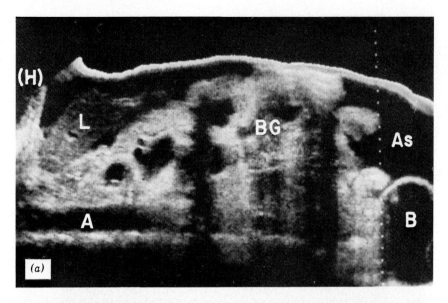

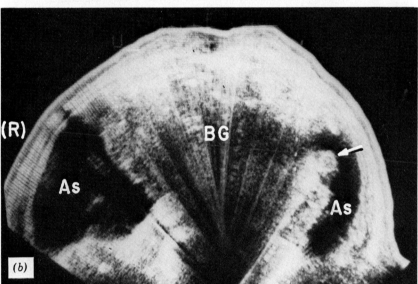

Figure 7-27 Extensive transudative ascites. (*a*) Longitudinal midline scan showing loops of gas-filled bowel (BG) floating anteriorly and freely in the ascitic fluid (As). B = partial distended urinary bladder; L = liver; A = aorta; (H) = toward patient's head. (*b*) Transverse scan of the lower abdomen in a different patient demonstrating loops of gas-filled bowel (BG) floating anteriorly and midline in ascites (As). Arrow denotes a partially collapsed loop of bowel. (R) = toward patient's right side.

Transudative ascites invariably demonstrates findings typical of anechoic fluid evenly dispersed throughout the abdomen. In a recent series, however, exudative ascites, either malignant or infected, demonstrated atypical findings in nearly 70 percent of cases.[64] These findings enabled the diagnosis of exudative ascites and included hyperechoic debris within the ascitic fluid, septations, matted bowel loops, loculation of the fluid (Fig. 7-31), as well as hepatic metastases associated with malignant ascites. Septations and debris appeared to be more common in infective ascites,[64,65] although both of these features have been demonstrated in malignant ascites.[64] Occasionally, the demonstration of peritoneal implants as solid rounded plaques on the parietal peritoneum and

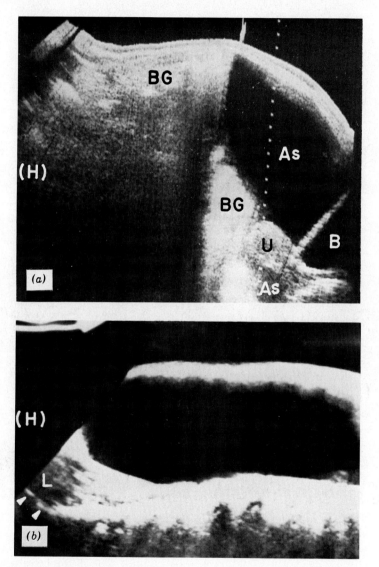

Figure 7-28 A comparison of tense ascites to a large ovarian cyst. (*a*) Longitudinal midline scan of a patient with tense ascites (As). The fluid is large in amount, collecting in the lower abdomen and pelvis, posterior to the uterus (U) in the cul-de-sac. Most of the bowel has been displaced to the midline by the fluid. BG = bowel gas; B = bladder. (*b*) Longitudinal scan in the midline of a patient with a large paraovarian cyst. The fluid-containing cyst has displaced bowel away from the midline and has compressed the liver (L). The degree of organ displacement by the cystic structure is evidenced by the high position of the diaphragm (arrowheads). (H) = toward patient's head.

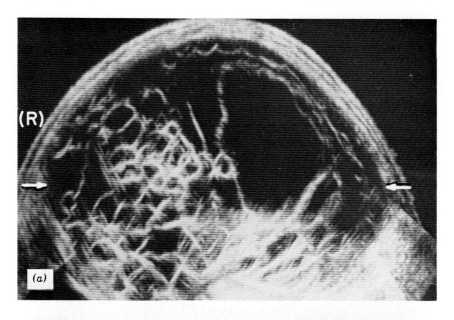

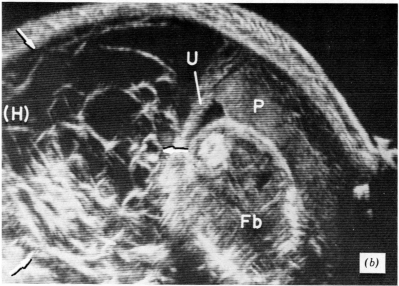

Figure 7-29 Intrauterine pregnancy with a cystadenoma. (*a*) The transverse and (*b*) the longitudinal scans in a patient with a 28-week pregnancy coexistent with a large ovarian cystadenoma (arrows). The multiple loculations and extent of this tumor could be confused with ascites, but it would have to be assumed that all the bowel loops were fluid-containing, an unlikely possibility. U = uterus; P = placenta; Fb = fetal body; (R) = toward patient's right side; (H) = toward patient's head.

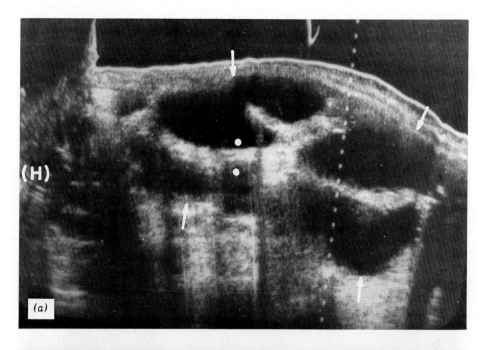

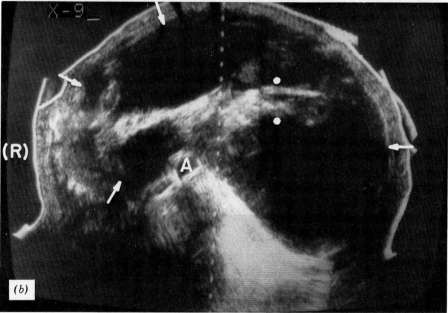

Figure 7-30 Pseudomyxoma peritonei. (*a*) Longitudinal and (*b*) transverse scan in a patient with multiple thick septations (dots) dividing the irregular loculations (arrows). A = aorta; (R) = toward patient's right side; (H) = toward patient's head.

the mesentery has permitted the diagnosis of malignancy (Fig. 7-32). In a series of 14 patients with exudative ascites, these features allowed the differentiation from transudative ascites in all four cases of the infected ascites but in only six of 10 cases with malignant ascites.[64] Therefore, while any abnormality within the ascites allows the diagnosis of an exudate, the imaging of anechoic,

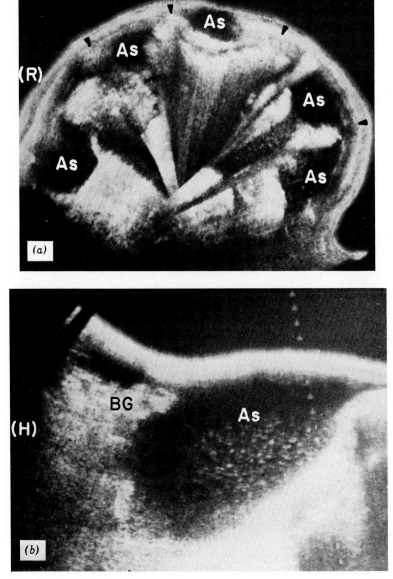

Figure 7-31 Exudative (malignant) ascites. (*a*) Transverse scan in the midabdomen of a patient with malignant ascites (As) demonstrating the multiple loculations of fluid and adherence of bowel loops (arrowheads). (*b*) Longitudinal scan in the same patient to the right of midline demonstrating hyperechoic debris within the ascites (As). BG = bowel gas; (H) = toward patient's head; (R) = toward patient's right side.

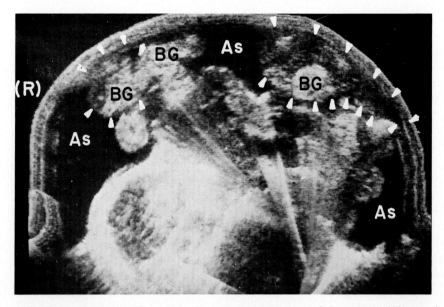

Figure 7-32 Exudative (malignant) ascites. Transverse scan of the upper abdomen in a patient with malignant ascites (As) demonstrating gas-filled bowel (BG) adherent to the anterior abdominal wall. In addition, there are mass lesions (arrowheads) along the parietal peritoneum, indicative of peritoneal metastatic implants. (R) = toward patient's right side.

nonseptated, nonloculated fluid does not exclude the diagnosis of malignancy. Infrequently, there may be a difficulty with diagnosis when transudative ascites is associated with preexisting bowel adhesions. In addition, problems may occur in the differentiation of complicated ascites from the ill-understood entity pseudomyxoma peritonei (Fig. 7-30). This unusual, disseminated intraabdominal neoplasm produces a mucinous ascites and intraperitoneal tumor deposits. Ultrasound features include solid intraperitoneal masses,[66] a peripheral band of fluid with low-level echoes displacing bowel posteriorly,[67] the presence of septations in the fluid, and scalloping of the surface of the liver.[68] Of all these features, liver scalloping, if present, appears to be pathognomonic.

FLUID ASPIRATION AND DRAINAGE

Ultrasound can provide significant anatomic information with respect to the site, size, shape, and number of loculations of intraabdominal fluid. It can demonstrate the relationship of the fluid collection to intraabdominal organs. As has been discussed, however, although certain inferences can be drawn about the nature of the fluid from the ultrasound characteristics, the final arbiter is the obtaining of fluid for laboratory study. The use of the "skinny" or the Chiba needle for aspiration of small volumes of fluid has resulted in a technique that is without significant morbidity and mortality, even if the needle transgresses a solid or hollow viscus before the penetration of the fluid collection.

Ultrasound can localize the fluid collection for more accurate needle place-ment, and this procedure has become more specific with the introduction of first A-mode aspiration/biopsy transducers,[69,70] and more recently, real-time aspiration/biopsy transducers.[71-75] Having located the site of fluid collection, sampled the fluid, and determined its nature, treatment may be instituted.[76,77] Ultrasound can further be used to guide subsequent needling with a larger bore needle followed by guide-wire insertion and catheter exchange to allow not only sampling but also definitive percutaneous drainage. As more and more experience is achieved in the percutaneous drainage of intraabdominal abscesses, the application of this procedure is becoming more widespread. The technique now makes it feasible to insert wide-bored tubes capable of draining even very viscous fluid.[78,79,80]

It is suggested that the ideal approach to the drainage of an intraabdominal abscess should use both ultrasound and computed tomography.[79] Computed tomography is probably the most suitable method for planning the ideal route of drainage because of its unique ability to demonstrate the location of bowel loops with respect to an intraabdominal abscess or other fluid collection, as well as identifying the position of other organs. This allows a drainage route to be planned that does not pass through any of these organs, and, once chosen, real-time ultrasound biopsy transducers may be used to guide the initial needle placement.

Because of the increased feasibility and applicability of ultrasound-guided aspiration and drainage procedures in intraabdominal abscesses, the role of surgical drainage may become restricted to certain specific indications: (1) where there is a multiloculated abscess not amenable to drainage by a single percutaneous tube (although more than one percutaneous drainage tube can be easily inserted); (2) where percutaneous drainage has failed to resolve the abscess; and (3) where percutaneous drainage was used as a holding maneuver before definitive surgical drainage in an attempt to improve the patient's condition sufficiently to withstand an operation.

COMPARISON OF ULTRASOUND WITH OTHER TECHNIQUES FOR DETECTION OF INTRAABDOMINAL FLUID

Conventional radiography, radionuclide imaging, ultrasound, and computed tomography are all used in the diagnosis and assessment of intraabdominal fluid. Each of these relies on different physical principles. It is difficult to compare the role of each modality in every clinical situation. Since the diagnosis of intraabdominal pus provides perhaps the most common and challenging diagnostic problem, it is in this situation that most comparative studies have been undertaken.

The use of isotope imaging, either with gallium 67 or with the more recently introduced indium-111-labeled leukocyte, relies on the uptake of the radioactive tracer by an inflammatory focus within the body. While each radionuclide has advantages and disadvantages, both can detect inflammatory foci not confined to the abdomen. Both require a single injection of radionuclide and then one or two gamma-camera images depicting the entire thorax and abdomen. Disadvantages of indium-labeled leukocytes are that it is expensive, difficult to prepare, and not universally available. Gallium may produce false-positive results because of accumulation in bowel, within recent wounds, and also because of accumulation within malignant as well as inflammatory lesions. Furthermore, it is not just "an inflammatory focus" that the surgeon is looking for, but rather a well-defined collection of pus.

Computed tomography depends on the differential attenuation of an x-ray beam as it passes through the body; the reconstructed image being derived from the information obtained by multiple x-ray detectors. The technique is noninvasive, easy to perform, and provides accurate anatomic delineation of intraabdominal organs, including the bowel, following administration of dilute oral contrast medium. Similarly, computed tomography is not restricted to the examination of the abdomen in the search for an abscess or other fluid collection. However, disadvantages include the high cost of equipment, the need for patient mobility, and, at least until the advent of fast scanners, the incidence of motion (including bowel) artifact, and surgical clip streaking. Hope that computed tomography would provide a specific diagnosis for intraabdominal fluid collections has not been borne out by clinical studies, since the attenuation values for many fluids overlap.[81] Indeed, experimental work by Filly et al. has suggested that in certain circumstances, some fluids may be isodense with a tissue model on CT, whereas they remained anechoic to ultrasound examination.[30]

Ultrasound is a rapid, noninvasive procedure, relying for image production on sound propagation and on differential reflection and scattering by tissues and organs. The problem created by bowel for imaging the midabdomen has been described. Similarly, fluid/feces-filled bowel may produce pseudolesions resembling abscess formation.[82,83] Meticulous technique and expertise in interpretation are essential to avoid confusion of normal anatomy with an abnormal fluid collection (Figs. 7-33 and 7-34).[84,85]

In comparing the various imaging techniques, Norton et al. reported an overall accuracy rate of only 67 percent for CT scanning, 57 percent for ultrasound, and 54 percent for gallium radionuclide scanning.[4] However, he agreed that his patient population might have been unusual. Further, his criteria for the definition of false-positive and false-negative results are also somewhat unusual. Other workers have stressed the advantages of isotope imaging,[86] computed tomography,[2] and ultrasound.[3] Current opinion, however, suggests that if computed tomography, ultrasound, and radionuclide scanning techniques are compared, the differences in diagnostic accuracy among them are not statistically significant.[87–89] In one of these series, the accuracy was reported as 96 percent for CT, 90 percent for ultrasound, and 92 percent for indium 111.[89] Other workers have reported a sensitivity of between 86 percent and 93 percent for ultrasound with a specificity of between 96 percent and 100 percent.[3]

While every work-up for possible abdominal abscess should be individualized, a generalized approach to this difficult problem is proposed (Fig. 7-35). The flow chart starts with the appropriate history, a physical examination, and an abdominal radiograph. When localizing signs are present, ultrasound of that

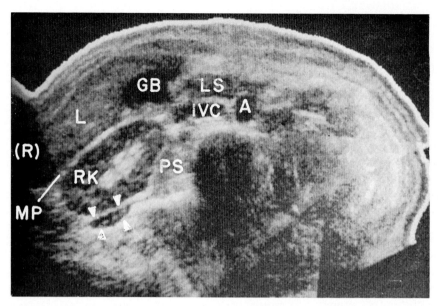

Figure 7-33 Normal anatomy. Transverse scan of the upper abdomen demonstrating lentiform appearance of a hypoechoic quadratus lumborum muscle (arrowheads). RK = right kidney; PS = psoas; IVC = inferior vena cava; A = aorta; LS = lesser sac; GB = gallbladder; L = liver; MP = Morrison's pouch; (R) = toward right side of patient.

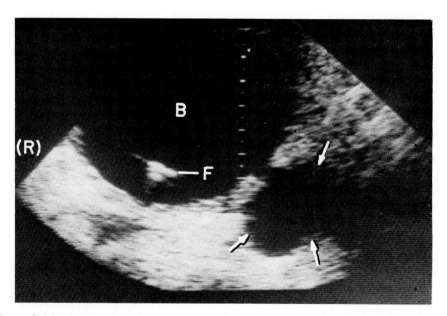

Figure 7-34 Bladder diverticulum. Transverse pelvic scan demonstrating the anechoic bladder, containing the bright echo of a Foley catheter (F). A fluid collection, obviously communicating through a narrow neck with the bladder and outlined by arrows, is the diverticulum. (R) = toward patient's right side.

280

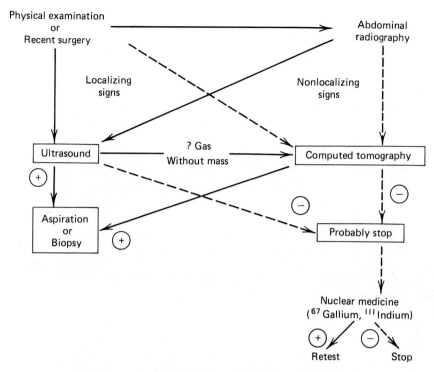

Figure 7-35 Proposed algorithm for suspected abscess.

region should be undertaken and, if a well-defined mass is imaged, aspiration or biopsy performed. If ultrasound is negative, computed tomography might be used if there remains a high index of suspicion of an abscess. Computed tomography may be the investigation of first choice when there are no localizing signs on clinical examination or plain radiography. When both tests fail to image a mass, isotope imaging may be used, but probably only if clinical suspicion remains high. A positive nuclear image could be either diffuse inflammation or a well-defined mass, and in this situation, ultrasound or computed tomography would have to be repeated in an attempt to image a well-defined and, therefore, treatable abscess.

Certainly it appears that ultrasound is a very sensitive examination method for intraabdominal fluid collections. It is also clear, however, that a high degree of expertise is necessary to perform and interpret the scans, and careful attention to technique is mandatory to achieve accurate information. When performed in the correct manner by experienced personnel, ultrasound provides a relatively cheap, noninvasive, rapid, and mobile method of examining the patient for suspected intraabdominal fluid. It is therefore, suggested that ultrasound be used as part of a wider spectrum of imaging modalities as demonstrated in the proposed algorithm. If ultrasound is used as part of a combined diagnostic approach in concert with the information available from clinical history, physical examination, and subsequent aspiration or biopsy, an accurate diagnosis may be achieved in the majority of patients.

REFERENCES

1. Connell TR, Stephens DH, Carlson HC, Brown ML: Upper abdominal abscess: A continuing and deadly problem. *AJR* 134:759–765, 1980.

2. Halber MD, Daffner RH, Morgan CL, et al: Intraabdominal abscess: Current concepts in radiologic evaluation. *AJR* 133:9–13, 1979.

3. Taylor KJW, Sullivan DC, Wasson JS McI, Rosenfield AT: Ultrasound and gallium for the diagnosis of abdominal and pelvic abscesses. *Gastrointest Radiol* 3:281–286, 1978.

4. Norton L, Eule J, Burdick D: Accuracy of techniques to detect intraperitoneal abscess. *Surgery* 84:370–378, 1978.

5. Eiseman B, Beart R, Norton L: Multiple organ failure. *Surg Gynaecol Obstet* 144:323, 1977.

6. Norton L, Moore G, Eiseman D: Liver failure in the post-operative patient: The role of sepsis and immunologic insufficiency. *Surgery* 78:6, 1975.

7. Mancuso AA: Ultrasonography of the general abdomen: Peritoneal cavity, bowel and mesentery and abdominal wall, in Sarti, Sample WS (eds): *Diagnostic Ultrasound: Text and Cases*. Boston, G.K. Hall & Co., 1980. pp. 412–451.

8. Bearman S, Snaders RC, and Oh K: B-scan ultrasound in the evaluation of pediatric abdominal masses. *Radiology* 108:111–117, 1973.

9. Kangarloo H, Sukov R, Sample WS, et al: Ultrasonographic evaluation of juxta diaphragmatic masses in children. *Radiology* 125:785–787, 1977.

10. Leopold GR, Asher WM: Diagnosis of extra-organ retroperitoneal space lesion by B-scan ultrasonography. *Radiology* 103:133–138, 1972.

11. Maklad NS, Doust BD, Baum JK: Ultrasonic diagnosis of post-operative intra-abdominal abscess. *Radiology* 113:417–422, 1974.

12. Wicks JD, Silver TM, Bree RL: Giant cystic abdominal masses in children and adolescents: ultrasonic differential diagnosis. *AJR* 130:853–857, 1978.

13. Hollinshead WH: *Textbook of Anatomy*, ed 3. Chapter 20:561–669; chapter 21: 677–699. New York, Harper & Row, 1974, pp 561–669, 677–699.

14. Meyers MA: The spread and localization of acute peritoneal effusions. *Radiology* 95:547–554, 1970.

15. Meyers MA; Dynamic radiology of the abdomen: Normal and pathologic anatomy. New York. *Heidelberg Springer* 113–194, 1976.

16. Meyers MA, Whalen JP, Teele K, Berne AS: Radiologic features of extra-peritoneal effusions: An anatomic approach. *Radiology* 104:249–257, 1972.

17. Love L, Meyers MA, Churchill RJ, et al: Computed tomography of extra-peritoneal spaces. *AJR* 136:781–789, 1981.

18. Doust BD, Thompson R: Ultrasonography of abdominal fluid collections. *Gastrointest Radiol* 3:273–279, 1978.

19. Leopold GR: Invited commentary to Ascher et al.: "Radio-labelled autologous leukocyte scanning in abscess detection," *World J Surg* 4:401–402, 1980.

20. Hill M, Sanders RC: Grey scale B-scan characteristics of intra-abdominal cystic masses. *J Clin Ultrasound* 6:214–294, 1978.

21. Doust BD, Quiroz S, Stewart JM: Ultrasonic distinction of abscesses from other intra-abdominal fluid collections. *Radiology* 125:213–218, 1977.

22. Bree RL, Silver TM: Differential diagnosis of hypo-echoic and an-echoic masses with grey scale sonography: A new observation. *J Clin Ultrasound* 7:249–254, 1979.

23. Thurber LA, Cooperberg PL, Clement JG, et al: Echogenic fluid: A pitfall in the ultrasonographic diagnosis of cystic lesions. *J Clin Ultrasound* 7:273–278, 1979.

24. Fleisher AC, James AE Jr: *Introduction to Diagnostic Sonography*: New York, John Wiley & Sons, 1980, p. 187.

25. Kaplan GN, Sanders RC: B-scan ultrasound in the management of patients with occult abdominal hematomas. *J Clin Ultrasound* 1:5–13, 1973.

26. Fleisher AC, Kulkarai M, Johnson K, et al: Diagnostic specificity of sonographic, scintigraphic, and clinical findings in peri-renal allograft masses. Paper presented at eighty-first annual meeting, The American Roentgen Ray Society, San Francisco, March 23–27, 1981.

27. Wicks JD, Silver TM, Bree RL: Grey scale features of hematomas: Ultrasonic spectrum. *AJR* 131:977–980, 1978.

28. Kressel HY, Filly RA: Ultrasonographic appearance of gas-containing abscesses in the abdomen. *AJR* 130:71–73, 1978.

29. Conrad MR, Bregman R, Killman WJ: Ultrasonic recognition of parenchymal gas. *AJR* 132:395–399, 1979.

30. Filly RA, Sommer SG, Minton MJ: Characterization of biological fluids by ultrasound and computed tomography. *Radiology* 134:167–171, 1980.

31. Itzchak Y, Rubinstein Z, Heyman Z, Gerzof S: Role of ultrasound in the diagnosis of abdominal hyatid disease. *J Clin Ultrasound* 8:341–345, 1980.

32. Ariel IM, Kazarian KK; *Diagnosis and Treatment of Abdominal Abscesses*. Baltimore, Williams & Wilkins, 1971, pp 174–206.

33. Whalen JP: *Radiology of the Abdomen: An Anatomic Basis*. Philadelphia, Lea & Febiger, 1976.

34. Miller WT, Tallman EA: Subphrenic abscess. *AJR* 101:961–969, 1967.

35. Rice RP, Masters SJ: Intra-abdominal abscess. *Semin Roentgen* 8:365–374, 1973.

36. Landay M, Harless W: Ultrasonic differentiation of right pleural effusion from subphrenic fluid on longitudinal scans on the right upper quadrant: The importance of recognizing the diaphragm. *Radiology* 123:155–158, 1977.

37. Haber K, Asher WM, Freimanis AK: Echographic evaluation of diaphragmatic motions in intra-abdominal diseases. *Radiology* 114:141–144, 1975.

38. Doust BD, Doust VL: Ultrasonic diagnosis of abdominal abscess. *Dig Dis* 21:569–575, 1976.

39. Mee TL, Forsberg FG, Koehler TR: Postsplenectomy: True mass and pseudo-mass ultrasound diagnosis. *Radiology* 134:707–711 1980.

40. Yeh HC, Wolf BS: Ultrasonic contrast study to identify stomach tap-water micro-bubbles. *J Clin Ultrasound* 5:170–174, 1976.

41. Crade M, Taylor K, Rosenfield A: Water distension of the gut in evaluation of the pancreas by ultrasound. *AJR* 131:348, 1978.

42. Sample WS: Pelvic inflammatory disease and endometriosis, in Sanders RC, James AE Jr (eds): *The Principles and Practice of Ultrasonography in Obstetrics and Gynecology*, New York, Appleton Century Crofts, 1980, pp 321–334.

43. Silver TM, Campbell B, Wicks JB, et al: Peri-transplant fluid collections: Ultrasound evaluation and clinical significance. *Radiology* 138:145–151, 1981.

44. Wyatt TM, Spitz HB: Ultrasound in the diagnosis of rectus sheath hematoma. *JAMA* 241(14):1,499–1,500, 1979.

45. Kaftori JK, Rosenberger A, Pollack S, Fish JH: Rectus sheath hematoma: Ultrasonographic diagnosis. *AJR* 128:283–285, 1977.

46. Laing FC, Jacobs RT: Value of ultrasonography in the detection of retroperitoneal inflammatory masses. *Radiology* 123:169–172, 1977.

47. Kumari S, Fulco JD, Karayalcin G, Lipton R: Gray scale ultrasound: Evaluation of ilio-psoas hematomas in hemophiliacs. *AJR* 133:103–106, 1979.

48. Thomas JL, Cunningham JJ: Echographic detection and characterization of abdominal hemmorhages. *Arch Intern Med* 138:1,392–1,393, 1978.

49. Adelman MI, Gishen P, Dubbins P, Mibashan RS: Localized intramesenteric hemorrhage: A recognizable syndrome in hemophilia? *Br Med J* 642–643, September 15, 1979.

50. Lee TG, Brickman SE, Avecilla, LS: Ultrasound diagnosis of intramural intestinal hematoma. *J Clin Ultrasound* 5:423–424, 1977.

51. Federle MP, Goldberg HI, Kiser JA, et al: Evaluation of abdominal trauma by computed tomography. *Radiology* 138:637–644, 1981.

52. Berger TE, Kuhn JP: Computed tomography of blunt abdominal trauma in childhood. *AJR* 136:105–110, 1981.

53. Kay CJ, Rosenfield AT, Armm M: Gray scale ultrasonography in the evaluation of renal trauma. *Radiology* 134:461–466, 1980.

54. Son GT, Hunter TB, Haber K: Utility of ultrasound for diagnosis of mesenteric hematoma. *AJR* 134:381–384, 1980.

55. Foley LC, Teele RL: Ultrasound of epigastric injuries after blunt trauma. *AJR* 132:593–598, 1979.

56. Wilson RL, Rogers WS, Shaub MS, Birnbaum W: Splenic subcapsular hematoma: Ultrasonic diagnosis. *West J Med* 128:6–8, 1978.

57. Johnson MA, Cooperberg TL, Boisvert J, et al: Spontaneous splenic rupture in infectious mononucleosis: Sonographic diagnosis and follow-up. *AJR* 136:111–114, 1981.

58. Goldberg BB: Ultrasonic evaluation of intra-peritoneal fluid. *JAMA* 235:2,427–2,430, 1976.

59. Yeh C, Wolf BS: Ultrasonography in ascites. *Radiology* 124:783–790, 1977.

60. Proto AV, Lane EJ, Marangola JP: A new concept of ascitic fluid distribution. *AJR* 126:974–980, 1976.

61. Goldberg BB, Goodman GA, Clearfield HR: Evaluation of ascites by ultrasound. *Radiology* 96:15–22, 1970.

62. Sanders RC: The significance of sonographic gallbladder wall thickening. *J Clin Ultrasound* 8:143–146, 1980.

63. Nelson LH, Weeks L, McCune B: Ultrasound in the differential diagnosis of abdominal fluid. *South Med J* 72:1,216–1,218, 1979.

64. Edell SL, Gefter WB: Ultrasonic differentiation of type of ascitic fluid. *AJR* 133:111–114, 1979.

65. Gompels BM, Darlington LG: Ultrasonic diagnosis of tuberculous peritonitis. *Br J Radiol* 51:1,018–1,019, 1978.

66. Merrit CB, Williams SM: Ultrasound findings in a patient with pseudomyxoma peritonei. *J Clin Ultrasound* 6:417–418, 1978.

67. Tavsek EJ, Lewin JR: Diagnosis of pseudomyxoma peritonei combining ultrasound and computed tomography. *Pennsylvania Med* 34–35, December 1980.

68. Seshul MB, Coulam CM: Pseudomyxoma peritonei: Computed tomography and sonography. *AJR* 136:803–806, 1981.

69. Goldberg T, Pollack H: Ultrasound aspiration transducer. *Radiology* 102:187, 1972.

70. Holm H, Kristensen J, Rasmussen S, et al: Ultrasound as a guide in percutaneous puncture techniques. *Ultrasonics* 10:83, 1972.

71. Goldberg BB, Cole-Beuglet C, Kurtz AB, Rubin CS: Real-time aspiration biopsy transducer. *J Clin Ultrasound* 8:107–112, 1980.

72. Holm HH, Petersen JS, Kristensen JK, et al: Ultrasonically-guided percutaneous puncture. *Radiol Clin N Am* 13: 493–503, 1975.

73. Saitoh M, Watanabe H, Ohe H, et al: Ultrasonic real-time guidance for percutaneous puncture. *J Clin Ultrasound* 7:269–272, 1979.

74. Otto R, Deyhle P: Guided puncture under real-time sonographic control. *Radiology* 134:784–785, 1980.

75. Lindegren PG: Ultrasonically-guided punctures: A modified technique. *Radiology* 137:235–237, 1980.

76. Elyaderani MK, Skolnick ML, Weinstein BJ: Ultrasonic detection and aspiration confirmation of intra-abdominal collection of fluid. *Surg Gynaecol Obstet* 149:1,529–1,533, 1979.

77. Pedersen JS, Hancke S, Kristensen JK: Renal carbuncle: Antibiotic therapy governed by ultrasonic aspiration. *J Urol* 109:777, 1973.

78. Haaga JR, Alfidi RJ, Havrilla TR, et al: CT detection and aspiration of abdominal abscesses, *AJR* 128:465–474, 1977.

79. Gerzof SG, Robbins AH, Birkett DH, et al: Percutaneous catheter drainage of abdominal abscesses guided by ultrasound and computed tomography. *AJR* 133:1–8, 1979.

80. Gerzof SG, Spira R, Robbins AH: Percutaneous abscess drainage. *Semin Roentgen* 16(1):62–71, 1981.

81. Bydder TM, Kreel L: Attenuation values of fluid collections within the abdomen. *J Comput Assist Tomog* 4:145–150, 1980.

82. Cunningham JA: False-positive gray scale ultrasonography for intra-abdominal abscesses. *Arch Surg* 111:810–811, 1976.

83. Teele RL, Rosenfield AT, Freedman GS: The anatomic splenic flexture: An ultrasonic renal imposter. *AJR* 128:115–120, 1977.

84. Callen PW, Filly RA, Marks WM: The quadratus lumborum muscle: A possible source of confusion in a sonographic evaluation of the retro-peritoneum. *J Clin Ultrasound* 7:349–352, 1979.

85. Rao KG, Woodlief RM: Excessive right subdiaphragmatic fat: A potential diagnostic pitfall. *Radiology* 138:15–18, 1981.

86. Ascher NL, Forstrom L, Simmons RL: Radiolabelled autologous leucocyte scanning in abscess detection. *World J Surg* 4:395–400, 1980.

87. Korobkin M, Callen TW, Filly RA, et al: Comparison of computed tomography, ultrasonography and gallium 67 scanning in the evaluation of suspected abdominal abscess. *Radiology* 129:89–93, 1978.

88. McNeil BJ, Sanders R, Alderson PO, et al: A prospective study of computed tomography, ultrasound and gallium imaging in patients with fever. *Radiology* 139:647–653, 1981.

89. Knochel JQ, Koehler PR, Lee PG, Welch DM: Diagnosis of abdominal abscesses with computed tomography, ultrasound and indium 111 leucocyte scans. *Radiology* 137:425–432, 1980.

8

Normal
and Abnormal Bowel

Paul A. Dubbins
Alfred B. Kurtz

INTRODUCTION

Until recently the effect of the bowel on abdominal imaging was felt to be always deleterious. This opinion was held primarily because bowel gas caused significant scattering of the ultrasound beam, thus obscuring deeper structures. In addition, considerable difficulty was encountered in the accurate identification of collapsed and fluid-filled bowel.

While the problem of gas persists, several factors have contributed to better appreciation of the varied ultrasound appearances of the normal and abnormal bowel: (*a*) Technological advances have improved the resolution and versatility of ultrasound instrumentation. (*b*) Greater experience has allowed recognition of certain typical sonographic bowel patterns. (*c*) Real-time scanning has permitted continuous monitoring and visualization of movement within bowel loops. (*d*) The use of fluid distension of the upper and lower gastrointestinal tracts has decreased bowel gas, has eliminated bowel pseudotumors as a possible source of error, and has allowed better visualization of adjacent structures.[1-5]

NORMAL BOWEL PATTERNS

The ultrasound appearance of the normal stomach and the small and large bowel depends on whether the bowel is collapsed or distended, and if distended, whether filled with fluid, gas, or both. Usually, the bowel exists simultaneously in all these states and, therefore, appears as a mixture of all three patterns.[6] In addition, the large bowel and, the rectosigmoid colon in particular, may contain varying amounts of fecal material, further complicating these patterns.[5]

Recently, specific normal values for the thickness of the bowel wall in both distended and nondistended states have been reported.[7] While slight differences were noted for the stomach and the small and large bowel, the average bowel wall thickness for the nondistended bowel was always normal if less than 5 mm, although one normal transverse colon wall measured 9 mm.[7,8] In the distended state, the mean thickness of the bowel wall decreased to 3 mm.[7]

Mucus Pattern

In the collapsed state, the mucosa of the bowel is lined by varying amounts of mucus. The ultrasound appearance is described as a *target*, consisting of an hyperechoic core of mucus and trapped gas surrounded by a hypoechoic halo of mucosa. While all the bowel in the collapsed state exhibits this appearance, it is most commonly recognized at the esophagogastric junction, at the pyloric antrum of the stomach, and in the transverse colon (Fig. 8-1). While the target pattern is the most characteristic of the normal bowel patterns, slight variations exist depending on the degree of bowel collapse and the presence or absence of small amounts of trapped gas and fluid (Fig. 8-1).

Fluid Distension of Bowel

Fluid distension in the normal bowel produces different appearances, tubular and circular (cystic), depending on whether the bowel is imaged along its long or short axis (Figs. 8-2, 8-3, and 8-4). Retained fluid and/or food in the stomach may on occasion mimic a midabdominal or left upper quadrant mass (Fig. 8-2). However, changes induced by a shift in the patient's position or by ingestion of fluid with gas microbubbles often identifies the stomach.[9] In addition, structural features within the bowel lumen often allow not only the specific identification of large and small bowel, but also further differentiation of jejunum from ileum. In the small bowel, the valvulae conniventes produce regular repeating interfaces characteristic of the "key board sign" of normal jejunum (Fig. 8-3), while the ileum has typically smooth, featureless borders.[10,11] In the large bowel, irregular luminal projections corresponding to colonic haustrations can be identified (Fig. 8-4).

Gas Pattern

Gas contained within the bowel produces a brightly hyperechoic pattern (Figs. 8-1a and 8-3a). Not infrequently, a distal acoustic shadow is also imaged, classically described as "dirty" in contradistinction to the sharp acoustic shadowing associated with calculi (Figs. 8-3b, 8-4b, and 8-5a).

Colon Pseudotumor patterns

While the ultrasound patterns created by admixtures of fecal matter, fluid, and gas within the large bowel (pseudotumors) are not one of the three classic bowel patterns, they nevertheless commonly occur in the normal colon. These pseudotumors may be initially analyzed in terms of their anatomic placement and echogenicity.

Position

Any tubular structure in the paracolic gutters should be considered as possibly originating from the ascending or descending colon (Fig. 8-4). The transverse colon, however, is more difficult to analyze because of its variable position. The

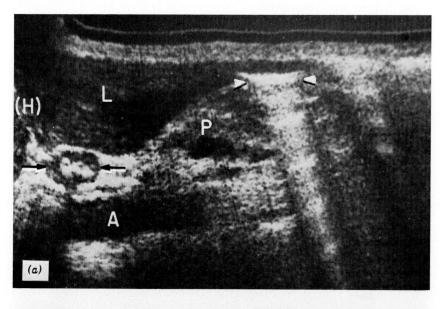

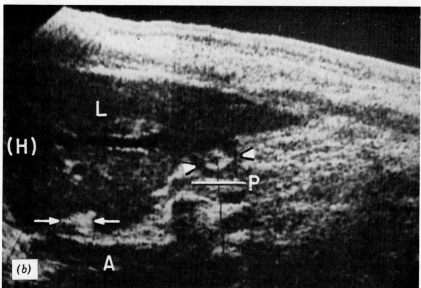

Figure 8-1 Longitudinal midline ultrasound scans in four different patients. Note the changes in the esophagogastric junction (arrows) and antrum of the stomach (dots). P = pancreatic body; A = aorta; L = liver. (*a*) The esophagogastric junction has the classic "target" appearance, whereas the antrum is gas-filled. (*b*) The esophagogastric junction, while slightly atypical, is still a normal "target." The antrum has fluid in the center of the "target." (*c*) The esophagogastric junction has a very small mucus center, while this feature is very prominent in the antrum. (*d*) The esophagogastric junction is the classic "target," slightly more prominent than in part *a*. There is no central mucus in the antrum. (H) = toward patient's head.

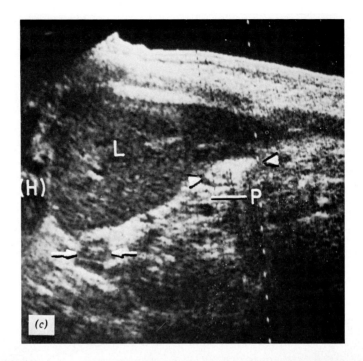

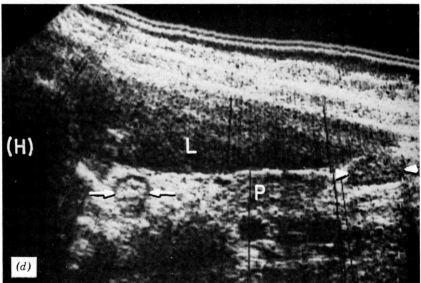

Figure 8-1 *(continued)*

rectosigmoid colon, while anatomically located within the pelvis, occupies the
same position as do pelvic masses (Figs. 8-6 and 8-7).[4,5]

Echo Patterns
The echo patterns are variable, ranging from completely anechoic to hyperechoic (Figs. 8-4, 8-6a, 8-7a).[5] Therefore, for the accurate identification of the

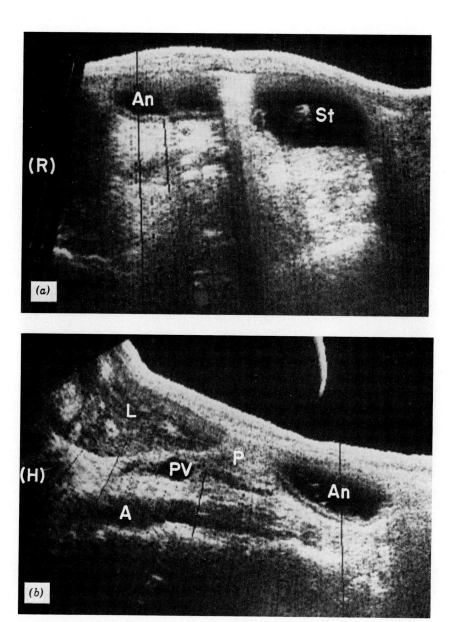

Figure 8-2 Normal fluid-filled stomach. (*a*) The transverse and (*b*) the longitudinal scan of the upper midabdomen. The body (St) and antrum (An) of the stomach are fluid-filled, more tubular on transverse and more ovoid in longitudinal. These anechoic areas should not be confused for cystic masses of the midabdomen and left upper quadrants. Note the brightly hyperechoic wall, presumably representing the partially distended rugae. The hyperechoic areas within the liver (L) are metastases from a colon primary. PV = portal vein; P = pancreatic body; A = aorta; (H) = toward patient's head; (R) = toward patient's right side.

291

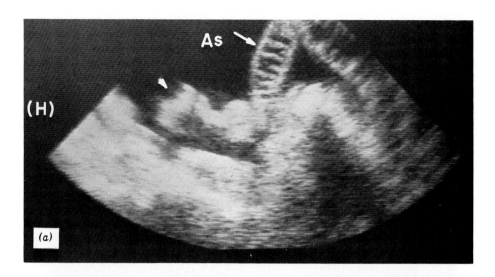

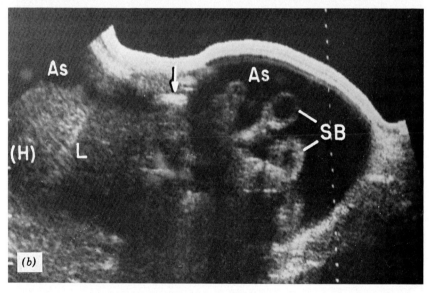

Figure 8-3 Normal fluid-filled small bowel, floating within ascites (As) in two different patients. (*a*) Longitudinal real-time sector scan of the left midabdomen showing the long-axis tubular appearance of a loop of jejunum with the typical stepladder "keyboard sign" (arrow). Note the collapsed loop of bowel containing gas and mucus (arrowhead). (*b*) Longitudinal scan to the right of the midline showing the short-axis circular appearance of fluid-filled loops of ileum (SB) on their mesenteric stalks. Note the hyperechoic gas-filled bowel (arrow) with its indistinct "dirty" distal shadow. L = liver; (H) = toward patient's head.

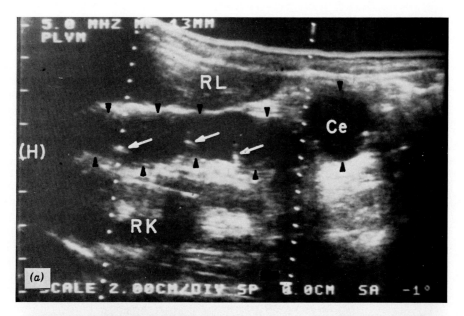

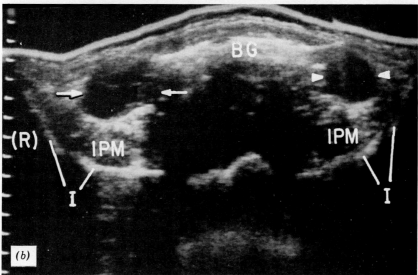

Figure 8-4 Normal fluid-filled large bowel in two different patients. (*a*) Longitudinal coronal scan of the right lower quadrant, scanned in the left lateral decubitus position, demonstrating the long-axis tubular appearance of the ascending colon (arrowheads) and cecum (Ce) between a prominent Reidel's lobe of the liver (RL) and the right kidney (RK). Note the echoes from the colon haustral markings (arrows). (*b*) Transverse image of the lower abdomen-upper pelvis showing two cystic structures, the ascending colon (arrows) and descending colon (arrowheads), directly anterior to the iliopsoas muscles (IPM). Note the hyperechoic gas-filled small bowel (BG) with indistinct "dirty" distal shadow. I = iliac bone; (H) = toward patient's head; (R) = toward patient's right side.

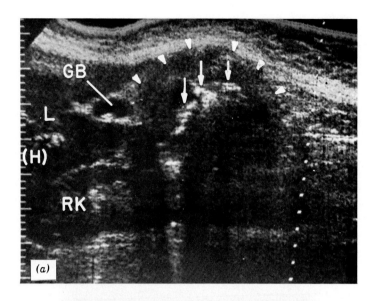

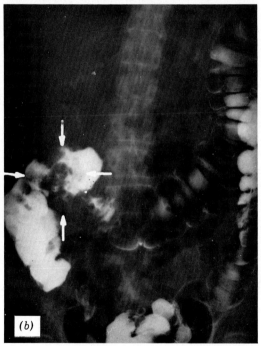

Figure 8-5 Carcinoma of the colon (hepatic flexure). (*a*) Longitudinal scan to the right of midline, demonstrating an irregularly thickened bowel wall (arrowheads) with central hyperechoic mucus and gas (arrows). Note the indistinct "dirty" shadow distal to the gas. This mass is in the region of the hepatic flexure of the colon, just inferior to the gallbladder (GB) and liver (L) and anterior to the right kidney (RK). (H) = toward patient's head. (*b*) Anteroposterior radiograph of a barium enema in the same patient, demonstrating a carcinoma of the hepatic flexure (arrows).

294

large bowel and particularly the rectosigmoid colon, a small amount of fluid should be introduced into the rectum. The examination should be continuously monitored using real-time. As fluid passes into the colon, it may create three appearances: (*a*) complete displacement of the abnormality (pseudotumor), thus defining the normal colon (Fig. 8-7*b*), (*b*) only partial displacement of the abnormality, thus suggesting that the abnormality is related to the colon (Fig. 8-8), and (*c*) identification of the normal colon next to the abnormality, thus suggesting that the abnormality is related either to the bowel wall or more commonly to the adjacent structures.

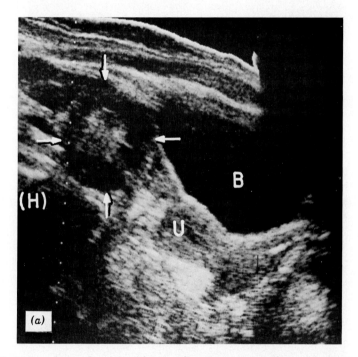

Figure 8-6 Comparison of a sigmoid "pseudotumor" to two dermoids. (*a*) Longitudinal pelvic scan 1 cm to left of midline showing an atypical enlarged "target" area (arrows) superior to the urinary bladder (B) and uterus (U). The abnormality does not indent the bladder and is in the anatomic position of the sigmoid colon. A subsequent water enema demonstrated water flowing through and completely changing this area, thus confirming the diagnosis of pseudotumor. (*b*) Longitudinal pelvic scan 3 cm to left of midline in another patient showing an atypical enlarged "target" area (arrows), superior to the urinary bladder (B), with questionably minimal bladder indentation. While its appearance is not dissimilar to that of the sigmoid pseudotumor, part *a*, a water enema demonstrated the normal sigmoid colon posterior to the mass. Subsequent partial emptying of the bladder showed more bladder indentation by the mass. A dermoid was found at surgery. (*c*) Longitudinal pelvic scan 4 cm to left to midline in a third patient showing a hyperechoic mass with thin hypoechoic rim (arrows), an atypical "target" lesion, indenting the urinary bladder (B). This indentation suggested a true space-occupying lesion, and a dermoid was found at surgery. (H) = toward patient's head.

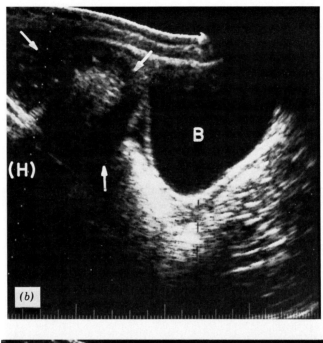

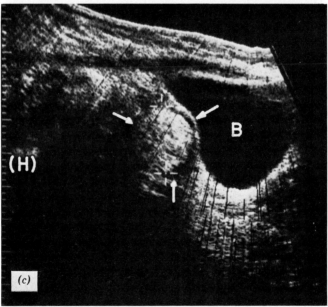

Figure 8-6 (*continued*)

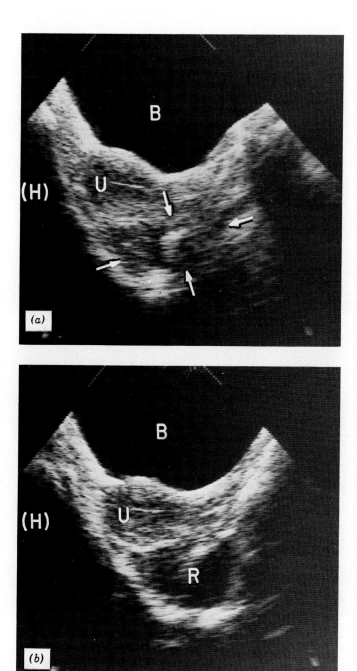

Figure 8-7 Rectal pseudotumor (fluid, feces and gas). (*a*) Real-time sector longitudinal midline pelvic scan demonstrating an irregularly shaped complex mass (arrows) posterior to the uterus (U). (*b*) Real-time sector longitudinal midline pelvic scan in the same patient following administration of water into the rectum (R) showing a complete change in the suspected mass, thereby confirming a pseudotumor. B = urinary bladder; (H) = toward patient's head.

297

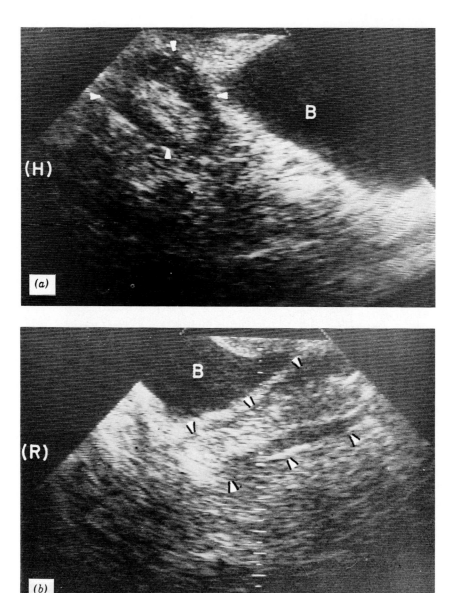

Figure 8-8 Sigmoid diverticulitis. (*a*) The longitudinal pelvic scan 3 cm to the left of midline, and (*b*) the transverse scan 5 cm above the pubic symphysis showing a long thickened segment of bowel wall (arrowheads) posterior, superior, and to the left lateral aspect of the urinary bladder (B). The bowel pattern demonstrates the "pseudokidney" sign in the anatomic region of the sigmoid colon with an enlarged hyperechoic center representing mucus and trapped air. A water enema failed to alter the overall appearance of the colon, with only minimal change noted in the hyperechoic center. (*c*) The CT scan of the same region as part *b* demonstrates intraluminal water-soluble contrast passing through the diffusely thickened bowel wall (arrowheads). Diverticulitis was confirmed on barium enema. (H) = toward patient's head; (R) = toward patient's right side.

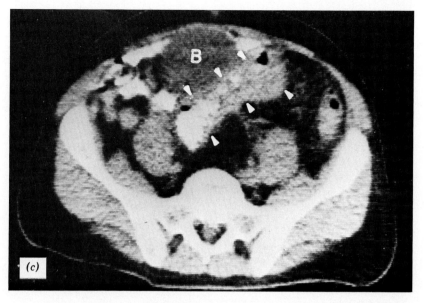

Figure 8-8 (*continued*)

ABNORMAL BOWEL

Ultrasound patterns seen in the abnormal bowel are often characteristic, representing variations on the appearances of the normal bowel. Any unusual distribution of bowel gas, any persistent fluid-filled loop of bowel, or any thickening of the normal target appearance should be considered abnormal, and these abnormal patterns may be analyzed by employing the same three basic categories that are used for normal bowel, that is, mucus pattern, fluid pattern, and gas pattern.

Mucus Pattern

The extent of thickening of the bowel wall, whether due to inflammatory disease or to primary or secondary malignancy, depends on the amount of bowel wall infiltration. Concentric bowel wall thickening produces an ultrasound appearance variously described as the *cockade sign*, the *atypical target configuration*, the *bulls-eye configuration*, and the *pseudokidney sign* (Figs. 8-8 and 8-9).[9,11–13]Measurement of bowel wall adds a quantitative dimension to these patterns, with reported wall thicknesses of abnormal bowel varying from 5 to 30 mm and averaging 23 mm.[7,8]

While bowel wall thickening has been described in gastrointestinal tumors (Fig. 8-5), inflammatory lesions (Fig. 8-8), intussusception (Fig. 8-9), lymphoma (Fig. 8-10), intramural hematoma, and hypertrophic pyloric stenosis,[8,14] at present it does not appear possible to distinguish differing causes solely on the basis of the ultrasound appearances.[9,15–20] Although it has been suggested that asymmetric target lesions are more likely to be related to secondary rather than

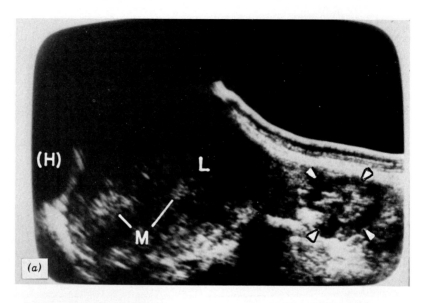

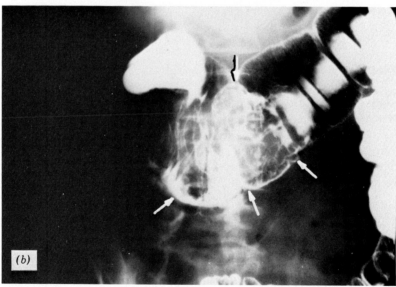

Figure 8-9 Transverse colon intussusception, secondary to a polypoid carcinoma. (*a*) Longitudinal scan 2 cm to the right of the midline demonstrating a complex "target" lesion (arrowheads) just caudal to the liver (L). Note the thickened outer halo, representing edematous intussuscipiens, surrounding a hyperechoic area of apposed bowel wall with associated mucus and trapped air. In the center is the irregularly shaped, hypoechoic area of the polypoid intussuscepting carcinoma. L = liver; M = liver metastases; (H) = toward patient's head. (*b*) Anteroposterior radiograph of a barium enema showing the polypoid carcinoma of the transverse colon (arrows).

300

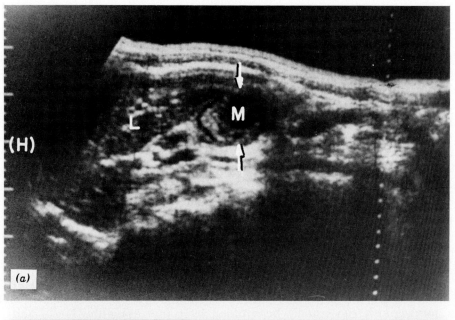

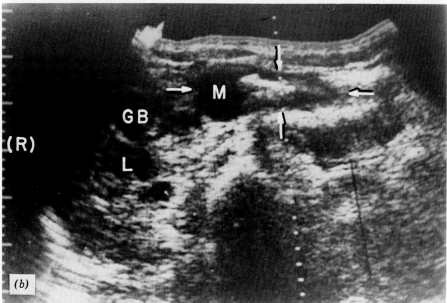

Figure 8-10 Gastric lymphoma. (*a*) The longitudinal and (*b*) transverse scans of the upper midabdomen, demonstrating asymetrical thickening of the stomach wall (arrows) with an anechoic solid mass (M) within. L = liver; GB = gallbladder; (H) = toward patient's head; (R) = toward patient's right side.

primary neoplasia, presumably due to involvement of the local mesentery, certain primary bowel lesions are also eccentric in growth, for example, leiomyosarcoma and lymphoma (Fig. 8-10). In addition, it is doubtful that the thickness of the halo can be used to differentiate benign from malignant diseases as two separate studies yielded entirely different results, that is, one suggesting that inflammatory lesions produce the greater increase in bowel wall thickness, while the other suggesting that increases in bowel wall thickness were more marked in malignancy.[7,9]

If a long length of bowel is thickened, however, it is more likely due to inflammatory disease (Fig. 8-8). Similarly, an intussusception may on occasion be identified as intussuscipiens and intussusceptum (Fig. 8-9).[21] In addition, the anatomic location of the abnormality, when considered with the patient's age and clinical status, may aid in establishing the correct diagnosis. This has been found helpful in the diagnosis of infantile hypertrophic pyloric stenosis when a concentrically enlarged target area is imaged on longitudinal midline scan at the most caudad anterior margin of the liver, the anatomic position of the normal distal stomach (Figs. 8-1b–d).[8,14]

Occasionally, coils consisting of fluid-filled loops of bowel folded on themselves may give the appearance of an enlarged pseudokidney or target lesion. A misdiagnosis can usually be avoided by compressing the bowel and by observing peristalsis during real-time examination. Similarly, in the pelvis, dermoids with their variable and unusual echo patterns may mimic bowel abnormalities (Fig. 8-6). Frequently, however, dermoids may be differentiated from the normal bowel if there is (a) significant change in the dermoid's position when the urinary bladder is emptied,[22] (b) indentation of the urinary bladder since bowel, except in the case of fecal impaction, usually does not, and (c) failure to change size and shape when fluid is administered per rectum.[4,5]

Fluid Pattern

In cases of bowel obstruction, the bowel is commonly distended with both gas and fluid. While this combination does not usually constitute a diagnostic problem on plain abdominal radiographs, the ultrasound picture is frequently confusing and nondiagnostic. On occasion, though, in cases of paralytic ileus and closed loop obstruction, only fluid may be present within the bowel.[10,23] When this occurs, abdominal radiographs and even barium studies may frequently be nondiagnostic, while ultrasound, despite the frequent absence of peristalsis, rapidly identifies the fluid-filled loops of bowel (Fig. 8-11).[23,24] In addition, specific bowel features such as the key board sign or a haustral pattern may allow the recognition of involved bowel and the identification of the level of obstruction (Fig. 8-11).[7,9,23]

Abnormal Gas Pattern

An unusual distribution of bowel gas, particularly if unchanged during real-time examination, is suggestive evidence of bowel obstruction or a gas-containing mass (Fig. 8-5). If ultrasound is the first examination performed in such a patient, confirmation should be obtained by follow-up abdominal radiographs or possibly computed tomography.

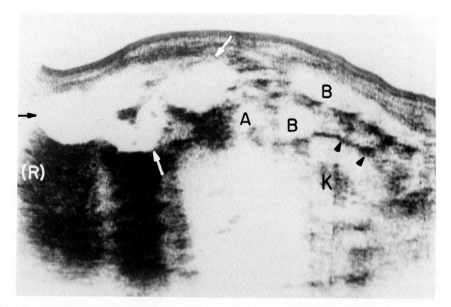

Figure 8-11 Pancreatic pseudocysts with associated small bowel paralytic ileus. Transverse scan of the midabdomen below the level of the pancreas showing multiple anechoic cystic areas (arrows) to the right of the midline, representing pseudocysts in a patient with chronic relapsing pancreatitis. Note the tubular, relatively anechoic structures to the left of the midline, representing fluid-filled bowel (B). The valvulae conniventes (arrowheads) are seen proving the bowel to be jejunum. A = aorta; K = left kidney; (R) = toward patient's right side.

Other Appearances

Certain other unusual bowel-related pathologies produce suggestive appearances. Typically, intramural tumors such as gastric leiomyomas and leiomyosarcomas may produce masses that are closely related to the bowel with either displacement or distortion of the bowel pattern.[25] Similarly, gastrointestinal tract duplication abnormalities, while not producing the typical bowel-associated lesions, appear as cystic, complex, or solid mass lesions that are in close anatomic relationship to the bowel both ultrasonographically and on correlative gastrointestinal contrast studies.[26,27] Finally, with the increasing use of the fluid-filled stomach and rectum for identification of other pathologies, it has become clear that it is possible to recognize polypoid lesions of the bowel mucosa, such as mucosal gastric polyps.[28]

SUMMARY

Barium studies combined with endoscopic techniques remain the method of choice in the evaluation of bowel pathology. However, as ultrasound becomes more commonly used in the investigation of intraabdominal masses, abdominal pain, and weight loss, bowel pathologies will be encountered with increasing frequency. It is therefore important that normal and abnormal bowel patterns be recognized and that the appropriate follow-up investigation be recommended. A more complete knowledge of the normal ultrasound bowel patterns, an understanding of the bowel's appearance during ultrasound fluid distension studies, and an appreciation of peristalsis on real-time examination permit more accurate diagnoses of bowel pathology.

REFERENCES

1. Crade M, Taylor K, Rosenfield A: Water distention of the gut in evaluation of the pancreas by ultrasound. *AJR* 131:348–349, 1978.
2. MacMahon H, Bowie JD, Beezhold C: Erect scanning of pancreas using a gastric window. *AJR* 132:587–591, 1979.
3. Warren PS, Garrett W, Phil D, Kossoff G: The liquid-filled stomach: An ultrasonic window to the upper abdomen. *J Clin Ultrasound* 6:295–382, 1978.
4. Rubin CS, Kurtz AB, Goldberg BB: Water enema: A new ultrasonic technique in defining pelvic anatomy. *J Clin Ultrasound* 6:28, 1978.
5. Kurtz AB, Rubin CS, Kramer SL, Goldberg BB: Ultrasound evaluation of the posterior pelvic compartment. *Radiology* 132:677–682, 1979.
6. Sample W, Sarti D: Computed tomography and gray scale ultrasonography: Anatomic correlation and pitfalls in the upper abdomen. *Gastrointest Radiol*, 3:243, 1978.
7. Fleischer AC, Muhletaler CA, James AE Jr: Sonographic assessment of the bowel wall. *AJR* 136:887–891, 1981.
8. Blumhagen JD, Coombs JB: Ultrasound in the diagnosis of hypertrophic pyloric stenosis. *J Clin Ultrasound* 9:289–292, 1981.
9. Morgan CL, Trought WS, Oddson TA, et al: Ultrasound patterns of disorders affecting the gastrointestinal tract. *Radiology* 135:129–135, 1980.
10. Fleischer AC, Dowling A, Weinstein M, et al: Sonographic patterns of distended, fluid-filled small and large bowel: Anatomic-radiographic correlation. *Radiology* 133:681, 1979.
11. Fleischer AC, Muhletaler CA, James AE Jr: Sonographic patterns arising from normal and abnormal bowel. *Radiol Clin North Am* 18(1):145–149, 1980.
12. Kremer H, Kellner E, Schierl W, et al: Ultrasonic diagnosis in infiltrative gastrointestinal diseases. *Dtsch Med Wochenschr* 103:965, 1978.
13. Bluth EI, Merritt CRB, Sullivan MA; Ultrasonic evaluation of the stomach, small bowel and colon. *Radiology* 133:677–680, 1979.
14. Strauss S, Itzchak Y, Manor A, et al: Sonography of hypertrophic pyloric stenosis. *AJR* 136:1,057–1,058, 1981.
15. Schwerk W. Braun B, Dombrowski H: Real-time ultrasound examination in the diagnosis of gastro-intestinal tumors. *J Clin Ultrasound* 7:425–431, 1979.
16. Mascatello VJ, Carrera GS, Telle RL, et al: The ultrasonic demonstration of gastric lesions. *J Clin Ultrasound* 5:383–387, 1977.
17. Peterson LR, Cooperberg PL: Ultrasound demonstration of lesions of the gastrointestinal tract. *Gastrointest Radiol* 3:303–306, 1978.
18. Burke LF, Clark E: Ilio-colic intussusception: A case report. *J Clin Ultrasound* 5:346–347, 1977.

19. Miller JH, Hindman BW, Lam AHK: Ultrasound in the evaluation of small bowel lymphoma in children. *Radiology* 135:409–414, 1980.

20. Lee TC, Brickman FE, Avecilla LS: Ultrasound diagnosis of intramural intestinal hematoma. *J Clin Ultrasound* 5:423–424, 1977.

21. Parienty RA, Lepreux JF, Gruson B: Sonographic and CT features of ileocolic intussusception. *AJR* 136:608–610, 1981.

22. Kurtz AB, Ashman FC, Dubbins PA, et al: Ultrasound evaluation of palpable ovarian masses: A comparison of filled and partially emptied urinary bladder techniques. *Appl Radiol*, JAN/FEB, 1982.

23. Scheible W, Goldberger LE: Diagnosis of small bowel obstruction: The contribution of diagnostic ultrasound. *AJR*: 136:608–610, 1981.

24. Pon MS, Scudamore C, Harrison RC, Cooperberg PL: Ultrasound demonstration of radiographically obscure small bowel obstruction. *AJR* 133:145–146, 1979.

25. Sandler M, Tatanatrakarf S, Madrazo B: Ultrasonic findings in intramural extra gastric lesions. *Radiology* 128:189, 1978.

26. Kangarloo H, Sample WF, Hansen G, et al: Ultrasonic evaluation of abdominal gastro-intestinal tract duplication in children. *Radiology* 131:191–194, 1979.

27. Teekem RL, Henschke CI, Tapper D: The radiographic and ultrasonographic evaluation of enteric duplication cysts. *Peadiatr Radiol* 10:9–14, 1980.

28. Kremer H, Grobner W: Sonography of polypoid gastric lesions by the fluid-filled stomach method. *J Clin Ultrasound* 9:51–54, 1981.

9

Kidney

Howard M. Pollack
Barry B. Goldberg

INTRODUCTION

Ultrasonography provides an important dimension in the diagnosis and treatment of renal disorders. Within a relatively short period, this modality has achieved an almost indispensible status in the assessment of both medical and surgical diseases of the kidney.[1] In certain clinical situations, such as uremia of undetermined origin, ultrasound is usually the first diagnostic procedure employed in the patient's evaluation. Its ability to evaluate the size, shape, and internal architecture of the kidney, provides an immediate clue as to whether uremia is most likely to be treated on a medical or surgical basis. Moreover, ultrasound has the unique attribute that its imaging properties are independent of renal function. This is not true of other methods of renal visualization such as radionuclide or roentgenographic procedures. Even computed tomography requires the injection of iodinated contrast material for maximal information even though pertinent information is obtainable without contrast. Thus, in the presence of poor renal function, ultrasound appears to be the most satisfactory noninvasive method of examining the kidneys.

There are several other advantages of ultrasound. It emits no radiation and thereby becomes an important study in pregnancy as well as in children and in women of child-bearing age. It is portable; thus real-time equipment can be used to perform ultrasonography at the bedside if necessary, or it can be brought to the fluoroscopic suite where it may be used to guide the placement of needles and catheters into the kidney. Ultrasound and procedures employing ionizing radiation are not competitive methods of examination. In fact, the methods are most often complementary. Ultrasound does have properties not offered by other modalities, and whenever clinically indicated, full advantage of these attributes should be taken.

Not only can ultrasound provide excellent two-dimensional static images in shades of gray, but with real-time techniques, it also can be used to evaluate dynamic changes such as renal mobility. Real-time imaging can be used to guide needles into renal masses, both cystic and solid, for aspiration, biopsy, or percutaneous nephrostomy. These techniques are discussed in greater detail in Chapter 12.

The future of ultrasound in renal evaluation appears quite promising. The likelihood of obtaining improved resolution is great, thus the depiction of smaller anatomic structures such as intrarenal blood vessels and small stones may be near at hand. Using pulsed Doppler ultrasound techniques in combination with two-dimensional imaging, renal blood flow has been measured.[2] With new developments in research, ultrasound is expected to expand its already important place in the diagnosis of retroperitoneal diseases, especially those involving the kidney.

NORMAL ULTRASONIC ANATOMY

The kidneys are paired retroperitoneal structures that, in the majority of cases, may be found between the levels of the first and third lumbar vertebrae. There is a range of normal variation, however, so that not infrequently the upper pole of a normal kidney may be found at the level of the twelfth thoracic vertebra, while the lower pole of another also normal kidney may be found at the level of the fourth lumbar vertebra. The upper pole of each kidney lies

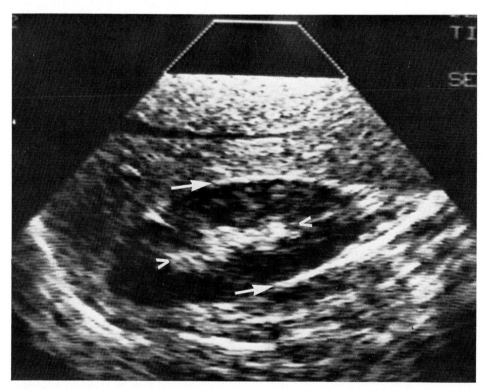

Figure 9-1 Supine longitudinal ultrasonogram of the right kidney demonstrates the typical characteristics of higher echogenicity arising from the capsule (arrows) and renal sinus (arrowheads) with less echogenicity of the parenchyma.

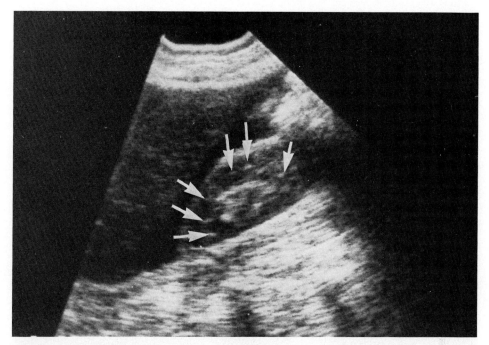

Figure 9-2 Supine longitudinal ultrasonogram demonstrates a normal kidney with the capsule well seen due to surrounding ascites. Multiple bright reflections are seen (arrows) arising from arcuate arteries. These arteries are located at the junction between the renal cortex and pyramid.

more medial than the lower pole resulting in the long axes having an oblique course that becomes a consideration in obtaining technically satisfactory longitudinal ultrasonograms. The average renal length in adults is approximately 11 to 12 cm, with the left kidney being slightly longer than the right in most persons. Normally, the kidneys are mobile and may move one or even two cm with respiration as well as with standing or sitting. This motion is easily detectable during sonography. The distance from the dorsal skin surface to the corresponding surface of the kidney is approximately 4 to 5 cm. It is this relatively short distance and the absence of interposed gas-filled structures that account for the ease with which ultrasonic images of the kidney may be obtained in the prone position. Laterally, the distance is approximately the same, so that lateral decubitus views for both the right and left kidneys are also extremely informative and are employed routinely in ultrasonic evaluation. The lateral decubitus (coronal) views along with the supine longitudinal view of the right kidney through the liver are usually the first images obtained in most renal studies, having all but supplanted the prone sagittal views for this purpose.[3] The anteroposterior thickness of the kidney measures approximately 4 cm in the normal adult. It is important to remember that since there is no magnification of the kidneys with ultrasound, they appear to be smaller than their roentgenographically determined size. Of course, there are considerable variations in size, position, and shape of the kidneys, all of which can be demonstrated easily by ultrasound.

The ultrasonic appearance of the normal kidney is quite characteristic and consists basically of two parts: (*1*) a central elliptical complex of strongly reflected echoes surrounded by (*2*) a thicker more sonolucent zone that is devoid of echoes except at high-gain settings (Fig. 9-1). The central complex of echoes (sometimes called the *renal sinus echoes*) is a composite produced by the renal collecting system (pelvis and calyces), renal vessels (arteries and veins), and renal sinus supporting tissue (fat and areolar tissue) The poorly echo-producing surrounding zone represents renal parenchyma. With high-resolution ultrasound, the parenchyma can be further separated into two divisions: (*1*) the more echogenic renal cortex and (*2*) the less echogenic medulla or renal pyramids. Occasionally, arcuate vessels may be recorded as bright echoes at the corticomedullary junction (Fig. 9-2).[4] Haller et al have noted that renal cortical echogenicity is increased in neonates and young infants, possibly as a result of immaturity of glomeruli and altered ratios of glomerular to supporting stromal tissues.[5] Scheible and Leopold have described the ultrasonic appearance of the neonatal kidney using a high-resolution (10 MHz) transducer.[6] Both authors

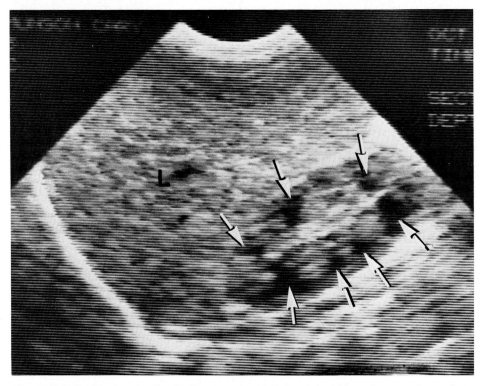

Figure 9-3 Supine longitudinal ultrasonogram of the right kidney in a newborn demonstrates prominence of the renal pyramids (arrows), as well as a slight increase in overall echogenicity of the surrounding cortex. This is normal for this age group. This pattern can also be seen in utero near term. L = liver.

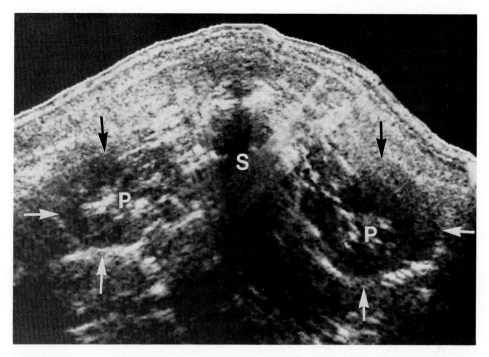

Figure 9-4 Prone transverse ultrasonogram demonstrates the parenchyma (arrows) along with the more echogenic medially located central echo complex. P = renal pelvis, S = spine.

have noted marked hypoechogenicity of the renal pyramids of this age group. Portions of the perinephric fat and the perinephric fascia (fascia of Gerota) also can be seen. The size and shape of the kidneys are anatomic in depiction. On saggital section, the central echoes are midline and centrally distributed, in keeping with their origin from the renal hilar structures. However, the central echoes tend to be more medially located when viewed on the transverse and coronal scans. In transverse mode, the renal parenchyma is distributed in a C-shaped configuration around the medial central echo complex (Fig. 9-4). Displacement, distortion, or fragmentation of the core of central echoes may be of great diagnostic significance. In similar fashion, displacement or distortion of the contour of the kidney parenchyma either by intrinsic or extrinsic masses, can be easily demonstrated (see Chapter 10).

The renal artery and vein are identifiable in many patients when the examination is performed in the supine position. Both structures appear grossly similar, but can be differentiated by means of their respective relationship to the aorta and vena cava (Fig. 9-5) (see Chapter 2). Duplex Doppler can also help to differentiate the vessels by flow determination (Fig. 9-6). Not infrequently, portions of the renal vessels may also be seen with coronal imaging in the lateral decubitus position. Occasionally, a segment of proximal ureter may also be seen in this way.

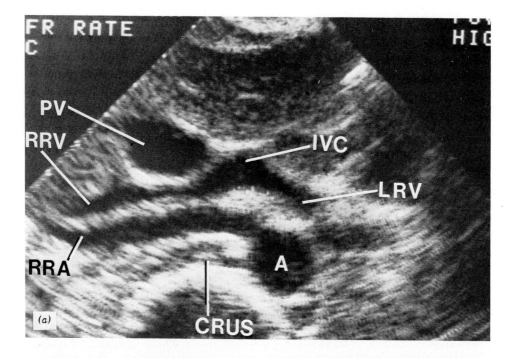

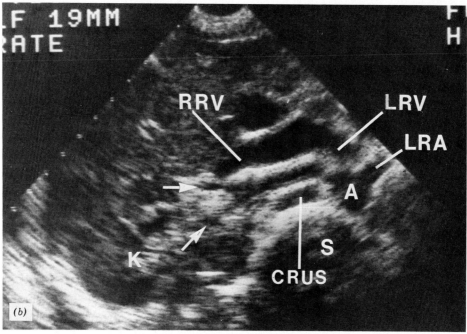

Figure 9-5 (*a* and *b*) Transverse ultrasonograms demonstrating various renal vessels, including the right renal vein (RRV), left renal vein (LRV), and the right renal artery (RRA). In transverse image (*b*), note the branching (arrows) of the right renal artery before its entrance into the right kidney (K). LRA = left renal artery; A = aorta; S = spine; PV = portal vein.

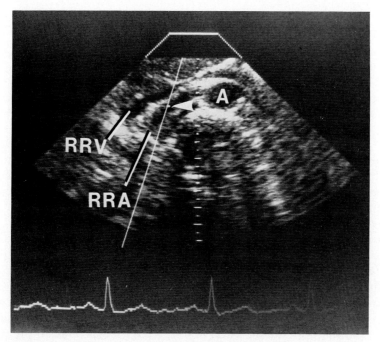

Figure 9-6 Real-time transverse supine ultrasonogram shows the right renal vein (RRV) and right renal artery (RRA). A pulsed Doppler sample volume was obtained with the bright dot (arrowhead) along the sample line seen to be in the region of the right renal artery. The structure immediately anterior is the right renal vein and posterior is a portion of the crus of the diaphragm. A = aorta.

TECHNIQUE

As with any diagnostic study, technique is all important and must be mastered thoroughly if credible results are to be achieved. Most mistakes in ultrasonic renal diagnosis occur not because of ignorance or misinterpretation, but because of poor technique. This in turn, leads to opinions based on images that are, in fact, uninterpretable.

Optimal demonstration of renal anatomy is accomplished when the highest ultrasonic frequency that will image the kidney without producing objectionable back scatter echoes in the renal parenchyma is used. This is usually 3.5 MHz for average-sized adults and 5 MHz for children and thin adults, especially those thin adults whose kidneys contain large amounts of fluid. Medium-focus transducers are best for scanning in the decubitus and prone positions. Long-focus transducers should be available for supine scanning and for any situations where the kidneys are 10 cm or more from the anterior abdominal wall.[7]

When examining the kidneys, it is helpful to scan the organ quickly in various positions with real time. High-resolution sector scanners are ideal for this purpose. In this fashion, not only can an initial impression of whether the kidneys are normal or diseased be obtained, but the most optimal position for further static (articulated arm) scanning can be quickly determined. As the resolution of modern real-time scanners improves, the number of patients in whom real-time renal images prove definitive is increasing rapidly. It is possible to begin and end a nephrosonographic examination with real-time imaging alone whenever these images appear to provide clear and unequivocal evidence of the information being sought. On occasion, real-time imaging of the kidneys may need to be supplemented by conventional (static) scanning.

Static, or articulated arm, scanning is begun first in the supine position with a series of saggital plane sweeps of the transducer over the liver in an effort to image the right kidney (Fig. 9-1). Following this, the patient is turned to the left decubitus position and transverse and coronal images of the right kidney are made. Finally, if needed, prone images of the right kidney in the sagittal and cross-sectional planes are made (Figs. 9-4 and 9-7). For the left kidney, the supine approach is usually inadequate because of interposed bowel gas. The right lateral decubitus position, therefore, is usually chosen to start, and a series of transverse and coronal sections is made (Fig. 9-8). As with the right kidney, prone imaging is done last. In general, we usually obtain prone longitudinal scans by moving the transducer in a sector fashion from cranial to caudal. With gray scale ultrasound, a single linear or sector scan (single-pass scanning) rather than compound sectoring usually produces the best image. Supine and coronal sector scans in the lateral decubitus position are made by sweeping the transducer in the opposite direction that is, from the iliac crest to the subcostal margin (caudocranial). Once the general area of the kidney including its upper

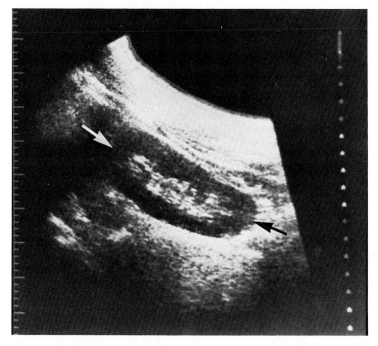

Figure 9-7 Prone longitudinal ultrasonogram of the kidney demonstrates the typical configuration, with bright central echoes and capsule as well as the weaker parenchymal echoes. Arrows designate limits of upper and lower poles.

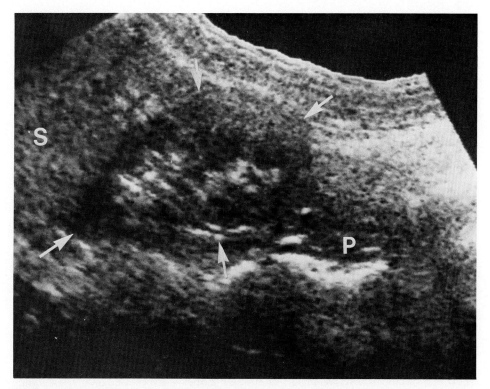

Figure 9-8 Coronal image of the left kidney (arrows) obtained by placing the patient in a right lateral decubitus position. S = spleen; P = psoas muscle.

and lower extent has been localized, transverse scans can be obtained. Real-time ultrasound is most useful in this task, since it can easily determine both the lateral and anterior angulations of the lower pole of the kidney and can thereby pinpoint its true axis in several planes. Transverse views may then be obtained at various locations along these axes in the supine, lateral decubitus, or prone positions as desired (Fig. 9-9). Transverse scans are made at 1-cm intervals proceeding from the lower pole of the kidney to the upper pole and just beyond.

In addition to real time, the true longitudinal axis of the kidney may be obtained in the following way. The examiner marks on the skin surface the maximum diameter of the kidney as shown on its transverse scan. These dots can then be connected at the completion of the transverse scanning process. The line thus made will indicate the axis of the longest diameter of the kidney. Longitudinal scans can then be obtained along this axis at set intervals of approximately 1 to 1.5 cm outlining the entire thickness of the kidney in this projection. An average of five to six sections are usually necessary to image the kidney adequately in the sagittal mode, while coronal sectioning can usually be accomplished with three to four passes. The number of transverse images is variable depending on the length of the kidney and the type of information being obtained. Generally, the diagnosis is apparent on the longitudinal images

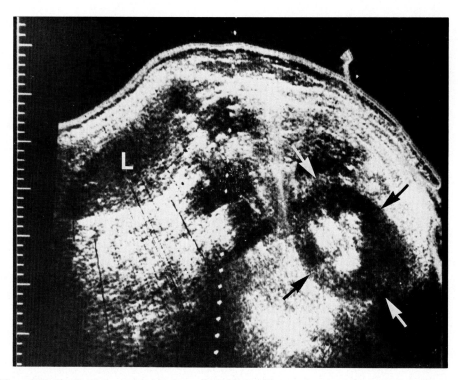

Figur 9-9 Supine transverse image of the left kidney (arrows) obtained by scanning anteriorly and laterally producing a cross-sectional image. In most cases, the ideal imaging is obtained by allowing the sound to be transmitted through the flank, since in the supine position the air-filled bowel usually prevents adequate penetration. L = liver.

making it unnecessary to make more than five or six renal images in the transverse plane.

Although it is relatively easy to outline the lower pole of the kidney unless it extends below the iliac crest, it sometimes may be difficult to outline the upper pole in the prone position. There are two major factors responsible for this: (1) Interposition of aerated lung between the transducer and the kidney, and (2) the presence of ribs overlying the kidney. This is one of the advantages of using the supine and lateral decubitus approaches. In the presence of overlying lung an image cannot be obtained, while ribs produce such attenuation of the ultrasonic beam that the chances of recording echoes from beneath it are poor. Reverberations from rib edges may also create difficulty in obtaining a satisfactory image and may produce artifacts as well. There are several methods of avoiding these problems; one, of course, is by the use of coronal sectioning in the lateral decubitus position. Another method is to obtain the scan in deep inspiration or expiration. With deep inspiration, the upper pole of the kidney may be displaced sufficiently caudad to allow a recording to be obtained. This does not always work, however, since the overinflated lung may accompany the kidney inferiorly and become superimposed. In such cases, an expiration study may allow a recording of the upper renal pole to be obtained. Another method is to perform scanning with the patient sitting or standing (Fig. 9-10). This usually brings out the kidney's maximum mobility. For documentation of degrees of ptosis, comparison recordings can be made between the prone and erect positions. Another technique of visualizing the upper pole of the kidney in the prone position is to angle the transducer cranially just as the lower rib is reached. In the supine position, changes in the degree of inspiration can also be helpful especially in moving the liver down over the kidney, which helps to displace any bowel gas from around the lower pole. The lower pole of a ptotic kidney that is partly obscured from ultrasonic evaluation because of the overlying iliac bone can sometimes be elevated out of the pelvis by placing a small sandbag or pillow beneath the lower pole of the kidney when imaging in the prone position. Supine and lateral decubitus views, of course, may obviate the need for this.

All ultrasonic renal scanning should be performed during suspended respiration. Since the kidney is normally mobile, motion occurs during scanning unless special pains are taken to avoid it. If careful attention is not given to this point, the resultant images could be blurred, and small structures or masses could easily be rendered indistinguishable.

When scanning in the supine position, both longitudinal and transverse scans of the right kidney are obtained through the liver using this structure as an

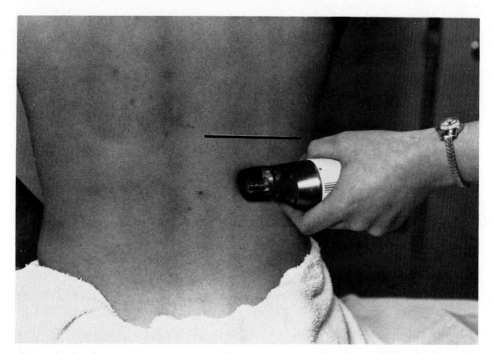

Figure 9-10 Ultrasound examination of a patient in the erect position to evaluate for ptosis of the kidney. Line on the skin of the patient notes the upper pole of the kidney before rescanning in the erect position.

acoustical window. Longitudinal sweeps usually are started from below the level of the umbilicus and swept upward until the costal margin is encountered by the transducer. At this point, the transducer is then angled cephalad without passing over the ribs. Again, to obtain maximum resolution the scans are obtained during suspended respiration. The scanning is initially linear in nature with sectoring under the rib cage. Once the upper and lower renal poles have been delineated by the longitudinal scans, transverse scanning may be begun, with care being taken to avoid interference from the anterior ribs. Satisfactory images of the left kidney are not usually obtainable in the supine position because of overlying bowel gas. Occasionally however, an interposed parenchymal structure such as a large left lobe of the liver, an enlarged spleen, or a fluid-filled stomach may displace the bowel and allow a sonic window through which the left kidney may be examined (Fig. 9-11).[8]

The best approach for evaluating the left kidney, therefore, is the coronal view. As indicated previously, this is also an extremely suitable approach for the right kidney as well. When imaging in this position, the patient lies on either the right or left side; that is, the side opposite the kidney of interest. Since a true lateral transducer sweep does not give an anatomic coronal representation of the kidney because of the normal dorsal angulation of this

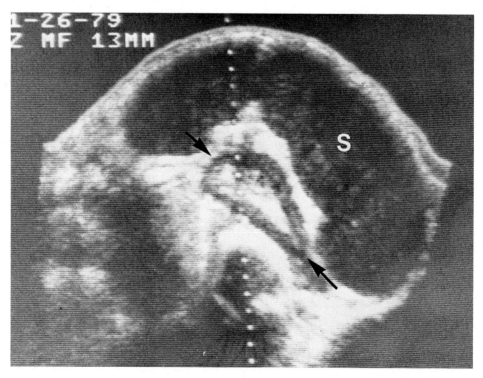

Figure 9-11 Supine transverse ultrasonogram shows the presence of a large spleen (S) extending laterally and anteriorly. The enlarged spleen has displaced the left kidney (arrows) from its normal location.

organ, a posterior oblique mode has been recommended.[9] Normally, the kidneys are dorsally angled approximately 30 to 40 degrees, but there is a wide range of normal. Angulation of the transducer by this amount intersects a more anatomic coronal plane through the kidney and gives a truer coronal image. The transducer is moved initially in a longitudinal direction. If ribs are interfering, the best approach is to place the transducer in the soft tissues between the superior aspect of the iliac crest and the inferior costal margin. Sector scans can then be obtained moving the transducer 1 cm at a time until the region of the kidney is recorded. Transverse scans are then obtained after the kidney has been demonstrated in the coronal view. Again, suspended respiration is needed for maximal detail. Scanning should be attempted in either sustained inspiration or expiration if initial studies do not provide adequate visualization.

If visualization of the main renal vessels is desired, scans are obtained in the supine position. The abdominal aorta is first localized in the longitudinal direction, and the level of the origin of the superior mesenteric artery (SMA) is demonstrated. The renal arteries usually originate just distal to this point. A mark is made on the skin at the level of the SMA aortic junction during longitudinal scanning, and the patient is then repositioned for transverse scanning. Recordings are obtained starting at the level of the SMA and moving in a generally caudad direction 3 mm at a time. The transducer sweep should be short over these areas without sectoring and with all scans obtained during suspended respiration. High-resolution real time has a distinct advantage here since the transducer can be easily and rapidly moved over the area of interest to determine the appropriate angle for best visualization of the renal vessels. In thin patients, it is also possible to obtain images of the kidney with the same technique, but obesity or the presence of bowel gas usually precludes this.[10] Demonstration of the renal arteries also allows measurement of their depth beneath the skin surface. By using gray scale B-scan or real-time gray scale in combination with pulsed Doppler ultrasound, the luminal diameter of these vessels can be obtained and the flow rate of blood within them may be calculated as well (Fig. 9-1).[11] In many cases, the renal veins can also be visualized. The left renal vein often is seen as it passes transversely between the abdominal aorta and superior mesenteric artery before entering the vena cava; the right renal vein enters directly into the vena cava.

Experience has suggested that, in general, the better hydrated the patient, the easier it is to depict that patient's kidneys ultrasonically. The reason for this is not clear, but may be related to the kidneys' increased fluid content during diuresis. The difference in the appearance of the hydrated and nonhydrated kidney is not vast, however, and even in the presence of severe dehydration adequate renal sonograms should be obtainable. If the renal images are not entirely satisfactory, repeating the examination with hydration should be considered. It should be noted that the use of iodinated water-soluble contrast agents does not interfere with renal sonography. When examining the kidneys, even though only one kidney may be under suspicion for the presence of disease, it is strongly recommended that both kidneys be scanned as a matter of routine.

RENAL MASSES

One of the earliest and perhaps still the most frequently employed urologic uses of ultrasound is the differential diagnosis of renal masses. Because of the relative frequency of asymptomatic masses, most of which are serous cysts, the development of a safe, reliable, and inexpensive method of investigating renal masses, based on ultrasound as the keystone study, has been a boon to patients, physicians, and third-party medical intermediaries alike. It has been estimated that as many as 600,000 new renal cysts occur each year in American adults.[12] In addition to simple serous cysts, there are many other masses that can involve the kidney including neoplasms, abscesses, hematomas, multilocular cysts, granulomas, and others. Table 9-1 represents a tabulation of all the ultrasonically examined renal masses in adults that we encountered in an 8-year period. The differentiation of these masses is based to a great extent on their sonographic patterns of which three main types are recognized: (*1*) The fluid pattern that is obtained from fluid-filled masses such as cysts, (*2*) the solid pattern that is obtained from parenchymatous lesions such as neoplasms, and (*3*) a complex or mixed pattern that is seen with masses having both fluid and solid components. There is further refinement of classification within these categories as is discussed in the following paragraphs.

Fluid-Filled Masses

The typically fluid-filled or cystic renal mass is seen as a sharply defined echo-free zone having strong far-wall echoes (Fig. 9-12). Since sound passing through a uniform fluid is not reflected, but sound encountering a fluid-solid interface is strongly reflected, both an echo-free zone and strong far-wall echoes are required to make the diagnosis of a cystic mass. Failure to adhere to this admonition results in mistakes in diagnosis. Since the distal wall of the cyst is seen as a smooth surface, the display of echoes from this area appears as a smooth line. Closer to the transducer, the proximal wall also presents a strong

Table 9-1 Types of Renal Masses Encountered in 775 Patients

Renal Mass	Number Encountered	Percent
Cysts	571	74
Neoplasms	70	9
Pseudotumors	62	8
Focal hydronephrosis	18	2
Abscesses	17	2
Hematomas	12	1.5
Polycystic disease	11	1.5
Urinoma	5	
Vascular malformations	5	
Focal pyelonephritis	3	2
Xanthogranuloma	1	

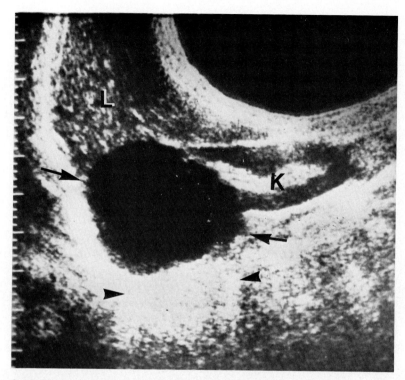

Figure 9-12 Supine longitudinal ultrasonogram demonstrates a large cyst (arrows) of the upper pole of the right kidney having the typical appearance of smooth walls with distal echo enhancement (arrowheads) and an echo-free central area. L = liver; K = kidney.

interface, but because of reverberation echoes, the near wall of the cyst frequently lacks the smooth, even contour of the far wall. As the sensitivity is increased, reverberation echoes are more likely to be recorded. Reverberation echoes or "false" echoes are present with solid masses as well as with cystic ones, but they are not normally recognized with the former because they are obscured by the true echoes. When there is a problem differentiating false from true echoes, scans should be obtained in two planes and compared. Echoes truly originating from within a mass do not change with changes in the direction of the ultrasound beam and they are stronger and more persistent than reverberation echoes (Fig. 9-13). In addition, an important finding in cystic masses is that the through transmission of sound is great, but with solid masses, the opposite is true (Fig. 9-14). Another characteristic of renal cysts is their tendency to be spherical or slightly ellipsoid. The marked transition between the enhanced sound transmission through the cyst and the partially attenuated zones on either side of it present as straight divergent lines that have been referred to by Sanders as the "lateral shades sign."[13] If there is any question about the strength of the through transmission, comparison can be made with the filled urinary bladder. In fact, the sonolucency of any mass can be compared with that of the equivalent-sized bladder. With masses smaller than the bladder,

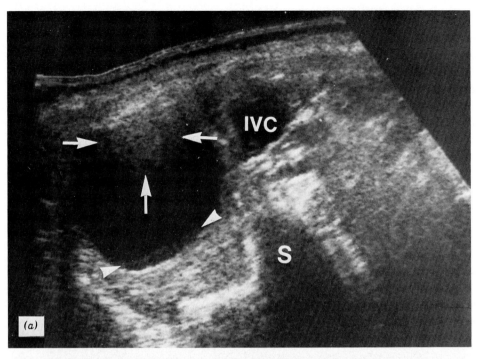

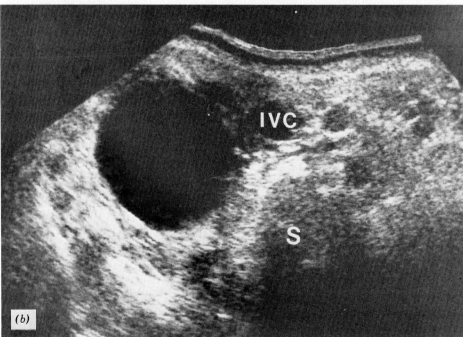

Figure 9-13 (*a*) Predominantly echo-free mass shows anterior echoes (arrows) that are due to reverberations and distal weak echoes (arrowheads) due to poor lateral resolution resulting in echoes arising from the walls of the cyst. (*b*) When the angle of the transducer was changed these echoes disappeared. IVC = inferior vena cava; S = spine.

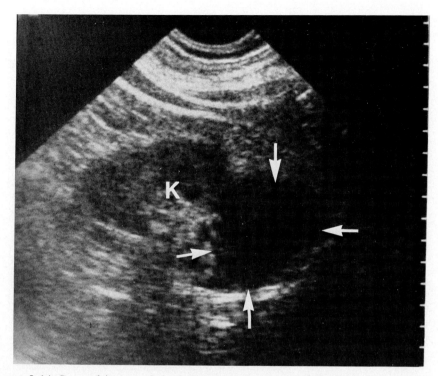

Figure 9-14 Coronal image of the left kidney (K) shows evidence of a hypoechogenic mass (arrows) of the lower pole with relatively poor through sound transmission compared to that which would be expected from a cyst (i.e., Figure 9-12). This was a renal cell carcinoma.

this viscus can be compressed until the diameter that lies in the path of the ultrasonic beam becomes roughly equal to that of the mass in question.

The minimum size of lesion that can be imaged reliably by ultrasound depends on both the frequency employed and the depth of the mass. Because of beam divergence, the deeper the mass, the larger it must be to allow satisfactory resolution. When a standard 3.5- to 5-MHz transducer is used, superficial masses less than 1 cm in diameter can be assessed accurately, while with deeper masses, at the approximate depth of the kidney, a diameter of approximately 1 to 1.5 cm is required to allow accurate evaluation (Fig. 9-15). By using higher frequency and appropriately focused transducers, masses much smaller than 1 cm in diameter can be differentiated, but the depth of penetration, of course, falls off as the frequency increases. The ability to differentiate a deeply placed mass is related to the width of the ultrasonic beam at the level of the mass and, therefore, to beam divergence. Since the lateral resolution is inversely proportional to the beam width, there is poor resolution of those structures smaller than the diameter of the beam itself. In such cases, echoes produced from structures immediately adjacent to the mass appear to originate from within the mass, thus imparting a complex quality to cystic masses (Fig. 9-13). With the use of electronic focusing and variable frequencies, however, it is possible to differentiate much smaller masses.

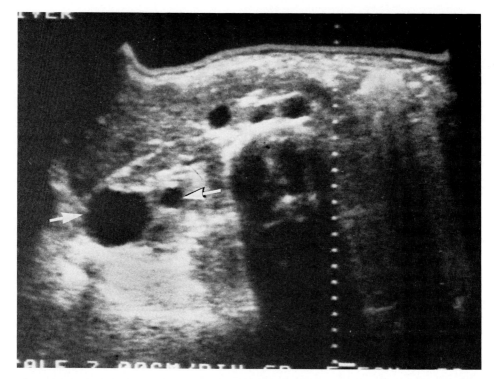

Figure 9-15 Supine transverse ultrasonogram of the right kidney shows evidence of two cysts (arrows), one measuring slightly greater than 2 cm in diameter and the other, 1 cm. A standard 3.5-MHz medium-focused transducer was used. Note that the enhancement behind the larger cyst is greater than that of the smaller cyst. This would be expected due to the laws of ultrasonic physics.

It must be emphasized that cystic patterns can be produced not only by liquids but by any tissue or substance that acoustically behaves like a liquid.[14] For example, uniform gelatin-like clots, abscesses consisting only of leukocytes without debris, and of course, unclotted blood, all show cystic patterns.[15] In addition, there are a few solid lesions that occasionally produce a pattern that so closely simulates a cystic one that only the most scrupulous and meticulous technique can be depended on to differentiate them. This is described in more detail in the section on solid masses. We have found it beneficial in the study of renal masses to confirm all gray scale images with a simple A-mode recording from the mass whenever there is any question as to its fluid nature. With A-mode, the pattern produced is only that contributed by passage of a sound beam through the mass. This is, of course, true also when real-time ultrasound is used.

In our hands, the accuracy with which a renal cyst can be identified by ultrasound is approximately 98 percent.[16] That is, approximately 2 percent of all renal cysts are misrepresented as tumors or overlooked completely. The reasons why some cysts are incorrectly diagnosed or completely missed are (*a*) the diameter is less than 1 to 2 cm, (*b*) the wall is calcified, (*c*) technical pitfalls, such as breathing, marked obesity, incorrect transducer, gain setting too low, etc., and (*d*) faulty interpretation. The most common lesions that may be most frequently misinterpreted as simple renal cysts are listed in Table 9-2. Some of these, such as calyceal diverticula may be impossible to differentiate unless they contain debris or other non-fluid material (Fig. 9-16). In contrast to the approximately 2 percent inaccuracy rate in diagnosing renal cysts by ultrasonography, the reliability of a typically cystic pattern obtained from a renal mass approaches a 100 percent confidence level when strict diagnostic parameters are met.[17-20] Pollack et al have broken down the patterns obtained from cystic renal masses into three subgroups.[17] In pattern I, all of the ultrasonographic criteria for a renal cyst are met, and this has proved unerringly accurate in their experience in allowing a definitive diagnosis of a renal cyst to be made. Routine renal cyst puncture with double-contrast cystography is unnecessary for diagnostic confirmation in pattern I lesions. Patterns II and III represented cystic lesions that lacked one or more of the qualities of a renal cyst, pattern III being more atypical than pattern II. In these two subgroups, they noted several cystic neoplasms. They recommended, therefore, that further studies

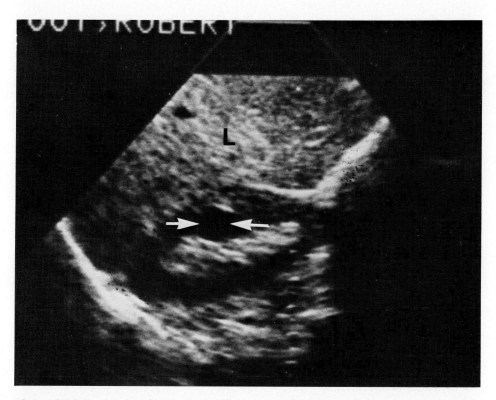

Figure 9-16 Supine longitudinal scan shows a small echo-free mass (arrows) located in the midportion of the right kidney adjacent to the central collecting system. While differentiation between calyceal diverticulum and renal cyst would be difficult, the most likely diagnosis would be renal cyst in terms of frequency. Intravenous urogram was needed to eliminate the possibility of a diverticulum. L = liver.

Table 9-2   Lesions That May Mimic Renal Cysts by Ultrasound

Intrarenal vascular malformations (i.e., AVMs, aneurysms)

Hematomas

Abscesses

Urine collections (i.e., localized hydronephrosis, urinoma)

Cysts containing small mural tumors[a]

Necrotic hemorrhagic tumors[a]

Lymphoma[a]

Renal pyramids[a]

[a] Rare causes.

be done in patients who had cystic patterns that were not prototypically those of an uncomplicated renal cyst, that is, patterns II and III.

Complex Masses

Complex masses may be considered to be essentially fluid-like masses that differ in that they contain echo-generating internal reflecting interfaces. These echoes, unlike reverberations, are persistent and constant in location if the position of the patient is changed. Free debris or clots within a mass change position with alteration of the patient's posture. Since complex masses are composed mainly of material that transmits sound well, their far-wall echoes are strong, although less so than cysts of the same size. The echoes are, however, discernibly stronger than the far-wall echoes emanating from typically solid masses (Fig. 9-17). This can be confirmed in most cases by comparing the far-wall echoes of the complex mass in question with the distal-wall echoes of the adjacent normal kidney. Normal kidneys transmit sound less well than complex masses. The most common renal lesions associated with complex patterns are listed in Table 9-3.

The most important mass yielding a complex pattern is a renal neoplasm. Although these lesions usually produce solid patterns, there are certain morphologic variants that are seen primarily as fluid-filled structures. Thus, those renal cell carcinomas that are partly cystic, as well as those associated with a great deal of hemorrhage take on fluid-like characteristics that acoustically may overshadow their basically solid nature. The same is true for neoplasms that have lost much of their blood supply and have become necrotic as a result (Fig. 9-18). The necrotic debris within the tumor becomes jelly-like and acts as a homogenous transmitting medium. If the internal echoes, sometimes sparse, are not recognized, the propensity for misdiagnosis is great. With meticulous technique, however, these low-level echoes are almost always detectable (Fig. 9-19). In questionable cases, needle aspiration of the mass, CT, or angiography should help to provide the correct diagnosis.

Cysts may produce complex patterns when they are multilocular or when they are multiple and placed very close together as in polycystic disease (Fig. 9-20). Here they may be seen as an overall complex mass, although each clear space actually represents an individual cyst. If the cysts are larger than 1 to 2 cm in diameter, as in most adult forms of polycystic disease, they are identifiable

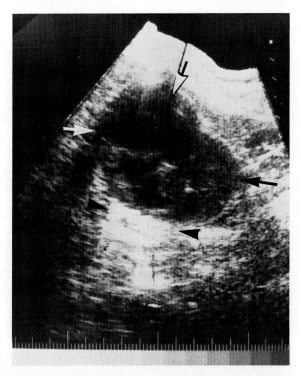

Figure 9-17 Supine longitudinal ultrasonogram shows evidence of a complex mass (arrows) of the upper pole of the kidney. Note the good through sound transmission (arrowheads). There are definite internal echoes mixed with the echo-free areas confirming the complex nature of the mass. This proved to be a necrotic renal cell carcinoma.

as individual lesions (Fig. 9-21). If, on the other hand, they are smaller than this as in infantile polycystic disease, they are not individually recognizable (Fig. 9-22). Cysts that contain either debris (infected cysts) or clot (hemorrhagic cysts) are also complex (Fig. 9-23). Hematomas may demonstrate fragments of clot, and abscesses may show fluid debris levels. Both of these lesions may be either complex or cystic depending on the physical state of their internal milieu. Often the walls of these lesions are not as smooth as the walls of uncomplicated renal cysts. Hemorrhagic infarcts, such as are seen in renal vein thrombosis, for example, also produce a complex pattern, expecially during the acute phase.

Table 9-3   Renal Lesions Producing Complex Sonographic Patterns

Neoplasms (i.e., cystic, hemorrhagic, or necrotic *only*)
Cystis (i.e., infected, multilocular, septated, bloody, or multiple)
Abscesses
Hematomas or hemorrhagic infarcts
Pyonephrosis

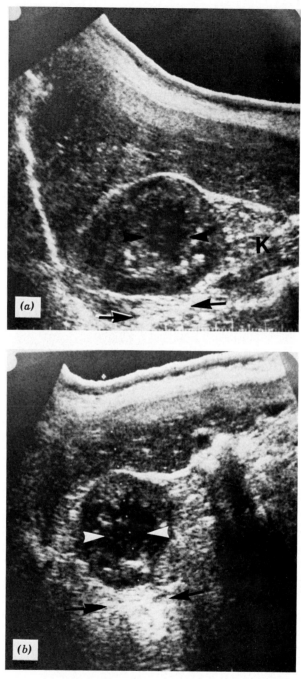

Figure 9-18 Longitudinal (*a*) and transverse (*b*) supine ultrasonograms show evidence of a mass of the upper pole of the kidney (K) with good through-transmission (arrows). The central area of decreased echoes (arrowheads) indicates the beginning necrosis of what proved to be a renal cell carcinoma. These changes are typical of early necrosis and/or hemorrhage within a tumor.

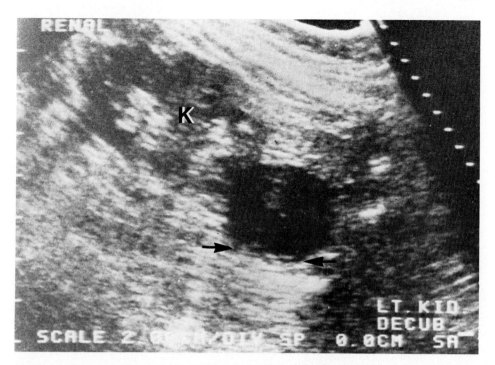

Figure 9-19 Longitudinal coronal image of the left kidney (K) shows evidence of a predominantly cystic mass of the lower pole that has irregular distal walls (arrows) and scattered internal echoes. This irregularity was enough to arouse suspicion. Aspiration confirmed the presence of a highly necrotic renal cell carcinoma.

This is due to areas of hemorrhage and necrosis. The kidney is usually swollen. In some cases, the thrombus may be seen within the renal vein (Fig. 9-24). In contrast, ischemic infarcts secondary to renal artery stenosis tend to look normal ultrasonically. Later, of course, there is some renal atrophy unless the blood supply is reestablished.

Internal echoes may occur from the edges of dilated calyceal rims and fornices converting the fluid pattern of hydronephrosis to an apparently complex one. When the urine in an obstructed kidney is heavily infected, as in pyonephrosis, echogenicity is increased.[21]

Parapelvic and central renal cysts may yield confusing appearances at times, since their central location places them into apposition with the larger renal vessels and the renal pelvis. As a result, extraneous echoes from these normal structures may appear to arise within the cyst, imparting a falsely complex quality to the ultrasonogram (Fig. 9-25). Central renal artery aneurysms can give a similar pattern, but often typical calcifications may be seen on the radiographs. Pulsed Doppler can also be used to detect flow within them. Xanthogranulomatous pyelonephritis may sometimes be detectable as a complex mass or a diffusely infiltrating process involving the entire kidney demonstrating complex characteristics. The mixed fluid-semisolid pattern in these cases, however, is usually attributable to the presence of infected hydronephrosis or even frank pyonephrosis.[22]

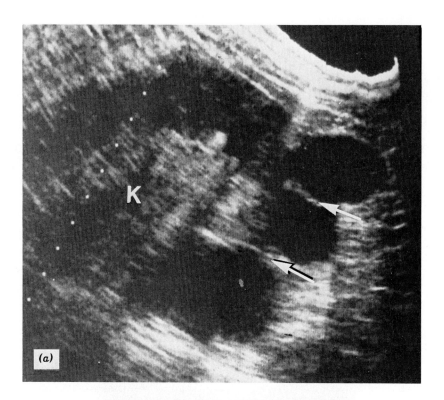

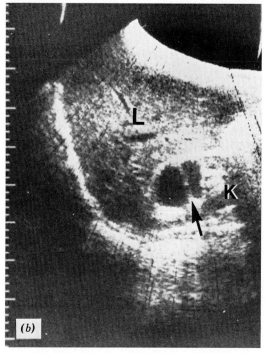

Figure 9-20 (*a*) Decubitus coronal image of the lower left kidney (K) shows evidence of multiple serous cysts of the lower pole. The clearly defined division between each cyst is noted (arrows). (*b*) In another patient, a supine view shows the presence of a cyst of the upper pole with an eccentrically located septum (arrow). L = liver.

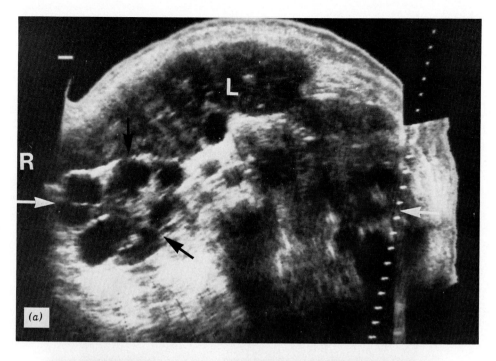

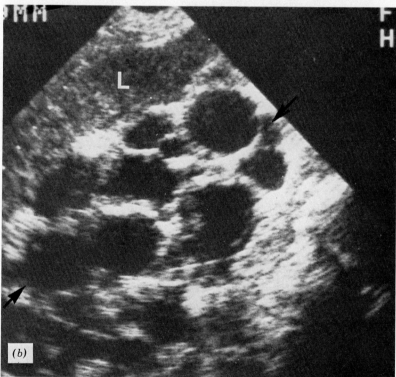

Figure 9-21 Supine transverse (*a*) and longitudinal (*b*) ultrasonograms demonstrate the adult form of polycystic kidney disease (arrows) with multiple cysts of various sizes clearly demonstrated. On the transverse view, a portion of the involved other kidney is also seen. L = liver.

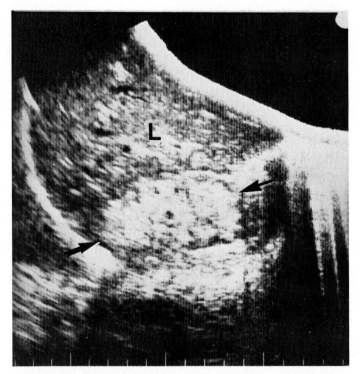

Figure 9-22 Supine longitudinal image of a large echogenic kidney (arrows) showing no discrete cysts. This pattern is typical of infantile polycystic disease. L = liver. (Courtesy of Herman Grossman, M.D., Professor of Radiology and Pediatrics, Duke University.)

Ultrasound has been of great value in differentiating parapelvic and central renal cysts from an entity frequently confused with them—sinus lipomatosis.[23] The latter is a condition characterized by the heavy deposition of fat in the renal sinus often seen in the nephrosclerotic or aging kidney. Although the roentgenographic picture of the two conditions is somewhat similar, they can be distinguished ultrasonically since a cystic or a complex pattern is seen with parapelvic and central cysts, while there is no sonographic evidence of fluid in sinus lipomatosis (Fig. 9-26). In fact, the echogenicity of the renal sinus may well be increased by the presence of abundant fat.

As discussed in the previous section, false complex patterns may occur with cysts smaller than the width of the ultrasonic beam. Such artifacts are hardly disastrous, however, since, if anything, they may cause cystic lesions to appear complex and, therefore, raise the clinician's index of suspicion rather than falsely lower it.

Solid Masses

There are two main features that characterize solid masses, and these may occur individually or together. First, solid masses have the capacity to generate internal echoes that increase in number and in intensity as instrument sensitivity is increased (Fig. 9-27). Second, the sound absorption within the mass is much

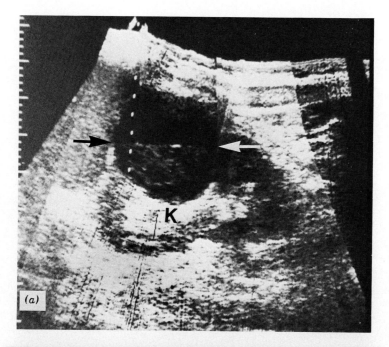

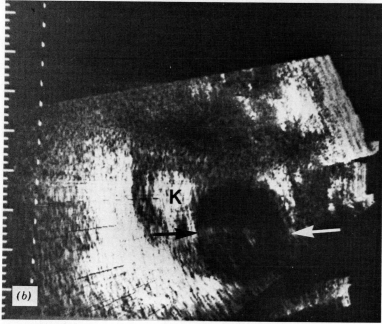

Figure 9-23 Coronal view of the left kidney (K) shows evidence of a predominantly cystic mass with dependent internal echoes that appear to layer (arrows). The presence of debris within what proved to be an infected cyst was confirmed by moving the patient (*b*). This resulted in a shift of the fluid-debris level (arrows).

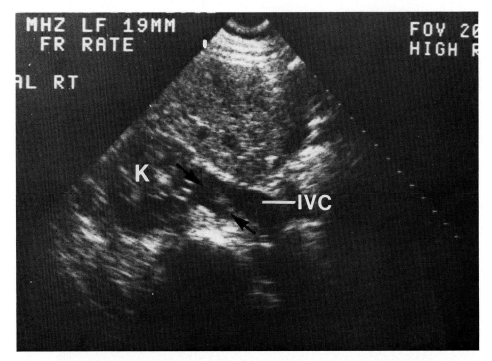

Figure 9-24 Ultrasound image of the right renal vein shows it to be engorged with definite internal echoes that proved to be due to the presence of thrombus (arrows). K = kidney, IVC = inferior vena cava.

greater than that seen with fluid-filled and complex masses, resulting in much weaker distal wall echoes (Fig. 9-28).When identifiable, the back wall is less smooth than in cystic lesions. When compared to the opposite kidney, the sound transmission is no greater; in fact, if the mass is larger than the kidney, the transmission through it is less than through the normal kidney, unless internal necrosis has occurred. In the same way, the urinary bladder may be used as a standard of comparison for the back wall of cystic lesions. Thus, if there is confusion in judging the nature of the far wall of any renal mass, comparison with these two readily available normal structures, the bladder and the opposite kidney, always provides a reliable background for comparison.

Not all masses in this category are uniformly solid; many have areas of hemorrhage or necrosis, and some have cystic components. It is possible to distinguish both the liquid and solid tissues so that a diagnosis of a predominately solid mass containing mixed elements can be made. Echoes need not originate uniformly from the entire mass, since there may be homogeneous areas containing very few reflecting interfaces. The most important quality of the solid mass is the absorption of sound within the mass and the resultant decrease in through transmission. Thus, the strength of the back wall becomes the key point in differentiating these masses from complex and cystic ones. Although the typical solid pattern includes multiple internal echoes, the examiner must not depend on these to make the diagnosis, for to do so is to invite diagnostic disaster (Fig. 9-29).

The reason for the variation in echo-generating properties between solid masses is not understood clearly, but several factors are thought to play a role. One factor is the size of the mass. The larger the mass, the more sound absorption, thus lessening the chances that the weaker echoes will reach the transducer for recording. Another is related to the tumor's vascularity. Although earlier claims[24] that hyperechoic tumors tended to be hypervascular were not entirely borne out by the work of Coleman et al,[25] these authors did find a rough correlation at the other end of the spectrum; that is, there was a slight tendency for the least echoic masses to be hypovascular. Hypovascularity occurs frequently in neoplasms of certain cell types. For example, papillary cystadenocarcinomas (a variant of renal cell carcinoma), lymphomas, sarcomas, and most metastatic tumors to the kidney are usually hypovascular. Still another factor related to the cause of anechoic masses is tissue homogeneity. If a mass is composed of tissue of fairly uniform type, the differences in specific acoustic

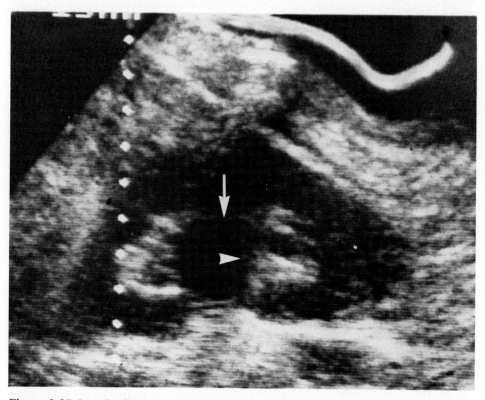

Figure 9-25 Longitudinal coronal view of the left kidney shows evidence of a predominantly cystic central renal mass (arrow) located within the central collecting system. Note that the inferior wall (arrowhead) is not quite as smooth with some minimal internal echoes, suggesting that it may be complex in nature. Aspiration and subsequent contrast filling confirmed the presence of a simple renal cyst.

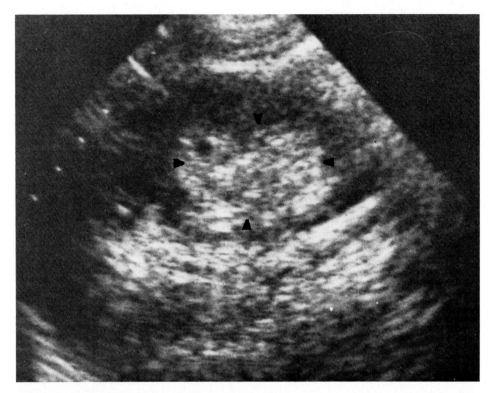

Figure 9-26 Coronal longitudinal image of the left kidney. The central renal sinus area (arrowheads) is markedly increased in its overall area compared to the parenchyma consistent with the diagnosis of renal sinus lipomatosis. Compared to Figure 9-25, it is obvious that cystic masses can be easily differentiated if present.

impedance between adjacent internal structures is slight, and the number and intensity of the echoes produced are diminished accordingly. Lymphomas in particular have been noted to exhibit this characteristic (Fig. 9-30).[26] At the opposite extreme, fat appears to impart a high degree of echogenicity to renal tissue including fat-containing renal masses such as angiomyolipomas (Fig. 9-31). Finally, large areas of hemorrhage, necrosis, or cystic degeneration within a neoplasm are associated within hypoechogeneity (Fig. 9-32). Flecks of calcium, on the other hand, produce increased echogenicity (Figs. 9-33 and 9-34). There are a number of other factors that control the degree of echogenicity within renal tumors, but at this time most of these factors remain unknown.

Rarely, a solid pattern is obtained from a renal mass other than a neoplasm. In our experience, this has happened most commonly in the presence of mural calcification, usually in the wall of a cyst, but occasionally in the wall of a hematoma or abscess. The marked reflection of sound produced by the calcium prevents the through transmission of enough sound to define the far wall (Fig. 9-35). It is important therefore, to correlate the ultrasonic findings with those seen on a roentgenogram at all times, lest obvious oversights such as failure to detect calcification occur. In the same vein, it cannot be overemphasized that

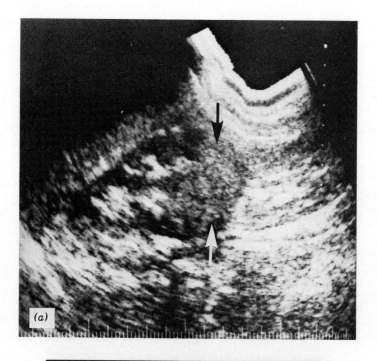

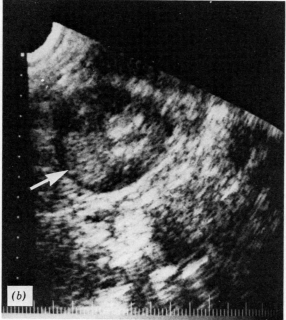

Figure 9-27 Supine longitudinal (*a*) and transverse (*b*) ultrasonograms demonstrate the presence of an echogenic renal tumor (arrows) disrupting the normal parenchymal architecture. This proved to be a renal adenoma.

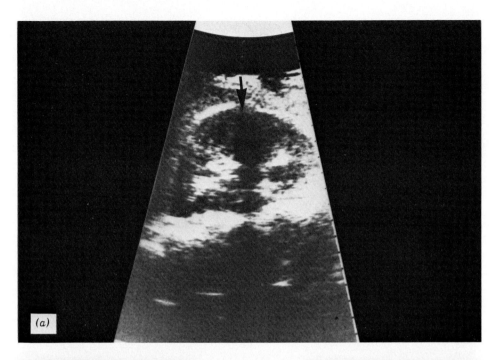

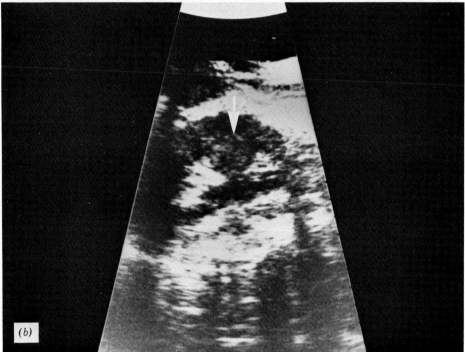

Figure 9-28 (*a*) Coronal view of the left kidney showed evidence of a poorly echogenic mass (arrow) with central acoustic shadowing. (*b*) With increased intensity, the internal echoes were clearly defined (arrow). The tumor can be seen involving the midportion of the renal pelvis and proved to be transitional cell carcinoma.

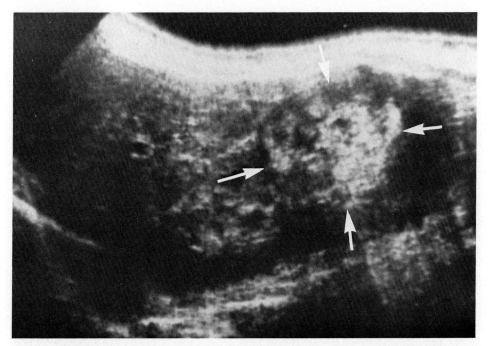

Figure 9-29 Supine longitudinal scan shows evidence of a large regular mass (arrows) of the lower pole with areas of increased and decreased echogenicity. Tumors can have a variety of patterns even within the same mass. This proved to be a renal cell carcinoma.

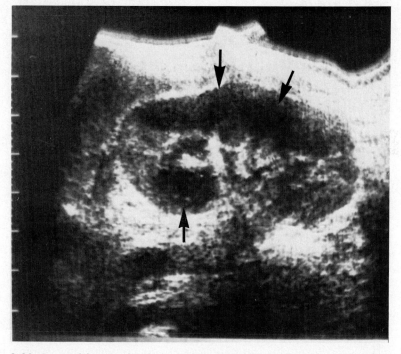

Figure 9-30 Coronal longitudinal view of the left kidney shows it to be enlarged with evidence of several areas of decreased echogenicity (arrows) having mass-like effect within the parenchyma. This is due to the presence of lymphoma.

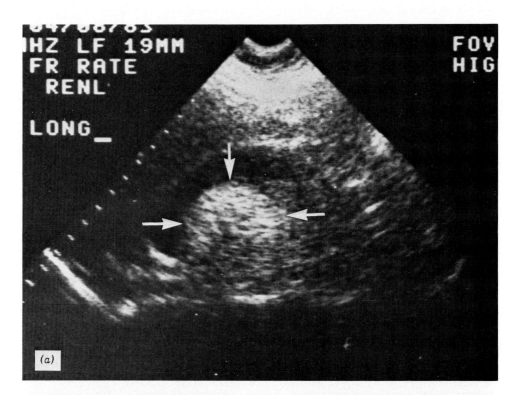

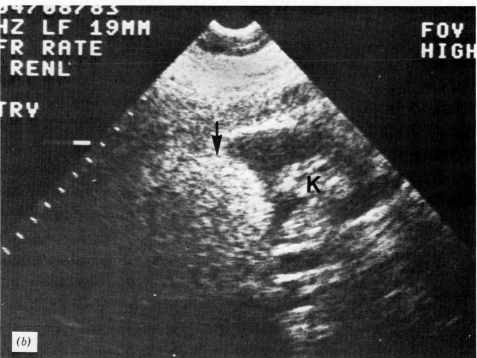

Figure 9-31 Supine longitudinal (*a*) and transverse (*b*) ultrasonograms showing involvement of the right kidney by a highly echogenic mass (arrows) with distal attentuation. These findings are quite typical for angiomyolipoma. K indicates the remaining portion of the kidney. (*c*) CT scan shows the typical changes of this fatty type tumor (arrows).

340

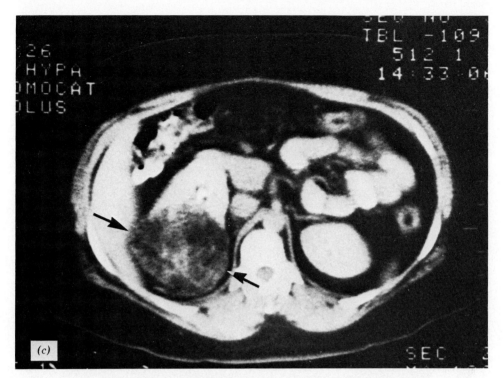

Figure 9-31 (*continued*)

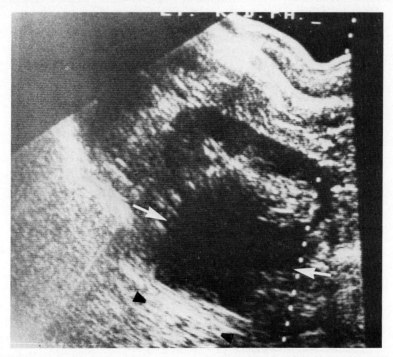

Figure 9-32 Longitudinal coronal image of the left kidney showed evidence of a large medially located irregular complex mass (arrows) with good through transmission (arrowheads) and scattered weak internal echoes. This proved to be a highly necrotic renal cell carcinoma.

341

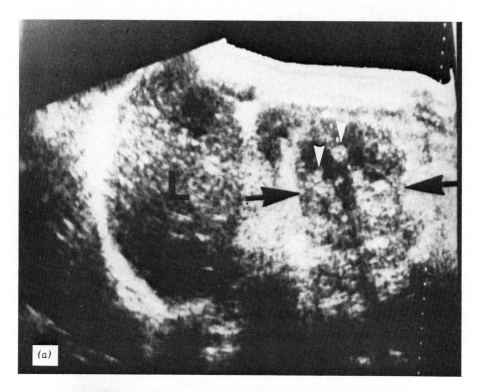

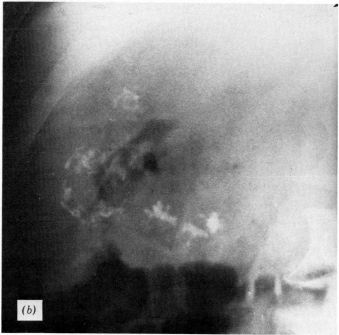

Figure 9-33 (a) Longitudinal supine ultrasonogram shows evidence of a large mass (arrows) distorting the right kidney with bright punctate echoes (arrowheads) producing acoustic shadowing. These proved to be areas of calcification within a renal cell carcinoma. (b) Confirmatory radiograph showed the presence of extensive tumor calcification.

342

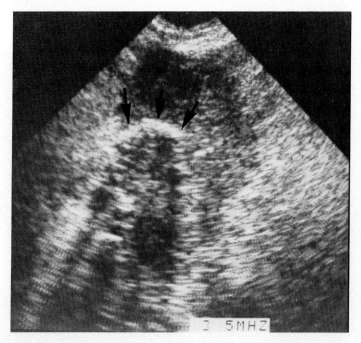

Figure 9-34 Longitudinal decubitus view of the left kidney shows the upper pole to be enlarged with bright curvilinear echoes (arrows) with distal acoustic shadowing highly suggestive of calcification.

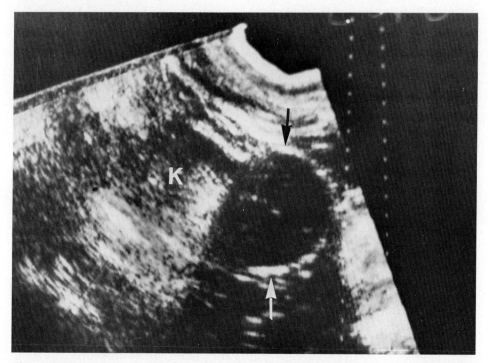

Figure 9-35 Prone longitudinal ultrasound of the right kidney (K) reveals a mass of the lower pole that has a bright rim (arrows) (best seen anteriorly and posteriorly) with distal acoustic shadowing simulating a solid mass. This, however, proved to be a cyst with a calcified wall, which accounts for the attenuation of the sound beam.

343

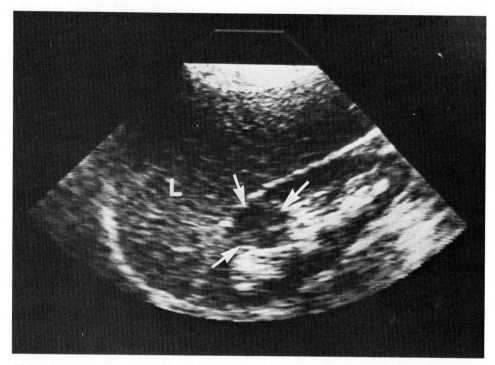

Figure 9-36 Supine longitudinal ultrasonogram of the right kidney shows evidence of what appears to be a mass (arrows) projecting into the central echo pattern. Note the similar echogenicity of the mass compared to the surrounding parenchyma. This was confirmed on isotope scan to be a prominent column of Bertin. L = liver.

ultrasound cannot always be depended on to diagnose solid tumors that are completely intrarenal and that do not bulge the renal contour. The presence or absence of a renal mass is best ascertained at the time of urography before the sonographic examination is performed. An intrarenal tumor may be difficult or impossible to distinguish sonographically from normal renal parenchyma. If, at urography, the presence or absence of a bona fide renal mass cannot be ascertained, then radionuclide scanning should be performed to differentiate between a pseudotumor—such as a column of Bertin (Fig. 9-36)—and a pathologic mass.[28] This differentiation can also be accomplished with CT. In many cases, however, an intrarenal tumor has a different echogenicity than the surrounding parenchyma (Fig. 9-37). In such cases, radionuclide scanning may not be necessary. Other nonneoplastic masses that may impart a solid ultrasonographic appearance are a solitary xanthogranuloma or malakoplakia.

Other characteristics of renal neoplasms include the presence of tumoral calcification (10–20 percent)[29] and tumor extension to the renal vein and the vena cava (4–6 percent).[30] Calcification in renal cell carcinoma may be peripheral and circumferential, punctate, or both. Peripheral calcification that, as mentioned above, produces technical problems in obtaining optimal ultrasonograms, may be seen with either cysts or tumors (Figs. 9-34 and 9-35). Punctate calcification, on the other hand, is almost exclusively seen with neoplasms and can often be recognized by ultrasonography (Fig. 9-33).[16] Venous extension of tumor is also readily detectable by ultrasound and is described further on. Total evaluation of solid renal masses, therefore, includes not only the assessment of the renal mass itself, but also careful evaluation of the vascular drainage of the kidney as well as the retroperitoneal nodes.[31]

Among the most highly echogenic of all renal masses is the angiomyolipoma (Fig. 9-31). The profound echogenicity within this tumor is thought to be attributable to the numerous fatty fibrous interfaces within the lesion. The echogenicity has, at times, been great enough to allow a presumptive diagnosis of angiomyolipoma to be made. However, this cannot be done with extreme reliability, since some highly echogenic renal cell carcinomas can overlap the spectrum of echo production seen with angiomyolipomas. In addition, angiomyolipomas frequently undergo hemorrhage, and a superimposition of blood within the lesion may significantly alter the sonographic characteristics.[32]

Renal masses in infants and children also may be assessed reliably by ultrasound.[33] As in adults, three basic types of patterns are encountered. A cystic pattern in a neonate, especially multiple cysts in the absence of parenchyma suggests multicystic dysplastic kidney (Fig. 9-38) or hydronephrosis.[35,36] These entities can be differentiated easily if a dilated renal pelvis or ureter is seen.[37]

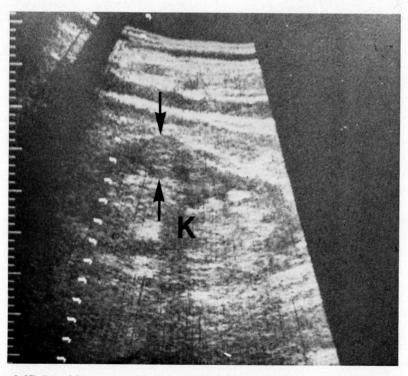

Figure 9-37 Decubitus coronal image of the left kidney shows the presence of a small mass (arrows) within the parenchyma that was slightly more echogenic than the surrounding tissue. The mass measured slightly less than 2 cm in diameter. At surgery it proved to be an oncocytoma. K = kidney.

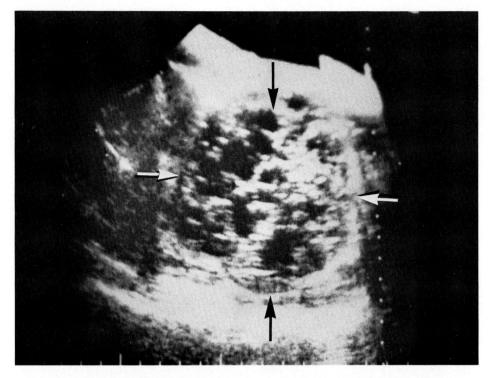

Figure 9-38 Prone longitudinal image of the right kidney (arrows) shows evidence of multiple cysts of varying sizes. These findings based on nonvisualization on intravenous urography suggested a diagnosis of multicystic dysplastic kidney. This was proven at surgery. (Courtesy of Herman Grossman, M.D., Professor of Radiology and Pediatrics, Duke University.)

Such a pattern is not seen with solid lesions. The sonogram of the Wilms' tumor or leiomyomatous hamartoma is solid or complex. Wilms' tumors are usually echogenically homogeneous, although they may contain discrete areas corresponding to areas of cystic necrosis (Fig. 9-39).[38] Echoes are plentiful and, in our experience, uniform and of low intensity. This serves to distinguish them from adrenal neuroblastomas with which they are occasionally confused radiographically. Neuroblastomas are less homogeneous in their appearance.[39] Ultrasonography can also aid in radiation therapy treatment planning of malignant tumors and in the periodic assessment of the renal bed and opposite kidney.

In children, when the presence of disease in one kidney presages the possible development of disease in the other, such as in the case of a Wilms' tumor, ultrasound can be used for follow-up evaluation of the remaining kidney for as long as desired. In a long-term setting, this approach has obvious advantages when compared to roentgenographic techniques, but more data regarding the comparative sensitivity of the two methods in detecting early abnormalities is required before ultrasound can be recommended confidently as a substitute

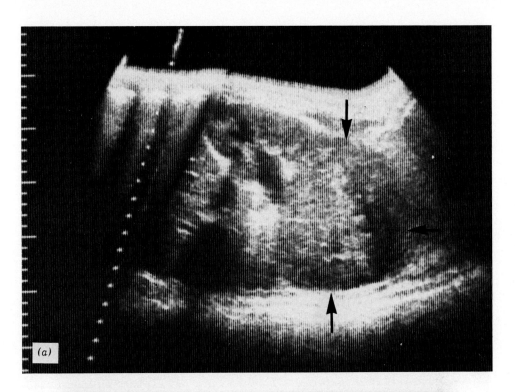

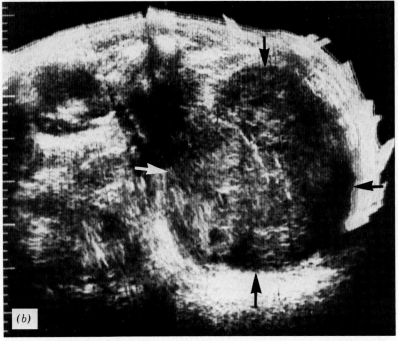

Figure 9-39 Prone longitudinal (*a*) and transverse (*b*) scans show a large mass (arrows) involving the lower pole of the left kidney. A few small areas of degeneration are shown by areas of decreased echogenicity, but the overall pattern is fairly uniform in texture. This was a Wilms' tumor. (Courtesy of Henrietta Rosenberg, M.D., Director, Subdivision of Ultrasound, Children's Hospital of Philadelphia.)

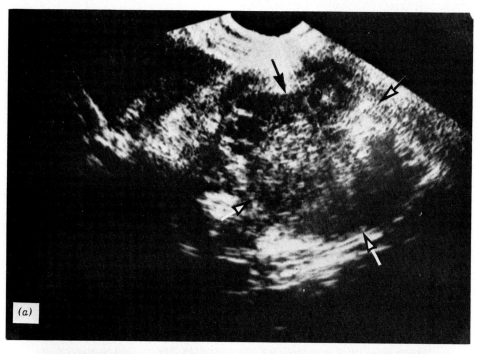

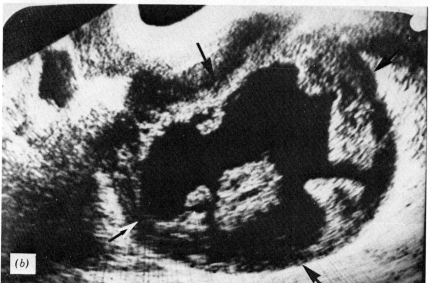

Figure 9-40 (*a*) Prone transverse ultrasonogram shows the presence of a large, predominantly solid, Wilms' tumor (arrows) involving the right kidney. Patient was undergoing radiation and chemotherapy treatment. (*b*) Follow-up examination obtained several months later demonstrated that the tumor had undergone extensive necrosis resulting in a complex pattern.

for urography in such situations. Similarly, children at risk for the development of renal tumors such as those with aniridia, hemihypertrophy, or the Beckwith-Weideman syndrome can be kept under surveillance for the appearance of a renal mass. Adults, too, with familial histories such as polycystic disease and tuberous sclerosis may be examined periodically by ultrasound to detect the appearance of renal masses. In fact, such renal monitoring can be extended to encompass innumerable clinical situations in which periodic reassessment is mandated. In this category are such diverse entities as patients with renal trauma who are being observed for the development of an expanding hematoma, patients with hydronephrosis, patients undergoing nonsurgical management of renal tumors (i.e., embolectomy, radiation therapy), and patients with renal and perinephric urine collections, to name only a few (Fig. 9-40). Leukemic infiltration of the kidneys may be encountered. Sonographically, such kidneys are diffusely enlarged and demonstrate a diffuse increase in echogenicity so that corticomedullary demarcation is lost and the renal sinus echoes are preserved (Fig. 9-41).

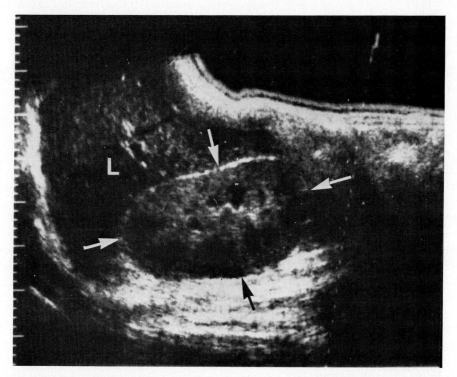

Figure 9-41 Supine longitudinal ultrasonogram of the right kidney shows it to be diffusely enlarged (arrows) with overall decreased echogenicity and loss of the normal bright central echo pattern with prominence of the renal pyramids. This pattern can be seen in type I renal disease. In this case, it was due to the diffuse infiltrative process of Burkett's lymphoma. L = liver.

ASSESSMENT OF RENAL ANATOMY

Ultrasonic renal imaging is of immense value when renal insufficiency precludes adequate depiction of the kidneys by excretory urography. Thus, in a uremic patient, about whom little else is known, an ultrasound examination may provide the necessary information to allow a therapeutic plan to be formulated or a presumptive diagnosis to be made.[12] It is thus the imaging procedure of choice in such a clinical setting.[40] With sonography, the following important facts about the status of the kidney may be ascertained: The number of kidneys present, their location, their size, their shape, the status of the renal pelvis, and to an extent, the presence or absence of certain parenchymal diseases. With these data, it is possible to assess accurately the likelihood of certain entities such as chronic end-stage renal disease, which produces bilaterally small, usually highly echogenic kidneys, with nondilated renal pelvises. It also can be used to rule out obstructive uropathy, polycystic disease, and various anomalies that produce distinctive sonographic patterns. Similar information is helpful when only one kidney is abnormal, such as in the case of a nonvisualized kidney on urography.[41,42] It is sometimes difficult to be certain whether such a kidney is even present. Ultrasound represents a quick relatively effortless and accurate way to find out.

Number of Kidneys

Unilateral renal agenesis occurs in approximately one in 1,000 persons.[43] Frequently, such people, as well as an occasional patient who has had a nephrectomy, are unaware that they have only one kidney. Even patients having this knowledge are sometimes too ill to impart it to their physician. Ultrasonic examination readily provides this information, although ordinarily urography would have detected it first. However, in severely uremic or traumatized patients or even under more normal conditions, urography may not prove definitive. Some patients with renal agenesis are initially suspected of having unilateral nonfunction. It is here that ultrasound achieves its maximum value, possibly obviating the need for retrograde pyelography or angiography. Obviously, the knowledge that patients in either of the above categories have only one kidney is of critical importance in their management. If a kidney cannot be imaged in the usual flank location, a search should be made for it in the pelvis. If not found there, the kidney must be either absent or so small as to be undetectable. The knowledge that a second kidney is present is equally important. We have seen several cases of newborns with hydronephrotic kidneys who were thought by urography to have only one kidney, but who were shown by sonography to have a small contralateral kidney. Ultrasonography is highly accurate in detecting absence of a kidney, although small nubbins of renal tissue may be overlooked. Not only is there a lack of any reniform structure in the renal fossa when the kidney is absent, but large or small bowel loops may be seen in this location instead.[41] Careful attention must be given to the anatomy of any structures seen in the flank lest such bowel loops be mistaken for a hydronephrotic kidney. In the neonate with renal agenesis, the adrenal gland has sometimes been mistaken for the kidney.[44]

Location of Kidneys

Although ectopically located kidneys usually are noted at urography, an occasional case is overlooked because of impaired function or perhaps because of obscurity by the underlying skeleton. Fortunately, it is possible to image pelvic kidneys by ultrasound in most instances, although, obviously, this must be done in the supine position and preferably with a filled urinary bladder (Fig. 9-42). Ectopic kidneys may be located at any point between the upper abdomen and the pelvis, and the search for them must be very purposeful and complete. The diagnosis is suspected when it is discovered that both kidneys are not present in their normal location. In the absence of prior nephrectomy, this observation mandates the need for immediate pelvic ultrasonography. The long axis of the pelvic kidney is frequently at an unconventional angle, making it difficult to obtain detailed visualization of the central echo complex by non-real-time techniques. With real-time ultrasound, of course, the long axis can be obtained rapidly. The detection of a pelvic kidney is especially important in female patients who are scheduled to undergo exploratory laparotomy for a "pelvic mass." Ectopic kidneys often exhibit associated pathology, such as ureteropelvic junction obstruction and calculi, and these complications also may be recognized. The location of kidneys that have been displaced from their normal locations by masses or other abnormalities also may be ascertained by ultrasound as well as by roentgenography. This is discussed further in Chapter 10.

Renal Size

The size of the kidneys is one of the most important determinants of prognosis in patients with renal failure. Generally speaking, those patients with small kidneys have a poor outlook, since they usually suffer from so-called "medical" renal disease, which is the contracted end-stage kidney of chronic glomerulonephritis, chronic pyelonephritis, nephrosclerosis, etc. or rarely, from bilateral congenital hypoplasia (Fig. 9-43). Surgery ordinarily plays little if any role in the management of such patients.

Patients in renal failure with normal-sized or even enlarged kidneys generally have a better prognosis, although there are notable exceptions to this such as renal cortical necrosis. Acute pyelonephritis, tubular necrosis, and amyloidosis are examples of renal disease accompanied by normal-sized or enlarged kidneys, although the former is a rare cause of renal failure. Those who can be helped surgically by stone removal or release of obstruction are usually also found in this category. Renal vein thrombosis, adult and infantile polycystic disease, xanthogranulomatous pyelonephritis, and leukemic infiltration usually cause renal enlargement. Duplicated kidneys and compensatory hypertrophy are the most common causes of unilateral global renal enlargement.

Renal size can be accurately estimated by ultrasonography. Brandt et al found the mean right renal length to be 10.74 cm and the left 11.10 cm, values approximately 1 cm less than those obtained by radiographic measurement. They attributed this to a lack of geometric magnification and osmotic diuretic renal swelling when ultrasound is used.[45]

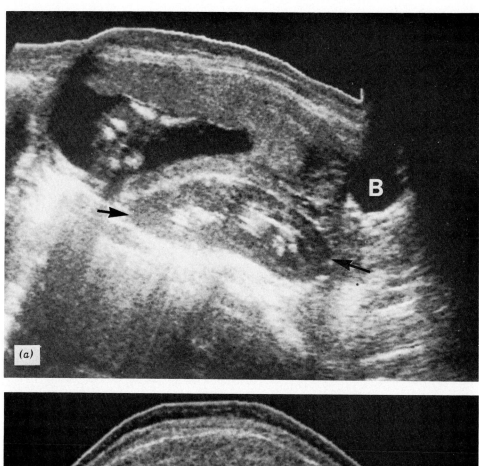

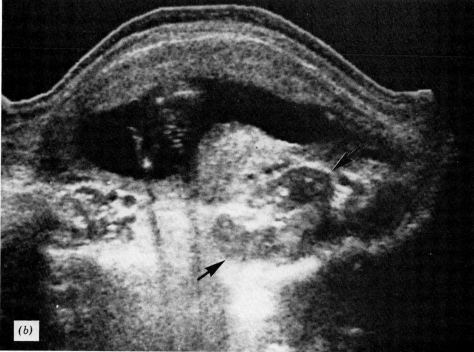

Figure 9-42 Supine longitudinal (*a*) and transverse (*b*) ultrasonograms of the pelvis show the presence of a left-sided ectopic kidney (arrows) posterior to the pregnant uterus. Obviously with this pregnancy the need for a full urinary bladder to visualize the kidney was not necessary. B = urinary bladder.

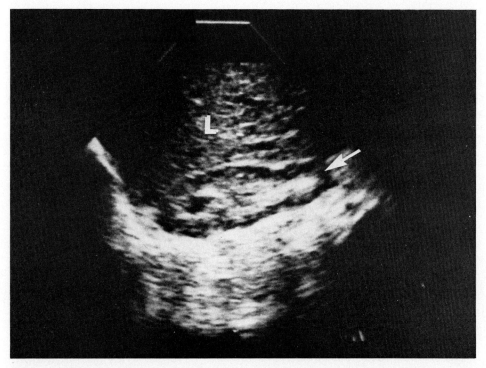

Figure 9-43 Supine longitudinal ultrasonogram delineates a small right kidney. Note the irregularity and volume loss of the lower pole (arrow). L = liver.

The volume of the kidney can be estimated accurately by ultrasonography.[46] Techniques for measuring both the volume and renal length have been developed.[47] Sonographically determined renal length appears to be more accurate than radiographically determined length, although this is not necessarily true for volume determinations.[46] Ultrasonically determined renal dimensions are generally 15 to 20 percent less than their roentgenographically determined counterparts, even allowing for magnification. This is the result of magnification of the long axis of the kidneys on radiographs.

Renal Shape

Abnormalities in the shape of kidneys occur primarily as a result of congenital anomalies. Polycystic and multicystic disease, which have been discussed previously, are examples of disturbances in morphology that can be evaluated nicely by ultrasound. While the shape of the kidney in infantile polycystic disease is generally reniform, gross distortion in the renal outline is commonly encountered in the adult variety. The ultrasonographic pattern of adult polycystic disease, which reveals innumerable large and small cysts, is pathognomonic in addition to being highly sensitive. In fact sonography is the most sensitive noninvasive method available for detecting this lesion. Many authors have shown that this disease—which invariably involves both kidneys sooner or later—can be detected sonographically before it becomes manifest by urography.[48,49] In addition, involvement of the liver, spleen, and pancreas can be identified if present. Liver involvement is estimated to occur in as many as 25 percent of all affected adults.

Fusion anomalies such as horseshoe kidney can also be depicted sonographically. The isthmus usually can be identified as it crosses anterior to the aorta and vena cava by scanning transversely in a supine position (Fig. 9-44). Duplex kidneys can be detected although they must be distinguished from artifacts simulating duplication (pseudoduplication).[50,51]

Renal Parenchyma

As previously described, the renal cortex is not a highly echogenic structure compared to other viscera. Normally it produces low-level echoes, much less intense than those produced, for example, by the liver or spleen. The renal medulla is even less echogenic and is classified as a basically sonolucent tissue.

Diseases of the renal parenchyma have been classified into those that increase cortical echogenicity while preserving medullary sonolucency (type I) and those that distort normal anatomy and eliminate corticomedullary definition (type II).[52] In type I diseases, the normal separation between cortex and medulla is exaggerated, whereas, with type II disease, it is diminished or eliminated. This may be either focal or diffuse. The increased echogenicity of type I parenchyma disease is best appreciated when the images are recorded in white on a black background. There are many diseases that are capable of producing a type I pattern including acute glomerulonephritis,[53,54] lupus erythematosis, nephrosclerosis, diabetic nephropathy, acute tubular necrosis, Alport's disease, leukemic infiltration, amyloidosis,[55] and nephrocalcinosis.[56] Even this is by no means an exhaustive list.

While any renal cortex whose echogenicity is as great or greater than the liver or spleen is considered to be abnormal (Fig. 9-45), an attempt has been made to further subdivide increased cortical echogenicity into various subtypes depending on whether the echogenicity is merely greater than the spleen, greater than the spleen and liver, or as great as the renal sinus echoes, which are usually greater than all three of the above.[57] However, it was found that such a classification did not add specificity to the nephrosonogram, since most diseases could fall into more than a single ultrasonographic category. However, there was a definite relationship between the echogenicity and the degree of interstitial disease as seen on renal biopsy;[57] Factors responsible for the increased echogenicity of type I diseases are largely unknown, but are thought to be related to the deposition of collagen or calcium in the renal interstices.

It is important when type I findings are present not to mistake the sonolucent medullae for cysts or hydronephrosis. The echo amplitude of type I disease has been noted to decrease with the regression of the underlying acute renal glomerulointerstitial process. This may permit ultrasonography to be used in place of serial renal biopsies to assess the progress of certain diseases in this category. It should be pointed out, however, that some observers have failed to note any increase in renal echogenicity in as many as 40 percent of all patients with advanced renal parenchymal disease.[58]

Examples of renal diseases that produce type II lesions are focal acute bacterial nephritis (lobar nephronia),[59] chronic pyelonephritis,[60] healing infarct,

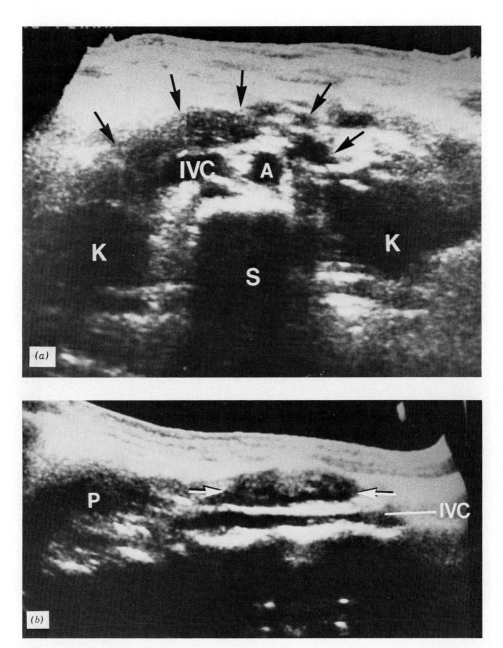

Figure 9-44 Supine transverse (*a*) and longitudinal (*b*) ultrasonograms demonstrate a horseshoe kidney (K) with the isthmus (arrows) seen extending anterior to the major vessels. IVC = inferior vena cava, A = aorta. On the longitudinal examination, the isthmus (arrows) is seen to be located inferior to the pancreas (P). S = spine.

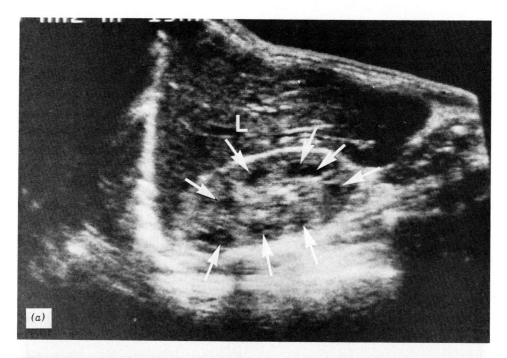

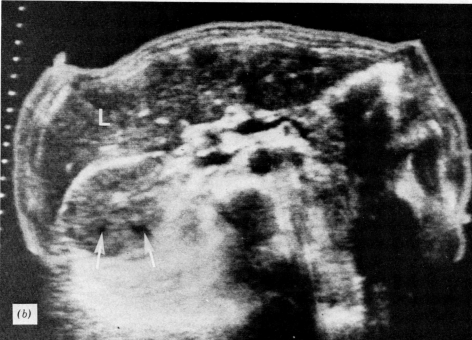

Figure 9-45 Supine longitudinal (*a*) and transverse (*b*) ultrasonograms of type I renal disease. Note the echogenicity of the cortex to be greater than that of the adjacent liver (L) and the relative prominence of the renal pyramids (arrows).

renal tubular ectasia,[61] and infantile polycystic disease. The two hallmarks of type II disease are focal disruption of parenchymal anatomy and diffuse loss of corticomedullary distinction (Fig. 9-46). Focal acute pyelonephritis (lobar nephronia) is a type II change that usually occurs focally.[62] The inflammatory infiltrate appears as a renal mass and displaces adjacent calyces. It is more sonolocent than renal cortical tissue, but does not have the accentuation of the far wall usually seen with an abscess. Unlike an abscess, no shifting debris is present within the lesion, and a sharp or rounded configuration to the lesion is lacking. Lobar nephronia is sometimes difficult to differentiate from an abscess, and, at times needle puncture or the test of time is required to allow a firm distinction between the two.[62] Focal increases in echogenicity can also be seen with chronic atrophic pyelonephritis or healing renal infarcts. Since the overlying parenchyma is thin, confusion may sometimes arise in the differential diagnosis between these diseases, and renal papillary necrosis or tuberculosis.[60]

Diffuse increase in echogenicity with a loss of normal corticomedullary boundary accompanies infantile polycystic diseases[63] and, to a lesser extent, tubular ectasia.[61] It should be noted that the end stage of some renal disorders originally classified as type I can occur as a type II abnormality when the kidney is small and demonstrates high-intensity echoes throughout its substance making

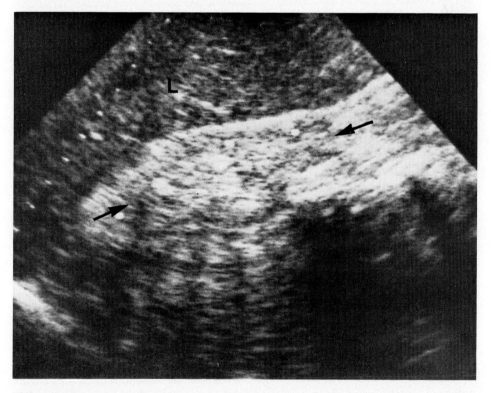

Figure 9-46 Supine longitudinal ultrasonogram shows evidence of a poorly delineated highly echogenic right kidney (arrows) with disruption of normal parenchymal anatomy. The renal sinus cannot be identified. This is typical of type II renal disease. L = liver.

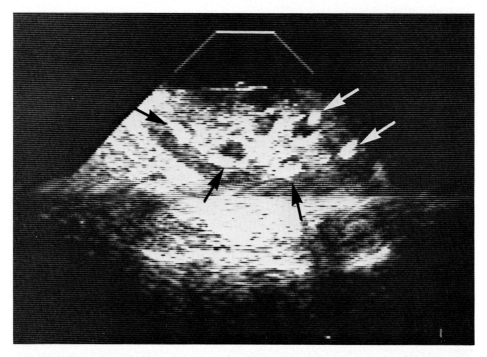

Figure 9-47 Coronal longitudinal view of the left kidney shows evidence of bright echoes (arrows) located in the region of the medulla representing changes of nephrocalcinosis.

differentiation between cortex and medulla, or for that matter, renal sinus no longer possible.

Because high-intensity echoes are created when sound is reflected by calcium, diffuse nephrocalcinosis produces intensely echogenic kidneys also (Fig. 9-47). Two patterns have been described. When the calcification is primarily cortical, an intense type I pattern with clearly distinguishable medullae is seen.[56] In medullary nephrocalcinosis, on the other hand, the pattern is reversed; that is, the medulla is extremely echogenic, while the cortex is not.[64] In severe cases, shadowing beyond the echogenic pyramids may be observed, in what may well be a distinctive sonographic pattern.

The sonographic appearance of the kidneys in acute diffuse pyelonephritis has been described only rarely. The kidneys are enlarged with an increased parenchymal mantle surrounding a normal central echo complex. Edell and Bonavita make no statement about the relative echogenicities of the renal cortex and medulla in acute pyelonephritis, stating only that the parenchyma appears uniformly enlarged with both components participating.[65] They feel that the parenchyma is decreased in its echogenic properties consistent with the presence of interstitial edema, but that scattered low-level echoes may be seen. It should be noted, however, that in their article, no supine or oblique sagittal views were obtained in either of their two patients. The enlarged kidneys returned to normal after treatment. They felt that ultrasonography was important in ruling out complications such as obstructive uropathy. To this might also be added the development of lobar nephronia, renal abscess, and perinephric abscess as well.[65] Renal abscesses are usually well marginated, round or oval masses that, since they contain fluid, are highly trans-sonic. Their internal debris, however, usually results in many internal echoes, which characteristically shift with changes in patient position. Their interior walls may be slightly irregular.[16,66] An interesting ultrasonographic pattern has been described in xanthogranulomatous pyelonephritis. The kidney is usually enlarged and contains scattered hypoechoic areas separated by thick islands of more echogenic renal tissue. The former are probably attributable to scattered collections of "pus," some of which represent dilated calyces, while the large more solid zones are presumably related to abundant infiltrating xanthomatous tissue, which characteristically replaces most if not all of the kidney in this disease (Fig. 9-48). Other sonographic features include the presence of highly echogenic foci with acoustic shadowing secondary to renal calculi.[67]

Ultrasonography may be helpful in renal trauma. In the case of a simple contusion, a hematoma may be identified within the renal parenchyma. Such a hematoma may appear as either a sonolucent or an echogenic mass depending on how soon after injury the patient is examined.[68] Liquifying hematomas may be extremely sonolucent and may contain small echogenic fragments repre-

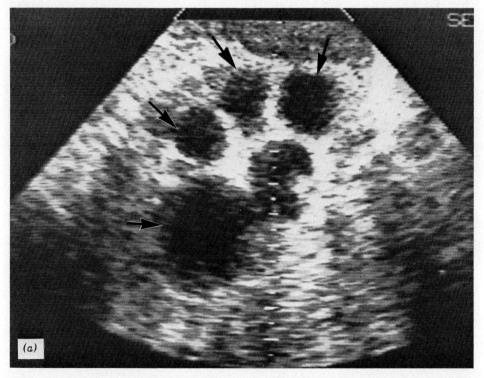

Figure 9-48 Series of coronal images of the left kidney taken at different levels show the typically mixed ultrasonic pattern that can be found with xanthogranulomatosis pyelonephritis. (*a*) A pattern of hydronephrosis (arrows denote dilated calyces). (*b*) A debris level (arrows) within a complex collection. (*c*) An area of increased echogenicity (arrows) perhaps related to infiltrating xanthogranulomatous tissue.

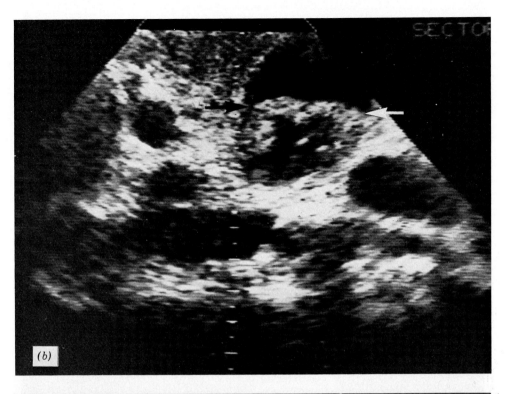

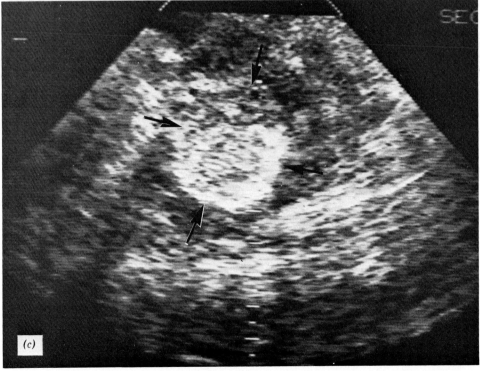

Figure 9-48 (*continued*)

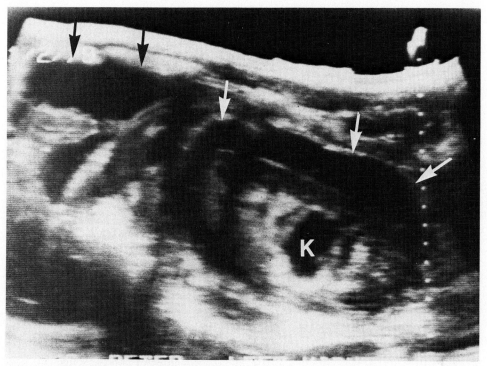

Figure 9-49 Prone longitudinal ultrasound study demonstrates several echo-free areas (arrows) surrounding and just superior to the kidney (K) representing urinomas.

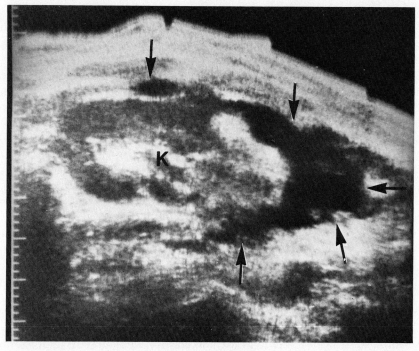

Figure 9-50 Supine longitudinal ultrasonogram demonstrates the presence of an irregular right kidney (K) with disruption of the normal parenchymal pattern in the lower pole secondary to traumatic laceration. There is also a perinephric hematoma (arrows).

senting clots. A consistent absence of echoes in a localized area suggests a laceration of the kidney. Renal lacerations may be associated with accumulation of blood beneath the renal capsule, in the perinephric space, or in both areas. Blood clots in the renal pelvis may also be identified. In the presence of a hematoma, be it either intrarenal or perinephric, serial ultrasonography may be helpful in following the resolution of the hematoma. This may be particularly helpful in patients who are suspected of bleeding following renal biopsy, for example. Extravasation of urine into the perinephric space (urinoma) often accompanies major renal injuries. These too, may be imaged clearly and their progress followed by ultrasonography (Fig. 9-49).[68] Finally, ultrasonography may suggest the presence of pre-existing renal disease predisposing to the renal injury. Schmoller et al encountered six such cases in their series of 27 patients with blunt renal trauma whom they examined with ultrasonography (Fig. 9-50).[68]

RENAL PELVIS AND COLLECTING SYSTEM

Hydronephrosis is the most important entity in this category. Hydronephrosis is a common and often unrecognized cause of renal failure. Since it is potentially one of the most remediable causes, it is crucial that its presence not be overlooked. Since hydronephrosis is relatively easy to detect by ultrasound,[70] it would seem reasonable to state that unless obstruction has been ruled out unequivocally by some other means, ultrasonic evaluation of the kidneys should be performed on all patients in renal failure. It is appropriate to note as well that ultrasound also may be employed to guide the procedure of percutaneous nephrostomy.[71] It has been found to be more accurate than fluoroscopy in localizing the dilated renal collecting system for puncture.

Ultrasound has proved to be very valuable and extremely reliable in the detection of hydronephrosis. This is most fortuitous, for often the hydronephrotic kidney is severely damaged and does not excrete urographic contrast agents well. Several sonographic patterns may be encountered.[72] The earliest sign is a ring-shaped echo-free area in the region of the renal pelvis surrounded by well-defined echoes from the walls of the renal pelvis. Thus, the normally homogeneous central echo complex takes on the configuration of a circular or elliptical sonolucent zone (Fig. 9-51). At times, dilated infundibula and calyces also may be identified (Fig. 9-52). Later, with progressive distention of the pelvis, the central echoes can no longer be seen, but instead strong echoes can be detected from compressed renal tissue surrounding the dilated pelvis. Finally, with advanced hydronephrosis, renal tissue can no longer be identified, the diseased area giving the appearance of a large cyst because of a fluid-filled sac that has developed (Fig. 9-53). The ureters should always be sought in hydronephrosis, since a dilated ureter suggests a distal ureteral obstruction. In cases of bilateral hydronephrosis, the urinary bladder should always be examined to rule out infravesical obstruction as a cause for the renal changes.

Attempts have been made to grade and classify the degree of hydronephrosis based on ultrasonic criteria. Finberg has done this in the hydronephrosis that develops during normal pregnancy.[73] In pregnant women who are symptomatic,

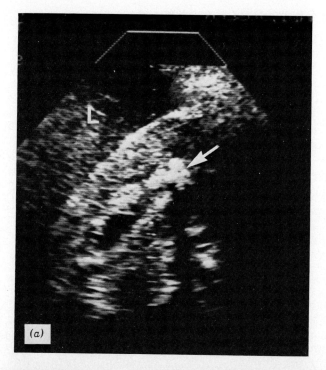

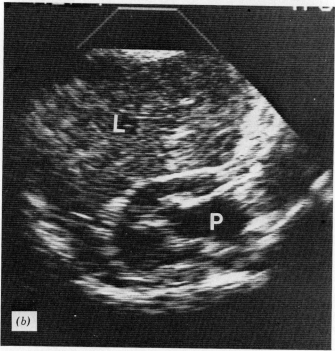

Figure 9-51 (*a*) Coronal longitudinal ultrasonogram of the right kidney shows evidence of minimal hydronephrosis (echo-free area located essentially in the upper portion of the kidney). The inferiorly bright echoes and accompanying acoustic shadowing is due to an associated calculus (arrow). (*b*) Transverse ultrasonogram of a different patient showing a more moderate dilatation of the renal pelvis (P). L = liver.

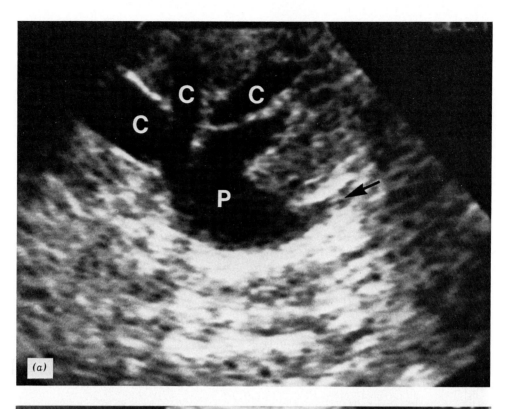

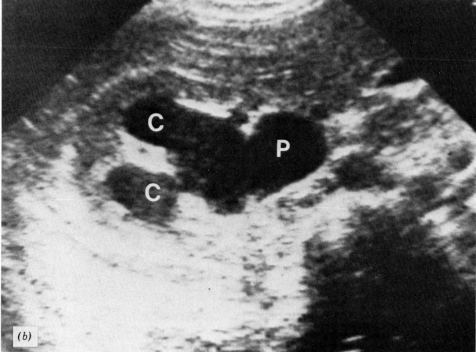

Figure 9-52 (*a*) Longitudinal coronal and (*b*) transverse supine images of a patient show moderate hydronephrosis. A renal pelvis is seen with it entering into a slightly prominent proximal ureter (arrow). In (*b*) echoes seen within the dilated calyces (C) may be due to floating debris. P = pelvis.

364

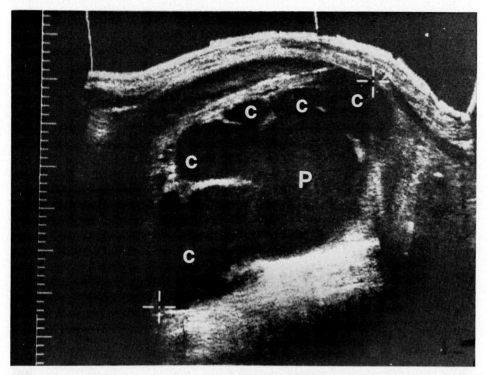

Figure 9-53 Longitudinal coronal ultrasonagram of the left kidney shows evidence of massive hydronephrosis with a markedly dilated renal pelvis (P) and calyces system (C). Almost no residual parenchyma was recorded.

and especially those with urinary tract infection, ultrasound can be used to assess as well as continually monitor the degree of hydronephrosis, thereby decreasing the need to use ionizing radiation in their investigation.

Hydronephrosis frequently occurs in duplicated kidneys (Fig. 9-54). Either the upper or the lower half may be involved. In such a setting, the focal nature of the hydronephrosis may be recognized by demonstrating a cystic mass in either the upper or lower half of a kidney in which a normal central echo complex remains in the uninvolved segment. The best position to demonstrate this is usually the decubitus position, which not only shows the hydronephrotic pelvis, but often shows the dilated ureter leading from it. The demonstration of a dilated ureter emanating from the sinus echo complex is also extremely useful in differentiating central renal cysts or parapelvic cysts from hydronephrosis. The demonstration of dilated infundibula and calyces may also be used for this distinction. Cross-sectional images are especially helpful in localizing a cyst-like fluid accumulation in the anatomic region of the renal pelvis. In addition to centrally located renal cysts, other entities in the differential diagnosis of hydronephrosis are listed in Table 9-4.

Care must be taken not to automatically equate the presence of a dilated collecting system with obstructive uropathy.[75] Table 9-5 lists circumstances under which a dilated collecting system may be seen in the absence of obstructive uropathy.

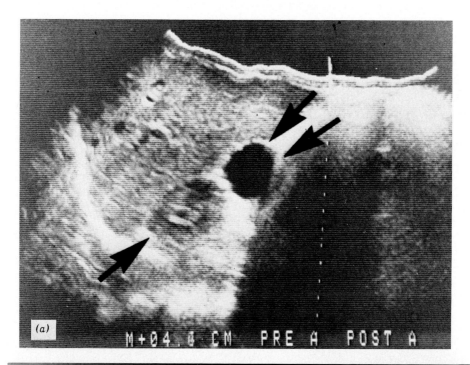

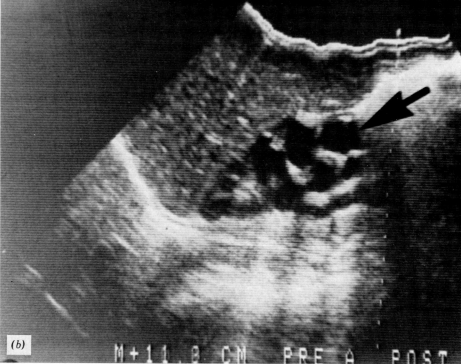

Figure 9-54 (*a*) Longitudinal ultrasonogram of the right kidney (arrow) shows what appears to be a cyst of the lower pole (double arrows). (*b*) A more lateral cut demonstrates what appears to be multiple cysts of the lower pole (arrow). (*c*) Transverse ultrasonogram demonstrates that, in fact, this represents hydronephrosis of the lower portion of a duplication. Note dilatation of a calyx (arrow). (*d*) Transverse image shows that the upper portion of the duplication (arrows) is not obstructed.

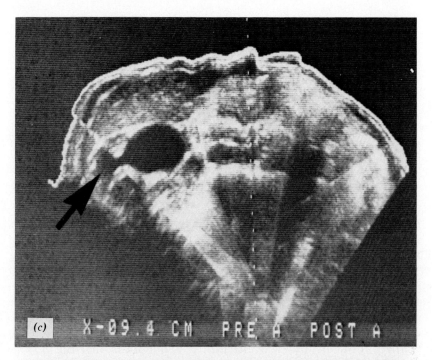

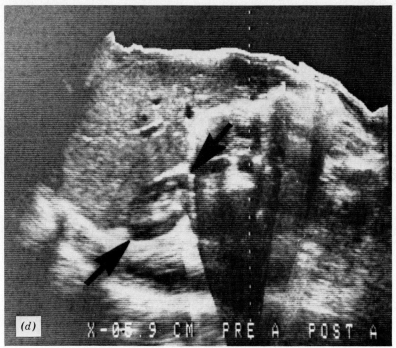

Figure 9-54 (*continued*)

367

Table 9-4   Lesions Confusable with
Hydronephrosis by Ultrasound

Central renal cysts
Multicystic kidney
Sinus lipomatosis
Parapelvic cysts
Lucent renal pyramids
Lumbar meningomyelocele
Pancreatic pseudocyst
Sonolucent masses (i.e., lymphoma)
Aneurysm and varices in renal hilum

While ultrasonography is extremely sensitive in detecting dilatation of the collecting system, false-negative and false-positive results do occur in approximately 7 percent of cases.[76] False-negative results may occur in the presence of staghorn calculi or those rare instances of hydronephrosis in which the dilatation is minimal.[77] This may be seen with retroperitoneal fibrosis or poorly obstructing ureteral calculi, for example. Since overhydration and a full urinary bladder may result in ureteropyelectasis, it is important that the bladder be empty during the examination and that the patient not be overly hydrated.[78] In equivocal cases of obstruction, scanning may be performed with the patient erect. If the dilatation is physiologic, the pelvis will drain in this position. Rosenfield has recommended a provocative test in the case of intermittent or partial obstructive uropathy. He recommends the use of the diuretic furosemide or the ingestion of large quantities of water with the examination being performed both before and after the administration of fluid challenge.[79] Lee et al, comparing real-time ultrasonography with static gray scale imaging, found that they were of similar accuracy in the diagnosis of hydronephrosis. They felt that, because of its greater flexibility and shorter scanning time, real-time ultrasonography was the procedure of choice in evaluating for hydronephrosis.[80]

Table 9-5   Causes of
Nonobstructive Dilatation[a]

Reflux
Infection
Diuresis
Distended bladder
Large extrarenal pelvis
Megacalyces
Papillary necrosis
Corrected obstruction

[a] False-positive results.

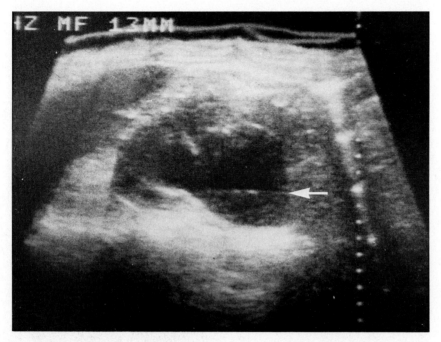

Figure 9-55 Longitudinal coronal image of the left kidney shows the presence of moderate hydronephrosis with echoes seen dependently in the dilated pelvis with a fluid-debris level (arrow). This was proven to be a pyonephrosis.

The sonographic appearance of hydronephrosis is altered considerably when the urine is infected especially in the presence of thick pus. This condition, known as pyonephrosis, produces persistent dependent echoes with a shifting urine-debris level dependent on the position of the patient (Fig. 9-55). When the renal pelvis is completely filled with thick tenacious pus, sound transmission is poor, and echoes may be seen completely filling the pelvis and calyces.[21] Complicating features such as renal calculi or abscesses may also be seen.

It is also possible to detect the presence of hydronephrosis in fetal kidneys using standard techniques of obstetric ultrasound.[81]

STONES, NEOPLASMS AND BLOOD CLOTS

Stones, neoplasms, and blood clots constitute the most common renal pelvic filling defects. Stones, whether opaque or nonopaque, can be satisfactorily imaged by ultrasound. The hallmarks of nephrolithiasis are the presence of a highly reflective structure within the collecting system accompanied by acoustical shadowing (Fig. 9-56). Stones produce stronger reflecting echoes and allow less sound transmission than soft tissue masses of the same size. Attempts to differentiate the chemical components of renal calculi on the basis of their ultrasonic behavior have as yet produced no clinically useful results. For example, nonopaque stones such as uric acid calculi appear to be equally

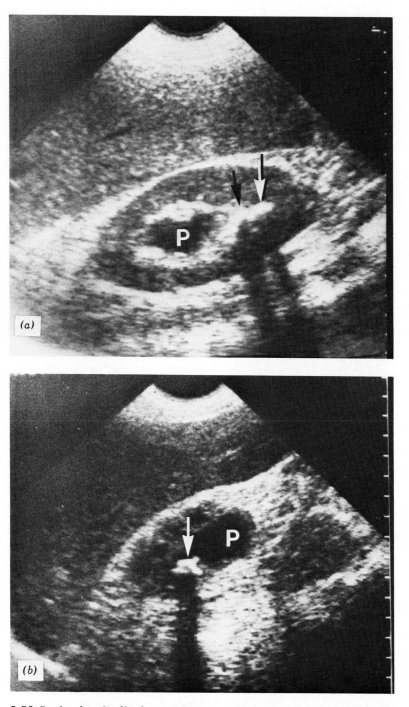

Figure 9-56 Supine longitudinal (*a*) and transverse (*b*) scans demonstrate the presence of renal calculi (arrows) appearing as bright areas of echogenicity with distal acoustic shadowing. There is associated moderate hydronephrosis with dilatation of the renal pelvis (P).

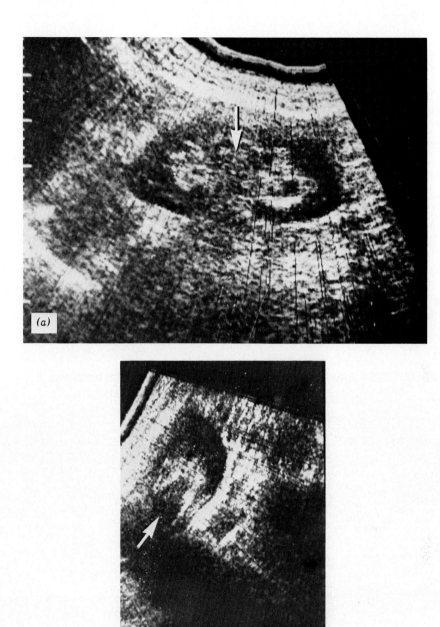

Figure 9-57 (*a*) Longitudinal image of the left kidney shows distortion of the central echo pattern by a weakly echogenic mass (arrow), which is also seen on the transverse image (*b*). This proved to be a transitional cell carcinoma.

reflective and produce as much acoustical shadowing as the more common opaque or calcium-containing renal calculi. Acoustical shadowing can be demonstrated beyond almost any renal calculus 5 to 7 mm in diameter or larger, but satisfactory visualization of this phenomenon is extremely dependent on technique and may, therefore, at times be difficult to produce. For the most part, the demonstration of shadowing is dependent on the use of a properly focused transducer and the use of optimal time-gain compensation settings. A high overall gain is to be avoided. The presence of hydronephrosis generally makes demonstration of calculi easier. With proper technique, stones as small as 7 mm have been imaged. The differential diagnosis of acoustical shadowing within the kidney is limited. Other than calculi, only internal gas—as in abscess— can produce acoustical shadowing.

The ultrasonographic findings in patients with transitional cell carcinoma of the renal pelvis consist of separation of the central renal echo complex by a collection of low-intensity echoes that do not change location with changes in the patient's position (Fig. 9-57). Hydronephrosis is often, but not invariably, present. Collecting system blood clots may have an echo pattern similar to urothelial neoplasms, but can usually be distinguished by their mobility and transitory nature.[84] Occasionally, a clot may produce a debris-fluid level.[79]

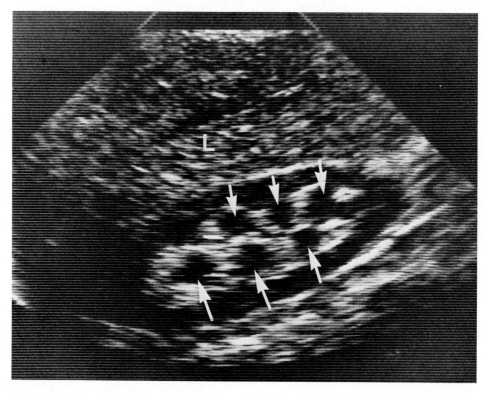

Figure 9-58 Longitudinal supine ultrasonogram of the right kidney revealed small echo-free areas (arrows) located centrally within the renal pelvis representing small cysts. L = liver.

Foreign bodies such as nephrostomy tubes also produce intrapelvic echoes, often allowing their recognition.

Sinus lipomatosis consists of a proliferation of fat in the renal sinus compressing the renal pelvis and calyces, often causing them to appear stretched. The cause of sinus lipomatosis is not known, but it is an exaggeration of the fat normally seen in the renal sinus. In very obese people, in patients with chronic atrophic renal disease, and in normal but aging kidneys, sinus lipomatosis may be seen. Since the same urographic appearance may be produced by multiple peripelvic cysts, ultrasonography is valuable in distinguishing between the two. With proliferation of peripelvic sinus fat, an echogenic renal sinus (Fig. 9-26) is seen, while with parapelvic cysts, a typical cystic appearance is imparted to the abnormal tissue masses filling the renal sinus (Fig. 9-58).[23]

RENAL BLOOD VESSELS

High-resolution gray scale ultrasound has allowed accurate identification of the renal vessels. In transverse section, the renal veins can be seen coursing to the vena cava and the renal arteries coursing to the kidneys from their origin in the aorta. Occasional normal variations may produce confusing patterns. Sometimes, the left renal vein may have a bulbous dilatation, often accompanied by an apparent focal defect in the aortic wall at approximately the same level. Kurtz et al have described this finding and pointed out how it may be easily mistaken for a left renal artery aneurysm.[85] Of course, using duplex Doppler, an aneurysm can be ruled out. Varicose enlargement of the left renal vein has also been confused with hydronephrosis as well as with pancreatic pseudocysts.[85] Enlargement of the renal vein, in association with a large ipsilateral renal artery suggests the diagnosis of a renal arteriovenous fistula. Such fistulas, when more than 2 cm in diameter, should be detectable by gray scale sonographic examination as anechoic masses.[87] The vascular nature of channels entering such anechoic masses can be confirmed by tracing them into the aorta or inferior vena cava or by use of real time or duplex Doppler studies. Enlargements of the renal artery are most often attributable to aneurysms. These can be detected readily by ultrasonography. They are not usually accompanied by dilatation of the ipsilateral renal vein, which helps to differentiate them from the enlarged renal arteries of arteriovenous fistulae. They may, however, be confused with renal cysts, especially if real-time or Doppler studies are not done.[15]

Renal vein thrombosis, which occurs in a variety of conditions in both children and adults, may be detected readily by ultrasonography.[88] The renal findings depend on the stage of the disease. Shortly after the onset of venous obstruction, decreased cortical echogenicity is seen, probably as a result of edema, and the kidney is enlarged. Later, increased echogenicity due to cellular infiltration follows, and the kidney may return to normal size or may even atrophy. The corticomedullary distinction is usually preserved. If the disease is not severe and especially if abundant collaterals develop, the echo texture of the kidney gradually returns to a more normal appearance. Chronic irreversible changes are accompanied by a decreased renal size, loss of corticomedullary definition,

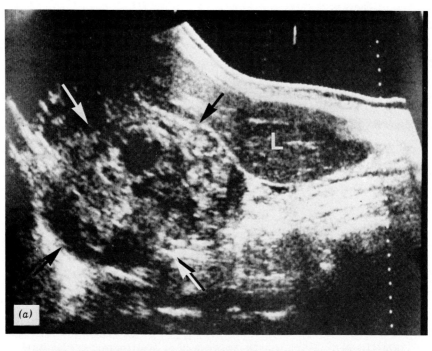

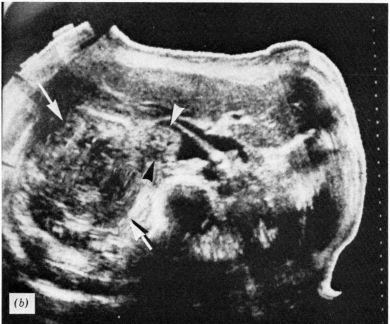

Figure 9-59 (*a*) Longitudinal ultrasonogram shows the presence of a large complex renal mass (arrows) that proved to be a renal cell carcinoma. (*b*) Transverse supine ultrasonogram shows the mass (arrows) and evidence of tumor (arrowhead) occupying the right renal vein and extending into a portion of the inferior vena cava.

374

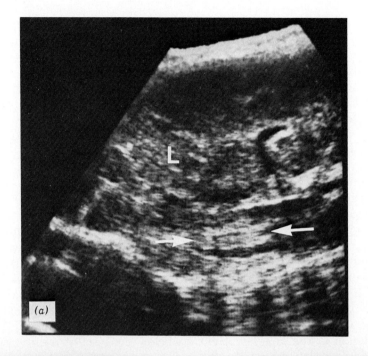

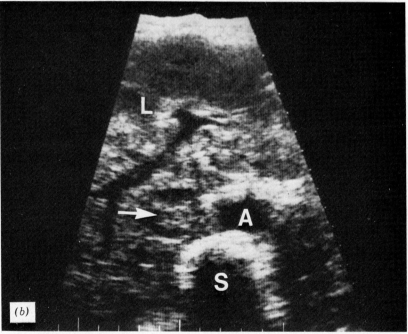

Figure 9-60 Longitudinal (*a*) and transverse (*b*) ultrasonograms demonstrate multiple echoes (arrows) within the inferior vena cava producing complete occlusion. This is the result of tumor thrombus extending in from the renal vein. A = aorta, S = spine, L = liver.

and increased parenchymal echogenicity. With real time, absence of normally transmitted venous pulsations is noted, and on Doppler, diminished or absent venous flow is seen.[89] The most distinctive feature of the disease, however, is the demonstration of the clot within the renal vein and, in some instances, the vena cava as well.[90] A common cause of renal vein thrombosis is extension of renal cell carcinoma. Extension begins first in the segmental renal veins from where it grows into the main renal vein (Fig. 9-59). As this becomes filled with tumor, it finally propagates into the vena cava and even beyond; that is, to the heart. Neoplastic renal vein and caval thrombosis is readily detectable by ultrasonography (Fig. 9-60). Extension into more remote vessels (e.g., the thyroid veins) has been recorded.[91] Since a renal neoplasm may produce renal vein enlargement by virtue of increased blood flow through the mass or by arteriovenous shunting, a diagnosis of renal vein tumor thrombus should not be made on the basis of an enlarged renal vein alone. Demonstration of the actual thrombus is necessary before this diagnosis can be invoked with certainty. Demonstration of renal vein tumor thrombus is ordinarily not difficult, since the thrombus tends to be a relatively hyperechoic structure situated within anechoic fluid. On rare occasions, however, tumor thrombus may be relatively echo-free, and occasionally, technical factors may result in low-level echoes occurring within a renal vein simulating tumor thrombus. It is helpful to recall that dilatation of the inferior vena cava below the level of the renal veins or abrupt narrowing of a dilated inferior vena cava, if present, usually bespeak obstruction.[92] Tumor thrombus in the inferior vena cava or renal vein appears as either a discrete echogenic mass or as diffuse echoes within the lumen. Renal artery thrombosis has also been demonstrated by ultrasonography.[97] Serial closely spaced transverse scans parallel to the long axis of the renal artery may reveal narrowing of the lumen with intraluminal low-intensity echoes. The optimal scanning plane is readily obtainable using real-time equipment. The arterial lumen is normally echo-free. Thrombosis leading to occlusion produces ultrasonic evidence of renal infarction either focal or diffuse. This appearance is characterized by scattered areas of sonolucency. Later, scarring may be seen as a focal area of parenchymal thinning.[94]

INTRAOPERATIVE NEPHROSONOGRAPHY

Using specially designed high-frequency transducers, intraoperative real-time renal ultrasonography has been employed in the detection and localization of renal calculi in the operating room.[95] The transducer and connecting cables may be sterilized and, where necessary, covered by sterile orthopedic type stockingette. A plastic bag with gel can be attached to the transducer head. Scanning of the intact renal surface with a 6 to 10 MHz transducer yields valuable information about the underlying kidney and any abnormalities that may be contained within it. Stones as small as 1 mm may be detected by the rather characteristic echo reflectivity and acoustical shadowing they produce. A reliable penetration to a depth of approximately 3 cm may be obtained by the type of equipment described. If a solitary calculus is to be located, it is best to commence the ultrasonic examination before the renal substance or collecting system has been incised so as to minimize the introduction of air within the collecting system. Stones remaining after the main stone fragments have been removed may also be detected. The pulsatile expansion of the intrarenal arteries may be visualized with these instruments. Ultrasonography may be employed alone for the localization of renal calculi or in conjunction with standard operative radiography if the stone cannot be located readily. It is sometimes helpful to mark its exact intrarenal location by means of a needle passed through a needle guide attached to the transducer, ensuring that the needle intersects in the approximate area of the stone.[95]

FETAL NEPHROSONOGRAPHY

Present ultrasonic equipment permits identification of the fetal kidneys as early as the fifteenth postmenstrual week. Almost all kidneys can be detected ultrasonically after the twentieth postmenstrual week.[96] The fetal kidneys have a sonographic appearance similar to that of adult kidneys, although the renal pyramids often appear more prominent (Fig. 9-61) than its adult counterpart. Many congenital anomalies of the kidney can be detected ultrasonically—most of these well within the period considered critical for genetic counseling.[81]

Bilateral renal agenesis can be detected by the twentieth postmenstrual

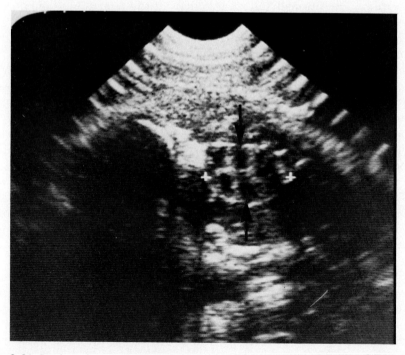

Figure 9-61 Supine ultrasonogram of pregnant uterus showed evidence of a term fetus. The fetal kidney (arrows) is well demonstrated. Its length can be easily measured (pluses). Note the prominence of the renal pyramids, which is normal near term and during the newborn period.

week.[81] Not only are the kidneys absent, but a fluid-filled urinary bladder cannot be demonstrated. As with all anomalies in which urine production is significantly reduced, there is oligohydramnios. Because of confusion produced by the fetal adrenal glands that may occasionally be mistaken for kidneys, it is suggested that the examination of the urinary tract in severe oligohydramnios be directed primarily toward the fetal urinary bladder when the diagnosis of bilateral renal agenesis is considered.[97]

Cystic lesions of the kidney are also detectable in utero with sonography. The most common of these is multicystic dysplastic kidney, which is, as previously described, a unilateral process. Rarely, it may be bilateral. An aggregate of many cysts of varying sizes is seen. This mass lacks a reniform configuration or a well-defined renal pelvis. In some cases, it is associated with contralateral hydronephrosis, in which case oligohydramnios is probably present.[80] Infantile polycystic disease can be recognized as early as the seventeenth postmenstrual week by the presence of bilateral massive nephromegaly without gross cyst formation or hydronephrosis.[98] The individual cysts are usually too small to be discretely imaged, although at times they may be seen. More often, the kidneys appear as highly echogenic masses that fill the fetal abdomen and are associated with oligohydramnios. The adult type of polycystic disease is extremely rare in the fetus or newborn. When present, the sonographic features can be easily confused with bilateral hydronephrosis. A family history of polycystic disease, however, can be extremely important in alerting clinicians to the possibility of this disorder. The normally lucent pyramids of the fetal kidney should not be confused with renal cysts or dilated calyces (Fig. 9-61).

One of the most common congenital anomalies of the urinary tract is hydronephrosis secondary to ureteropelvic junction obstruction (Fig. 9-62). This is usually unilateral and not hereditary. The sonographic findings depend on the severity of the obstruction, but usually a typical hydronephrotic pattern is observed in association with a large extrarenal pelvis.[81] The ureters are not abnormal and, therefore, are not visualized, and the bladder is normal when the disease is unilateral. Unilateral obstruction may also be produced by ureterovesical junction obstruction and primary megaureter, which can be detected ultrasonically.[72] Bilateral obstruction is usually a manifestation of infravesical disease, the most common cause being posterior urethral valves. This is a disease exclusively of men and results in a distended thickened urinary bladder. With more severe obstruction, the ureters are dilated and may be defined ultrasonically. The end result is bilateral hydronephrosis. The diagnosis of urethral obstruction in the male patient may be made on the basis of this constellation of findings. It is helpful to evaluate the urinary bladder under real time and note the completeness and regularity with which it empties. Infravesical obstruction is associated with poor or incomplete bladder emptying. In the more severe cases, the bladder will not empty at all. Far advanced hydronephrosis may be accompanied by tiny ruptures of the distended renal calyces leading to the gradual accumulation of extravasated urine in the retroperitoneum. Eventually, the urine may find its way into the peritoneal cavity. The resultant ascites is part of the spectrum of findings associated with severe urethral obstruction. Recent experiences with percutaneous in utero drainage techniques of the distended fetal bladder have been encouraging and

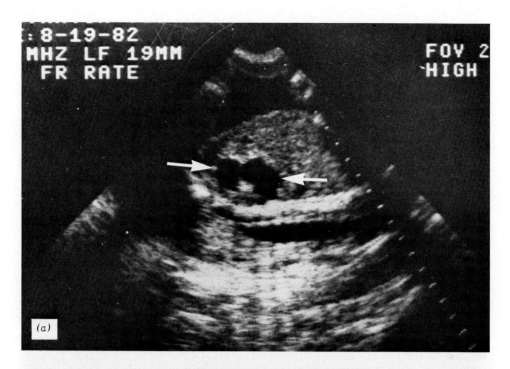

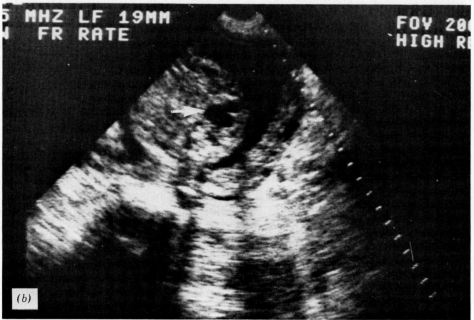

Figure 9-62 Ultrasonogram of the pregnant uterus demonstrates hydronephrosis (arrows) in utero due to unilateral uteropelvic obstruction. (*a*) Longitudinal view of fetus, and (*b*) transverse view of fetus.

indicate the potential value of careful ultrasonic evaluation of the anomalous fetal urinary tract and, further, careful evaluation of any pregnancy that is not proceeding as expected. Drainage of an obstructed bladder in utero may result in postpartum renal salvage.[99-101]

In prune belly syndrome, a triad consisting of deficient abdominal musculature, undescended testes, and various urinary tract anomalies, ultrasonography can frequently be helpful in early detection. Certain ancillary findings occurring in combination suggest the diagnosis. Almost invariably, the urinary bladder is dilated, and in most forms of the disease, the ureters are dilated as well. Not infrequently, they are massively enlarged and stand out in striking disproportion to the kidneys, which may not be proportionately hydronephrotic. In severe forms of the disease, however, the kidneys may show cystic dysplastic change.[102] It is occasionally possible to image the laxity of the anterior abdominal wall.[103]

To date, no reports of ultrasonic detection of tumors of the fetal kidneys have appeared, but, in view of the occurrence of congenital mesoblastic nephroma at birth, it may be expected that this lesion will be recognized in the near future.

THE TRANSPLANTED KIDNEY

Diagnostic ultrasound is one of the main techniques in the evaluation of patients with renal transplants. Ultrasound may be used both in the immediate postoperative period for evaluation of suspected complications and later for long-term serial follow-up as well.

If ultrasound is to be employed in the management of post-transplant patients, it has usually been found advisable to perform a routine baseline study as soon as possible after surgery, on all patients. This can usually be done at about the fifth postoperative day. The dressings can be removed and scanning performed adjacent to the healing surgical incision. The size, shape, and echo characteristics of the kidney as well as its volume are assessed at the time of the baseline examination. Volume measurements may be made by scanning the kidney longitudinally and transversely along the major axes and calculating the data by planimetry or an automated microprocessing system.[104]

The ultrasonic appearance of a normal renal transplant is similar to that of a normal nontransplanted kidney. Usually, architectural detail is more clearly depicted in the transplanted kidney probably because it is closer to the skin surface. Thus, the renal pyramids may be visualized more clearly than they are customarily seen, and the short specular reflections at the corticomedullary junction representing arcuate vessels are usually clearly visible. Minimal central separation of the central echo complex is often seen and should not be interpreted as evidence of obstructive uropathy. Nor should an extrarenal pelvis be mistaken for collecting system obstruction.[105]

After transplantation, the kidney begins to hypertrophy. Normally by the end of the second week, the average increase in renal volume is approximately 15 percent. By the end of the third week, renal volume increases on the average of 22 percent.[106] Increases in volume greater than this suggest rejection.

Acute failure of the transplanted kidney may be produced by acute tubular necrosis, acute rejection, or arterial obstruction. Acute rejection is a dynamic process with a spectrum of pathologic findings; therefore, the sonographic findings vary according to the stage.[106] Sonography reflects edema, congestion, and hemorrhage of the interstitium, largely as areas of sonolucency, while ischemic and cellular infiltration of the cortex may be expected to produce increases in echogenicity. Frank infarction and necrosis of the cortex may occur in severe cases.

The most common sign of rejection is an abnormal increase in renal volume (Fig. 9-63). This manifests itself as either a sudden increase (greater than 20 percent over a period of 5 days) or renal enlargement greater than 25 percent by the end of the second week.[106] The kidney also tends to take on a more globular shape with an increase in the ratio of the AP to craniocaudal diameter. The normal ratio of 0.36 to 0.54 may increase to as much as 0.7 in acute rejection.[107] A decrease in amplitude of the renal sinus echoes is commonly seen in rejection.[108] Also encountered are abnormal enlargement and increased transonicity of the renal pyramids causing enhanced definition of the cortico-medullary boundary (Fig. 9-64). The pyramids are considered enlarged when their height exceeds the thickness of the overlying cortex. The echogenicity of the renal cortex appears to be a variable finding in transplant rejection. In some patients undergoing rejection, cortical echogenicity increases, and, in others, it appears to decrease (Fig. 9-65). Hricak et al. found cortical echogenicity to be increased slightly more often than it was decreased.[108] A striking picture is often produced wherein sonolucent pyramids stand out in marked contrast to overlying and surrounding hyperechoic renal cortex. Decreased parenchymal echogenicity tended to occur as an early finding, while increased echogenicity often was not present on the first abnormal scan but occurred later.[106] Occasionally, sonolucency may be focal. In 58 percent of patients with acute rejection, crescentic perinephric fluid collections may also occur (Fig. 9-66). While rejection may occur at various intervals after transplant, it most commonly occurs in the first week or 4 to 5 weeks later (chronic rejection). The kidney's response to treatment can be followed easily with serial ultrasound examinations evaluating changes in volume and internal-echo pattern.

Unlike rejection, acute tubular necrosis produces few if any abnormal echogenic findings, and the renal volume usually remains within the range of normal.

With acute renal arterial occlusion, the sonographic anatomy remains grossly unaltered. However, duplex Doppler studies can reveal an absence or a diminution in flow.

Not infrequently, perinephric fluid collections occur around the transplanted kidney and ureter or around the urinary bladder. These may be due to lymphocele, urinoma, abscess, or hematoma singly or in combination (Fig. 9-67). It is usually not possible to differentiate these fluid collections consistently and with accuracy based on sonography alone, but certain characteristics may favor one type of collection over the others.[109] Hematomas usually occur in the early postoperative period. The ultrasonic appearance varies depending on the age of the hemorrhage as well as its location. Acute and chronic hematomas usually appear as well-defined echo-free masses with varying amounts of internal echogenicity depending on the number and size of remaining fragments of

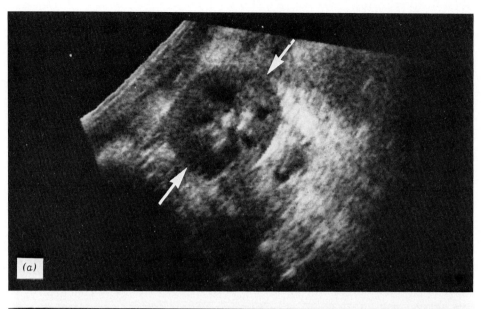

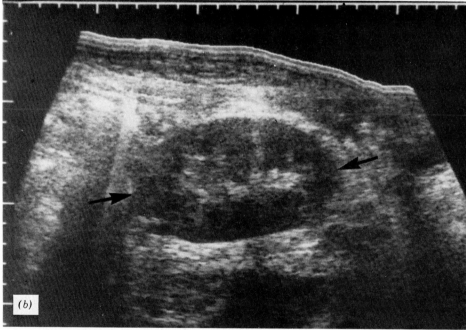

Figure 9-63 Transverse (*a*) and longitudinal (*b*) ultrasonograms show a recently transplanted kidney (arrows) with a relatively normal configuration. There is some prominence of the renal pyramids and slight overall swelling. A specific ultrasound diagnosis of abnormality was not possible in this patient who subsequently proved to have acute tubular necrosis.

382

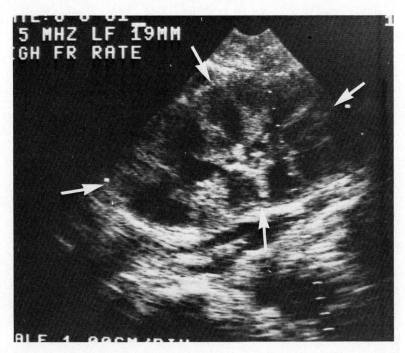

Figure 9-64 Supine longitudinal ultrasonogram of renal transplant (arrows) shows overall swelling and an increase in the parenchymal echogenicity with marked prominence of the renal pyramids and decrease in renal pelvic echoes. This patient was proven to have moderate changes of rejection.

clot. Septations may be present.[109] Urinomas usually occur within the first 2 postoperative weeks, but may occur later, especially if there is delayed necrosis of the ureter. Urinomas produce sonolucent masses, and there is often accompanying hydronephrosis secondary to compression of the ureter by the urinoma. Septations are usually not encountered. Confirmation of the diagnosis of urinoma is best made by urography, cystography, and/or radionuclide studies to determine the source of the urinary leak. Abscesses often have a fairly characteristic ultrasound pattern of numerous internal echoes caused by septae and debris. The borders are not as sharply defined as in other collections, probably because of inflammation and edema around the lesions. The debris in abscesses may often shift with changes in position of the patient. Abscesses usually occur in the immediate postoperative period.

The most common perinephric fluid collection is a lymphocele (lymphocyst), which occurs in approximately 12 percent of all transplant patients.[104] Lymphoceles occur from 2 weeks to 6 months after transplantation and are often asymptomatic and discovered incidentally. When symptoms occur, they are often due to pressure on adjacent organs such as the ureter, bladder, or kidney producing pain or hydronephrosis. Pressure on the iliac vessels may be associated with signs of venous stasis or thrombophlebitis. The ultrasonic characteristic of a lymphocele is that of a well-defined cystic area occasionally containing

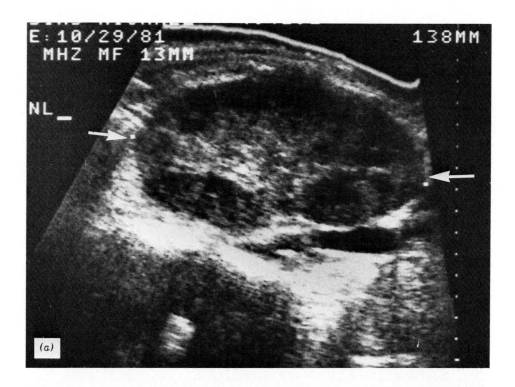

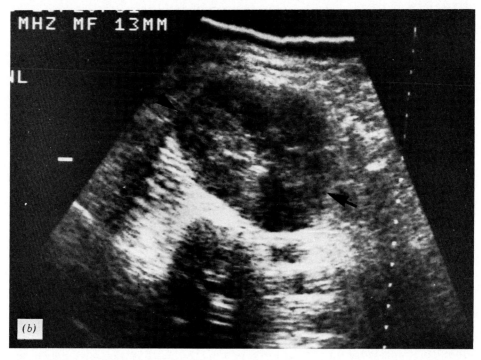

Figure 9-65 Longitudinal (*a*) and transverse (*b*) ultrasonograms of a renal transplant (arrows) show it to be enlarged with a relative decrease in the echogenicity of the renal pelvis and disruption of the parenchymal echo pattern. This is one of the typical findings reported in moderately advanced transplant rejection.

384

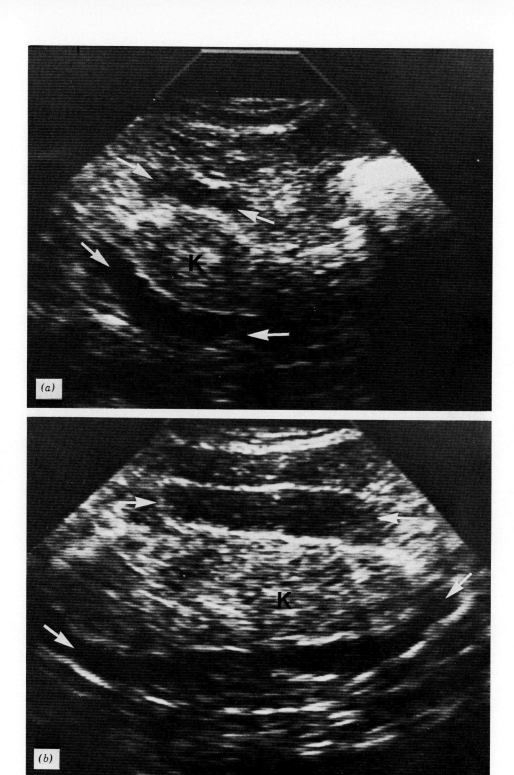

Figure 9-66 Transverse (*a*) and longitudinal (*b*) ultrasonograms of a renal transplant show evidence of a crescentic perinephric fluid collection (arrows) in this patient with known rejection. Note the loss of normal architecture of the kidney (K).

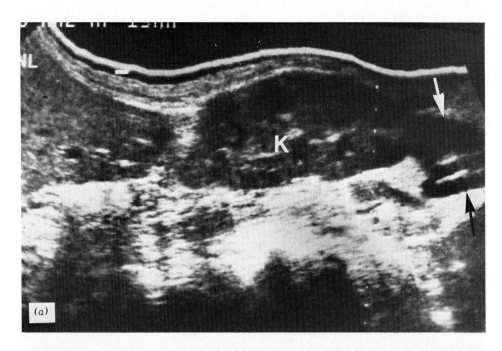

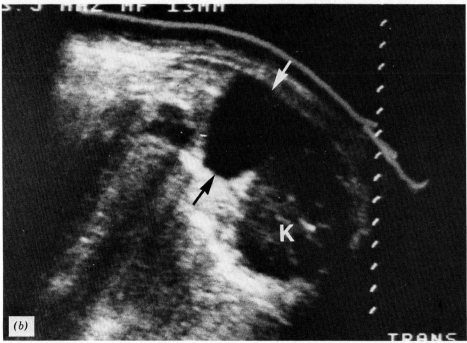

Figure 9-67 Supine longitudinal (*a*) and transverse (*b*) ultrasonograms show evidence of two fluid collections (arrows). These proved to be lymphoceles. K = transplanted kidney.

numerous septations. When serial studies have been performed, the differential diagnosis may be narrowed, since the possibility of an unrecognized abscess or gradually expanding hematoma would be unlikely. Lymphoceles are usually unilocular, but, occasionally, they occur as multiple masses or multilocular structures. Lymphoceles and urinomas are the fluid collections least likely to contain internal echoes. Most lymphoceles remain unchanged in size. If aspiration is deemed advisable, this can be accomplished readily using ultrasonic guidance. This has met with limited success with lymphoceles, since they tend to reaccumulate and there is a small but definite risk of infection. Ultrasound can also be used to guide the needles or drainage catheters into the other types of effusions described above.

Obstructive uropathy is not uncommon following renal transplantation and may be caused by a variety of factors including both intrinsic lesions, such as ureteral strictures, or extrinsic processes, such as lymphoceles. The clinical diagnosis is often first suggested by the detection of an escalating serum creatinine or BUN. Often, the patient has not detected any decrease in urinary output. However, since both oliguria and azotemia in the transplant patient may be caused by rejection as well as by obstruction, ultrasonography is ideally suited to serve as an early determinant in the differential diagnosis. Dilatation of the collecting system in an obstructed renal transplant is readily recognized by virtue of the classic findings in hydronephrosis, that is, dilatation of the calyces, separation of the renal sinus echoes, and/or visualization of a dilated ureter. When differentiation between nonobstructive dilatation and obstructive uropathy is a problem, a provocative diuresis established with an agent such as Lasix (furosimide) proves helpful. In the presence of obstruction, a forced diuresis accentuates the separation of the collecting system, whereas, in nonobstructive dilatation, the degree of dilatation is unchanged.

Finally, ultrasound has been used to localize the transplanted kidney for biopsy, particularly when there is suspicion of rejection. The depth of the kidney beneath the skin surface and the selection of the exact angle and site for placement of the needle are readily determined with ultrasound. After renal biopsy, ultrasound may be used to examine for the possibility of perinephric hematoma formation.

REFERENCES

1. Resnick MI, Sanders RC: *Ultrasound in Urology.* Baltimore, Williams & Wilkins Company, 1979, p vii.
2. Reid MH, MacKay RS, Lantz PM: Noninvasive blood flow measurements by Doppler ultrasound with applications to renal artery flow determination. *Invest Radiol* 15:323–331, 1980.
3. Weill FS, Bihr E, Rohmer P, Zeltner F: *Renal Sonography.* New York, Springer-Verlag, 1981, p 19.
4. Cook JH, III, Rosenfield AT, Taylor KJW: Ultrasonic demonstration of intrarenal anatomy. *AJR* 129:831–835, 1977.
5. Haller JO, Berdon WE, Friedman AP: Increased renal cortical echogenicity: A normal finding in enonates and infants. *Radiology* 142:173-n174, 1982.

6. Scheible W, Leopold GR: High resolution real-time ultrasonography of neonate kidneys. *J Ultra Med* 133–138, 1982.

7. Kossof G: in Watanabe H, Holmes JH, Holm HH, Goldberg BB (eds): *Diagnostic Ultrasound in Urology and Nephrology*. Tokyo, New York, Igaku-Shoin, 1981, p 17.

8. Warren PS, Garrett WJ, Kossoff G: The liquid-filled stomach: An ultrasonic window to the upper abdomen. *J Clin Ultrasound* 6:315–330, 1978.

9. Bazzocchi M, Rizzatto G: The value of the posterior oblique longitudinal scan in renal ultrasonography. *Urol Radiol* 1:221–225, 1980.

10. Isikoff MB, Hill MC: Sonography of the renal arteries: Left lateral decubitus position. *AJR* 134:1,177–1,179, 1980.

11. Kossoff G: in Watanabe H, Holmes JH, Holm HH, Goldberg BB (eds): *Diagnostic Ultrasound in Urology and Nephrology*. Tokyo, New York, Igaku-Shoin, 1981, p 20.

12. Rosenfield AT, Zeman RK, Cronan JJ, Kay CJ: Ultrasound in the evaluation of renal masses. *Connect Med* 44:1–5, 1980.

13. Sanders RD: Practical value of diagnostic ultrasound in urology. *J Urol* 126:283–287, 1981.

14. Filly RA, Sommer FG, Minton MJ: Characterization of biological fluids by ultrasound and computed tomography. *Radiology* 134:167–171, 1980.

15. Hantmann SS, Barie JJ, Glendening TB, et al: Giant renal artery anuerysm mimicking a simple cyst on ultrasound. *J Clin Ultrasound* 10:136–139, 1982.

16. Pollack HM, Banner MP, Arger PH, et al: Comparison of computed tomography and ultrasound in diagnosis of renal masses. *Clin Dia Ultrasound* 1:25–72, 1979.

17. Pollack HM, Banner MP, Arger PH, et al: The accuracy of gray scale ultrasonography in differentiating cystic renal neoplasms from benign renal cysts. *Radiology* 143:741–745, 1982.

18. Behan M. Wixson D, Pitts WR Jr, Kazam E: Sonographic evaluation of renal masses: Correlations with angiography. *Urol Radiol* 1:137–145, 1981.

19. Weill FS, Bihr E, Rohmer P, Zeltner F: *Renal Sonography*. New York, Springer-Verlag, 1981, p 72.

20. Lingard DA, Lawson TL: Accuracy of ultrasound in predicting the nature of renal masses. *J Urol* 122:724–727, 1979.

21. Coleman BG, Arger PH, Mulhern CB Jr, et al: Pyonephrosis: Sonography in the diagnosis and management. *AJR* 137:939–943, 1981.

22. VanKirk OC, Go RT, Wedel VJ: Sonographic features of xanthogranulomatous pyelonephritis. *AJR* 134:1,035–1,039, 1980.

23. Yeh HC, Mitty HA, Wolf B: Ultrasonography of renal sinus lipomatosis. *Radiology* 124:799–801, 1977.

24. Maklad NF, Chuang VP, Doust BP, et al: Ultrasonic characterization of solid renal lesions: Echogenic, angiographic and pathologic correlation. *Radiology* 123:733–739, 1977.

25. Coleman BG, Arger PH, Mulhern CB Jr, et al: Gray-scale sonographic spectrum of hypernephromas. *Radiology* 137:757–765, 1980.

26. Shirkhoda A, Staab EV, Mittelstaedt CA: Renal lymphoma imaged by ultrasound and Gallium-67. *Radiology* 137:175–180, 1980.

27. Yiu-Chiu V, Chow KC, Cjiu LC, Agrawal SK: Computed tomography and ultrasonography in the diagnosis of calcified renal masses. *CT: J Comput Tomogr* 5:51–61, 1981.

28. Pollack HM, Edell S, Morales JO; Radionuclide imaging in renal pseudotumors. *Radiology* 111:639–644, 1974.

29. Daniel WW Jr, Hartman GW, Witten DM, et al: Calcified renal masses: A review of 10 years experience at the Mayo Clinic. *Radiology* 103:503–508, 1972.

30. Schieble W, Talner LB: Gray scale ultrasound and the genito-urinary tract. *Radio Clin North Am* 17:281n300, 1979.

31. Green B, Goldstein HM, Weaber RM Jr: Abdominal pansonography in the evaluation of renal cancer. *Radiology* 132:421–424, 1979.

32. Hartman DS, Goldman SM, Friedman AC, et al: Angiomyolipoma: Ultrasonic-pathologic correlation. *Radiology* 139:451–458, 1981.

33. Harcke HT, Williams JL: Evaluation of neonatal renal disorders: A comparison of excretory urography wit scintigraphy and ultrasonography. *Ann Radiol* 23:109–113, 1980.

34. Wilson DA: Ultrasound screening for abdominal masses in the neonatal period. *Am J Dis Child* 136:147–151, 1982.

35. Ralls PW, Esensten ML, Boger D, Halls JM: Severe hydronephrosis and severe renal cystic disease: Ultrasonic differentiation. *AJR* 134:473–475, 1980.

36. Stuck KJ, Koff SA, Silver TM: Ultrasonic features of multicystic dysplastic kidney: Expanded diagnostic criteria. *Radiology* 143:217–222, 1982.

37. McInnis AN, Felman AH, Kaude JV, Walker RD: Renal ultrasound in the neonatal period. *Pediatr Radiol* 12:15–20, 1982.

38. Jaffee MH, White SJ, Silver TM, Heidelberger KP: Wilms' tumor: Ultrasonic features, pathologic correlation and diagnostic pitfalls. *Radiology* 140:147–152, 1981.

39. Hartman DS, Sanders R: Wilm's tumor versus neuroblastoma: Usefulness of ultrasound in differentiation. *J Ultrasound Med* 1:117–122, 1982.

40. Hennessy WT, Pollack HM, Banner MP, Wein AJ: Radiologic evaluation of anuric patient: A systematized approach. *Urol* 18:435–445, 1981.

41. Finberg HJ, Hillman B, Smith EH: Ultrasound in the evaluation of the non-functioning kidney. *Clin Dia Ultrasound* 2:105–123, 1979.

42. Behan M, Wixson D, Kazam E: Sonographic evaluation of the nonfunctioning kidney. *J Clin Ultrasound* 7:449–458, 1979.

43. Longo VJ, Thompson CJ: Congenital solitary kidney. *J Urol* 68:63–, 1952.

44. Silverman PM, Carroll BA, Moskowitz PS: Adrenal sonography in renal agenesis and dysplasia. *AJR* 134:600–602, 1980.

45. Brandt TB, Neiman HL, Dragowski MJ, et al: Ultrasound assessment of normal renal dimensions. *J Ultrasound Med* 1:49–52, 1982.

46. Moskowitz PS, Carroll BA, McCoy JM: Ultrasonic renal volumetry in children. *Radiology* 134:61–64, 1980.

47. Lewis E, Ritchie WGM: A simple ultrasonic method for assessing renal size. *J Clin Ultrasound* 8:417–420, 1980.

48. Rosenfield AT, Lipson MH, Eolf B, et al: Ultrasonography and nephrotomography in the presymptomatic diagnosis of dominantly inherited (adult-onset) polycystic disease. *Radiology* 135:424–427, 1980.

49. Kelsey JA, Bowie JD: Gray-scale ultrasonography in the diagnosis of polycystic kidney disease. *Radiology* 122:791–795, 1977.

50. Mascatello VJ, Smith EH, Carrera GF, et al: Ultrasonic evaluation of the duplex kidney. *AJR* 129:113–120, 1977.

51. Haller JO, Friedman AP, Lebensart DP: Pseudoduplication: A scanning artifact of renal ultrasonography. *Urol Radiol* 1:187–,

52. Rosenfield AT, Taylor KJW, Crade M, deGraaf CS: Anatomy and pathology of the kidney by gray scale ultrasound. Radiology 128:737–744, 1978.

53. LeQuesne GW: Ultrasonic detection of glomerular disease :opabstr). AJR 130:96, 1978.

54. Rochester D, Aronson AJ, Bowie JD, Kunzman A: Ultrasonic appearance of acute posstreptococcal glomerulonephritis. J Clin Ultrasound 6:49–50, 1978.

55. Subramanyam BR: Renal amyloidosis in juvenile rheumatoid arthritis sonographic features. AJR 136:411–412, 1981.

56. Shuman WP, Mack LA, Rogers JV; Diffuse nephrocalcinosis: Hyperechoic sonographic appearance. AJR 136:830–832, 1981.

57. Rosenfield AT, Siegel NJ: Renal parenchymal disease: Histopathologic sonographic correlation. AJR 137:793–799, 1981.

58. Hricak H, Cruz C, Madrazo BL, et al: Renal parenchymal disease: Sonographic-histological correlation. Paper read at the 66th Scientific Assembly and Annual Meeting of The Radiological Society of North America. Dallas, Texas, November 18, 1980.

59. Lee JKT, McClennan BL, Melson GL, Stanley RJ: Acute focal bacterial nephritis: Emphasis on gray scale sonography and computed tomography. AJR 135:87–92, 1980.

60. Kay CJ, Rosenfield AT, Taylor KJW, Rosenberg MA: Ultrasonic characteristics of chronic atrophic pyelonephritis. AJR 132:47–48, 1979.

61. Rosenfield AT, Siegel NJ, Kappelman NB, Taylor KJW: Gray scale ultrasonography in medullary cystic disease of the kidney and hepatic fibrosis with tubular ectasia: New observations. AJR 129:297–303, 1977.

62. Rosenfield AT, Glickman MG, Taylor, KJW, et al: Acute focal bacterial nephritis (acute lobar nephroma). Radiology 132:553–561, 1979.

63. Boal DK, Teele RL: Sonography of infantile polycystic kidney disease. AJR 135:575–580, 1980.

64. Glazer GM, Callen PW, Filly RA; Medullary nephrocalcinosis: sonographic evaluation. AJR 138–55–58, 1982.

65. Edell SL, Bonavita JA: The sonographic appearance of acute pyelonephritis. Radiology 132:683–685, 1979.

66. Gerzof SG, Gale ME: Computed tomography and ultrasonography for diagnosis and treatment of renal and retroperitoneal abscesses. Urol Clin North Am 9:185–193, 1982.

67. Subramanyam BR, Megibow AJ, Raghavendra BN, Bosniak MA: Diffuse and sonography. Urol Radiol 4:5–10, 1982.

68. Kay CJ, Rosenfield AT, Armm M: Gray-scale ultrasonography in the evaluation of renal trauma. Radiology 134:461–466, 1980.

69. Schmoller H, Kunit G, Frick J: Sonography in blunt renal trauma. Eur Urol 7:11–15, 1981.

70. Ellenbogen P, Scheible F, Talner L, et al: Sensitivity of gray scale ultrasound in detecting urinary tract obstruction. AJR 130:731–733, 1978.

71. Zegel HG, Pollack HM, Banner MP, et al: Percutaneous nephrostomy: Comparison of sonographic and fluoroscopic guidance. AJR 137:925–927, 1981.

72. Ralls PW, Halls J: Hydronephrosis, renal cystic disease and renal parenchymal disease. Semin Ultrasound 2:49–60, 1981.

73. Finberg H: Renal ultrasound: Anatomy and technique. Semin Ultrasound 2:7–20, 1981.

74. Marano GD, Elyaderani MK: Lateral lumbar meningocele: A possible pitfall in renal sonography. *J Clin Ultrasound* 9:334–335, 1981.

75. Amis ES, Cronan JJ, Pfister RC, Yoder IC: Ultrasonic inaccuracies in diagnosing renal obstruction. *Urology* 19:101–105, 1982.

76. Talner LB, Scheible W, Ellenbogen PH, et al: How accurate is ultrasonography in detecting hydronephrosis in azotemic patients? *Urol Radiol* 3:1–6, 1981.

77. Curry NS, Gobien, RP, Schabel SI: Minimal dilatation obstructive nephropathy. *Radiology* 143:531–534, 1982.

78. Morin ME, Baker DA: The influence of hydration and bladder distention on the sonographic diagnosis of hydronephrosis. *J Clin Ultrasound* 7:192–194, 1979.

79. Rosenfield AT, Taylor KJW, Dembner AG, Jacobson P: Ultrasound of renal sinus: New observations. *AJR* 133:441–448, 1979.

80. Lee JKT, Baron RL Melson GL, et al: Can real time ultrasonography replace static B-scanning in the diagnosis of renal obstruction? *Radiology* 139:161–165, 1981.

81. Hadlock FP, Deter RL, Carpenter R, et al: Sonography of fetal urinary tract anomalies. AJR 137:261–267, 1981.

82. Deter RL, Hadlock FP, Gonzales ET, Wait RB: Prenatal detection of primary megaureter using dynamic imaging ultrasonography. *Obstet Gynecol* 56:759–762, 1980.

83. Pollack HM, Arger PH, Goldberg BB, Mulholland SG: Ultrasonic detection of non-opaque renal calculi. *Radiology* 127:233–237, 1978.

84. Arger PH, Mulhern CB, Pollack HM, et al: Ultrasonic assessment of renal transitional cell carcinoma. *AJR* 132:407–411, 1979.

85. Kurtz AB, Dubbins PA, Zegel HG, et al: Normal left renal vein mimicking left renal artery aneurysm. *J Clin Ultrasound* 9:105–108, 1981.

86. Spira R, Kwan E, Gerzof SG, Widrich WC: Left renal vein varix simulating a pancreatic pseudocyst by sonography. *AJR* 138:149–150, 1982.

87. Thomas JL, Lymberis MEB, Hunt TH: Ultrasonic features of acquired renal arterivenous fistula. *AJR* 132:653–655, 1977.

88. Rosenberg ER, Trought WS, Kirks DR, et al: Ultrasonic diagnosis of renal vein thrombosis in neonates. *AJR* 134:35–38, 1980.

89. Rosenfield AT, Zeman RK, Cronan JJ, Taylor KJW: Ultrasound in experimental and clinical renal vein thrombosis. *Radiology* 137:735–741, 1980.

90. Braun B, Weilemann LS, Weigand W: Ultrasonographic demonstration of renal vein thrombosis. *Radiology* 138:157–158, 1981.

91. Chatzkel S, Cole-Beuglet C, Breckenridge JW, et al: Ultrasound diagnosis of a hypernephroma metastatic to the thyroid gland an external jugular vein. *Radiology* 142:165–166, 1982.

92. Thomas JL, Bernardino ME: Neoplastic induced renal vein enlargement: Sonographic detection. *AJR* 136:75–79, 1981.

93. Barber-Riley P, Patel AS: Ultrasonic demonstration of renal artery thrombosis. *Br J Radiol* 54:351–352, 1981.

94. Weill FS, Bihr E, Rohmer P, Zeltner F: *Renal Sonography*. New York, Springer-Verlag, 1981, p 93.

95. Cook JH, Lytton B: The practical use of ultrasound as an adjunct to renal calculus surgery. *Urol Clin North Am* 8:319–329, 1981.

96. Lawson TL, Foley DW, Berland LL, Clark KE: Ultrasonic evaluation of fetal kidneys. *Radiology* 138:153–156, 1981.

97. Dubbins PA, Kurtz AB, Wapner RJ, Goldberg BB: Renal agenesis: Spectrum of in utero findings. *J Clin Ultrasound* 9:189–193, 1981.

98. Habif DV Jr, Berdon WE, Yeh MN: Infantile polycystic disease: In utero sonographic diagnosis. *Radiology* 142:475–477, 1982.

99. Golbus MS, Harrison MR, Filly RA, et al: In utero treatment of urinary tract obstruction. *Am J Obstet Gynecol* 142:383–386, 1982.

100. Harrison MR, Golbus MS, Filly RA, et al: Fetal surgery for congenital hydronephrosis. *N Engl J Med* 306:591–593, 1982.

101. Harrison MR, Filly RA, Parer JT, et al: Management of the fetus with a urinary tract malformation. *JAMA* 246:635–639, 1981.

102. Garris J, Kangarloo H, Sarti D, et al: The ultrasound spectrum of prune-belly syndrome. *J Clin Ultrasound* 8:117–120, 1980.

103. Christopher CR, Spinelli A, Severt D: Ultrasonic diagnosis of prune-belly syndrome. *Obstet Gynec* 59:391–394, 1982.

104. Kurtz AB, Rubin CS, Cole-Beuglet C, et al: Ultrasound evaluation of the renal transplant. *JAMA* 243:2,429–2,431, 1980.

105. Maklad NF: Ultrasonic evaluation of renal transplants. *Semin Ultrasound* 2:88–96, 1981.

106. Hrick H, Cruz C, Eyler WR, et al: Acute post-transplantation renal failure: Differential diagnosis by ultrasound. *Radiology* 139:441–449, 1981.

107. Heckemann R, Rehwald U, Jakubowski HD, Donhuijsen K: Sonographic criteria for renal allograft rejection. *Urol Radiol* 4:15–18, 1982.

108. Hricak H, Romanski RN, Eyler WR: The renal sinus during allograft rejection: Sonographic and histopathologic findings. *Radiology* 142:693–700, 1982.

109. Silver TM, Campbell D, Wicks JD, et al: Peritransplant fluid collections. *Radiology* 138:145–151, 1981.

10

Retroperitoneum

Barry B. Goldberg
Howard M. Pollack

INTRODUCTION

Before the development of ultrasonography and CT, the retroperitoneum was the blind spot of abdominal diagnosis. The retroperitoneal space contains many structures and can give rise to many problems that are difficult to identify. Most roentgenographic studies that reflect disease in the retroperitoneum (for example, barium enemas and excretory urograms) provide evidence of an indirect nature, such as displacement or compression of a contiguous structure. Ultrasonography, on the other hand, permits direct visualization of such entities as primary retroperitoneal tumors, abscesses, and fluid collections.

With the exception of retroperitoneal fibrosis, most disease processes in the retroperitoneum are masses. They may occur anywhere in this relatively large space, and, in general, they produce displacement of adjacent structures, especially the kidneys. Ultrasound not only can detect such masses but also can show their relationship to other retroperitoneal structures in the majority of cases. The ureters, which are often displaced or obstructed by retroperitoneal disease, can sometimes be seen at their origin and at their site of insertion into the urinary bladder, if they are at all dilated. The urinary bladder provides a standard of reference to confirm the cystic or solid nature of a mass. Evaluation of the size of the bladder as well as detection of internal abnormalities such as tumors and stones can also be carried out. The prostate and adjacent structures may be visualized by any of several different approaches. The techniques used are discussed first in a general way in the following paragraphs and then more specifically in the appropriate sections of this chapter and Chapter 11.

TECHNIQUE

The techniques employed for evaluating the retroperitoneal area are similar to those discussed in the previous chapter. The evaluation of the upper retroperitoneal structures should be attempted with the patient in several positions including the supine, axillary (coronal), and prone approaches. First, the area of interest is located with reference to the kidney or other fixed normal retroperitoneal structures. Preliminary information is usually available through physical examination or on urography, demonstrating either a palpable mass or renal displacement. Thus, the kidneys initially are localized and the masses defined with reference to the ipsilateral kidney. For suprarenal and upper pole renal masses, several methods may be required to produce satisfactory imaging. These include sustained inspiration in an attempt to displace the mass downward or, if this results in interference by the lung, sustained expiration during each scan. Scanning with the patient erect also may be used if these two techniques fail to displace the mass sufficiently caudad. When the disease occurs on the right side, the supine position is excellent, allowing transhepatic scanning using the same techniques described in the earlier chapters with initial longitudinal scans followed by transverse scans during suspended respiration. Axillary coronal and cross-sectional views often add helpful information. When searching for the right adrenal gland, it should be recalled that its medial position extends behind the vena cava. For the left adrenal, a posterior oblique view is often best (Fig. 10-1).

When evaluating medially located masses or dilated ureters, longitudinal prone or supine scans are continued medial to the kidney. Here, the axillary view is often ideal. Masses located inferior to the kidney are usually very difficult to evaluate in the prone position because of the overlying iliac crest. Large masses that project intraabdominally displace the bowel, often allowing satisfactory imaging in the supine position. In this case, the techniques followed are similar to those used elsewhere in the abdomen. First, the area of interest is localized; then, scans are obtained at uniform increments in both longitudinal and transverse directions. The examiner must exercise care to avoid the overlying bowel, not only because of the deleterious effect of gas on the ultrasonic beam but also because similar effects may be produced by barium. Such interference is not a problem, of course, when examining in the prone

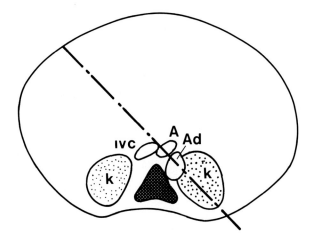

Figure 10-1 Diagram demonstrates ultrasonic pathway (dashed line) for obtaining images of the left adrenal gland. This approach has also been used to evaluate the right adrenal. IVC = inferior vena cava; A = aorta; K = kidneys; Ad = adrenal.

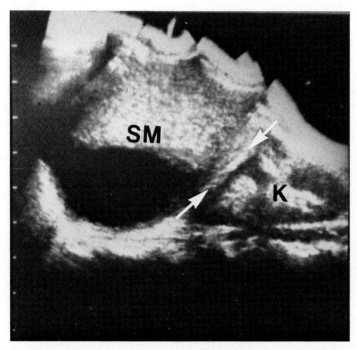

Figure 10-2 Longitudinal decubitus view producing a coronal image showing the kidney (K) with a suprarenal mass (SM) representing a large spleen containing a cystic area. The renal capsule (arrows) is clearly defined helping to establish that the mass is separated from the kidney.

position. Examination of the lower retroperitoneum is often facilitated by scanning through a filled urinary bladder.

The presence of normal structures capable of simulating masses must always be kept in mind. The spleen, for example, at times may show a large retroperitoneal surface, and, if care is not taken, this surface may be confused with a left suprarenal mass (Fig. 10-2). Usually, however, the spleen can be identified readily by its characteristic shape and complex ultrasonic pattern. On the right, a large caudate lobe of the liver may produce the same effect. Correlation with roentgenograms, radionuclide scans, or CT may be employed to assist in the anatomic localization of an unusually shaped liver or spleen.

Examination of the urinary bladder is performed in the supine position. Initial midline longitudinal scans are obtained extending from the pubis toward the umbilicus and beyond if necessary. Scans are then obtained at intervals of 1 to 2 cm on each side of the midline until the entire pelvic region has been examined. Next, transverse scans are obtained at set intervals, again starting at the level of the pubis and continuing upward to the umbilicus and beyond if needed. As with most gray scale techniques, there is little need for compound sectoring; linear or simple sector sweeps provide excellent results. A single sweep per scan is preferable to retracing areas already examined, as the latter procedure tends to produce falsely positioned echoes if there is any movement of structures within the body or change in the position of the transducer. Overscanning also increases reverberation echoes, producing confusing artifacts that may be mistaken for the anterior bladder wall or intraluminal pathology. Bowel gas is usually not a problem in urinary bladder evaluation since the bladder is anteriorly located and displaces the bowel as it distends. It is helpful if the sweeps that start at the pubis in both longitudinal and transverse planes are angled caudally into the pelvis so that the deep pelvic structures such as the bladder trigone, prostate, and posterior urethra in men, and the vagina and structures adjacent to the pouch of Douglas or cul de sac in women may be evaluated adequately. It is easy to do this when performing longitudinal sweeps by merely angling the transducer under the pubic bone. With transverse scans, the transducer arm must be angled.

Abnormalities of the urachus or cystic areas in the pelvis can be evaluated thoroughly using the same technique as that employed for the bladder. Similarly, the female pelvic organs and the prostate can be examined if the transducer is angulated steeply toward the pelvic floor in both the longitudinal and transverse scans. In general, it is a good rule to perform pelvic ultrasonography with a full urinary bladder. Not only does this practice provide information about the relationship of the bladder to contiguous pelvic masses but also serial examinations with controlled decreases in bladder volume through a catheter provide an estimate of the presence or absence of bladder wall fixation, which may accompany certain neoplastic and inflammatory processes. In addition, the sound-conducting properties of fluid allow the water- or urine-filled bladder to act as an excellent transmitting medium for ultrasonic evaluation of structures posterior or caudal to the bladder such as cul de sac collections, deep pelvic cysts, and even the prostate gland itself. Of course, the filled urinary bladder also serves as a standard against which to compare other masses for their sonographic properties. The urinary bladder may also be evaluated using an endoscanner. When all scans with a full bladder have been accomplished, the patient bladder should be emptied completely after which a repeat scan should be done. The repeat scan provides an estimate of the postvoid residual urine.

ADRENAL GLAND

Since the normal adult adrenal gland rarely measures more than 3 cm at its maximum diameter, special scanning techniques are usually required to record ultrasonic images of this structure. Although the normal adrenal gland can be imaged in most patients with careful technique, CT is generally recognized as being superior for the imaging of normal or only slightly enlarged adrenal glands.[1] Ultrasonography, on the other hand, offers clear advantages in children and very lean patients. Sample has reported an 80 to 90 percent success rate in obtaining satisfactory images of normal adrenal glands employing a technique based on a specific alignment of the left kidney with the aorta and the right kidney with either the aorta or inferior vena cava.[2,3] Yeh has developed a comparable meticulous scanning approach to the adrenals and reports that the right adrenal can be seen in 78 percent of patients, the left adrenal in 44 percent, and both glands in 31 percent.[4,5] When the adrenals are enlarged, ultrasound can be used effectively in not only establishing the presence of an adrenal mass, but also in determining its internal characteristics, such as, whether it is cystic, solid, or complex. Adrenal masses as small as 1.2 cm in diameter have been delineated ultrasonographically.[4]

The normal adrenals are triangular-shaped structures located just medial and superior to the kidneys with the left adrenal being slightly more medial and the right slightly more superior. Prone scans are almost never useful in demonstrating the adrenals unless there is considerable enlargement present. An effective technique is an oblique posterior approach in which the patient is placed in the decubitus position with the transducer moved both longitudinally and transversely, so that the adrenal gland and the aorta on the left and the opposite adrenal gland and vena cava on the right are recorded simultaneously (Fig. 10-3). Using the vena cava as a landmark and empirically employing various degrees of patient obliquity, ranging from supine to full left decubitus, the right adrenal gland, which tends to be located directly behind the inferior vena cava, can usually be imaged (Fig. 10-4). The left adrenal is more difficult to delineate. The posterior axillary oblique approach has proved to be the most useful.[1] It is Yeh's feeling that anterior transverse scanning is the best single method of scanning the adrenal gland and for detecting small masses.[5] Imaging in the erect position may be helpful when lung and rib interference render other positions unsatisfactory. The images should be made during suspended respiration. Changes in the normal triangular or lunate configuration of the adrenal (i.e., a rounded appearance) may indicate the presence of an adrenal mass. A pathologic process is also strongly suggested if the gland measures more than 3 cm in diameter or if its normal echogenicity is altered.

The adrenal lesions seen in clinical practice consist primarily of tumors and cysts, although large adrenal hematomas sometimes are encountered, especially in infants. The sonographic appearance of neonatal adrenal hemorrhage varies from a cystic to a complex pattern depending on the age of the hematoma (Fig. 10-5). In the acute phase, the pattern is cystic, but as clot fragmentation occurs, it becomes complex. Later, with absorption of the blood clot, the pattern may once again revert to the cystic type. The end stage of adrenal hemorrhage is accompanied by calcification, which on ultrasound is represented as linear areas of increased echogenicity with distal acoustic shadowing.[6] Adrenal cysts are occasionally encountered in adults, and these, too, are often calcified. It is conceivable that they represent the residual of undetected infantile or neonatal hemorrhage. Their ultrasonic characteristics are also variable just as are those seen in fresh adrenal hemorrhage (Fig. 10-6). Other benign conditions, such as abscesses, can also be defined in the adrenal region. The ultrasound pattern is that of either a complex or cystic mass depending on the exact mixture of fluid and solid (debris) components present. Usually a history of fever helps to make a more specific diagnosis of abscess possible. Urinomas may occasionally leak into the suprarenal region and have a cystic pattern.

While the most common adrenal lesions imaged by ultrasound are tumors, bilateral hyperplasia may be suspected when the adrenal glands are shown to be slightly enlarged and spherical in shape. Adrenal tumors may be either benign or malignant. Cortical adenomas, ganglioneuromas, and pheochromo-

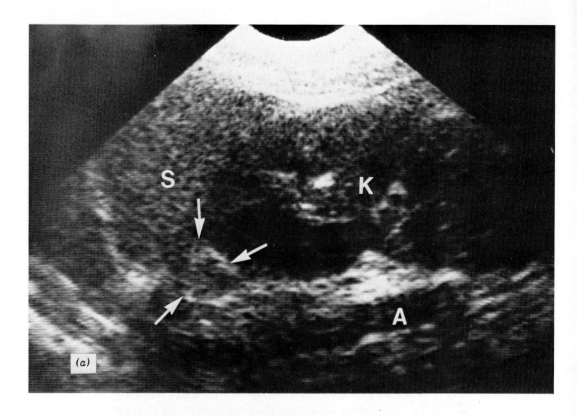

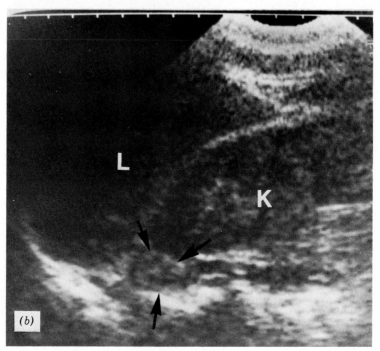

Figure 10-3 (*a*) Posterior coronal images of the left adrenal gland and (*b*) right adrenal gland (arrows). S = spleen; L = liver; A = aorta; K = kidney.

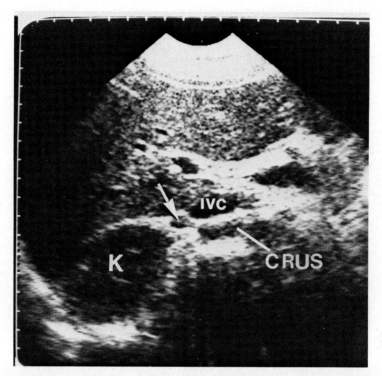

Figure 10-4 Supine transverse view of the right adrenal (arrow) demonstrates its location slightly posteromedial to the inferior vena cava (IVC) and anterior to the crus (line) of the diaphragm. K = kidney.

cytomas comprise most of the benign lesions and usually lend themselves well to ultrasonic imaging. Solid patterns are the rule in these cases, although cystic and complex patterns may be seen not infrequently (Figs. 10-7 and 10-8). With some pheochromocytomas and cortical adenomas, a well-defined capsule ("rind") may be identified as a highly echogenic area surrounding a fluid-filled or complex interior. Adrenal tumors are usually poorly echogenic. When there are focal zones of necrosis, areas containing strong echoes may appear. Some necrotic tumors may become almost totally anechoic. In patients with pheochromocytoma, careful attention should be given to the contralateral suprarenal area since, in 10 to 15 percent of cases, bilateral tumors are found.

The most common malignant lesions affecting the adult adrenal gland are metastatic tumors.[8] The sonographic appearance may be either solid or complex depending on the presence or absence of internal hemorrhage in the gland (Fig. 10-9). Of the two, the complex pattern is seen more often. Metastatic disease is usually bilateral (Fig. 10-10). Adrenal cortical carcinoma, which is much less common, may be seen as a solid or complex mass. In children, adrenal neuroblastoma is a relatively common malignant tumor and frequently grows to a large size before becoming clinically detectable. Ultrasonic visualization of this tumor presents few difficulties, and the pattern is that of a typically solid lesion.[9] Neuroblastomas exhibit more heterogenicity in their ultrasono-

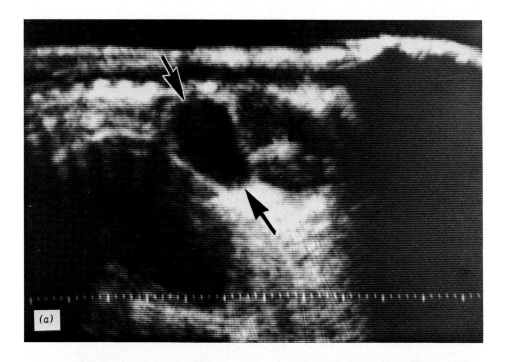

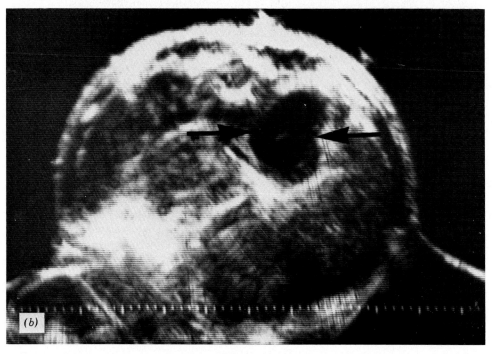

Figure 10-5 Prone longitudinal (*a*) and transverse (*b*) ultrasonograms demonstrate a predominantly cystic mass (arrows) representing adrenal hemorrhage in a neonate located superior to the kidney (K). On the transverse ultrasonogram, the few internal echoes are felt to represent clot.

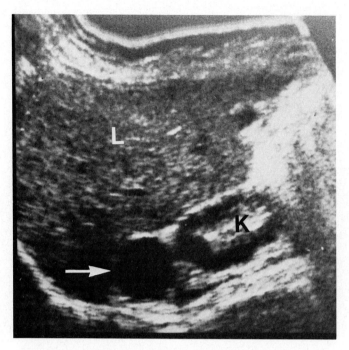

Figure 10-6 Supine longitudinal ultrasonogram shows evidence of a suprarenal cystic mass (arrow) seen to be separate from the kidney (K) and liver (L). This proved to be an adrenal cyst.

graphic appearance than do Wilms' tumors, a feature that often allows distinction between the two entities.[10] Adrenal neuroblastomas are diffusely highly echogenic and tend to absorb sound readily. Flecks of calcification may be seen within them (Fig. 10-11).

Occasionally, as with retroperitoneal tumors elsewhere, there may be difficulty in ascertaining the precise site of origin of a retroperitoneal tumor, especially an adrenal one. Tumors that originate in the kidney and invade the adrenal gland may be difficult to distinguish from large primary adrenal masses; the latter in turn may be difficult to distinguish from lesions in the caudoposterior aspect of the liver. To aid in this distinction, it is often helpful to analyze the appearance and configuration of the retroperitoneal fat—particularly that in the right upper quadrant. The fat may be displaced in a suggestive or characteristic manner by masses originating in this area, greatly assisting in the localization of such masses. Hepatic and subhepatic masses displace the highly echogenic and readily identifiable retroperitoneal fat posteriorly, while renal and adrenal lesions displace it anteriorly (Fig. 10-12).

In an attempt to compare the accuracy of ultrasonography versus CT in the diagnosis of adrenal masses, a multiinstitutional study encompassing 112 patients, of whom 51 had both ultrasonography and CT, was carried out. It was shown that CT had an accuracy of 90 percent compared to 70 percent for ultrasonography, indicating strong support for the diagnostic superiority of

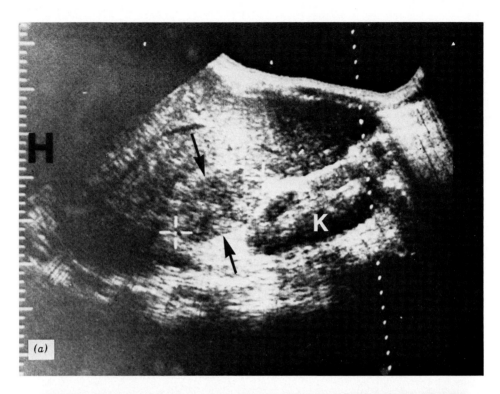

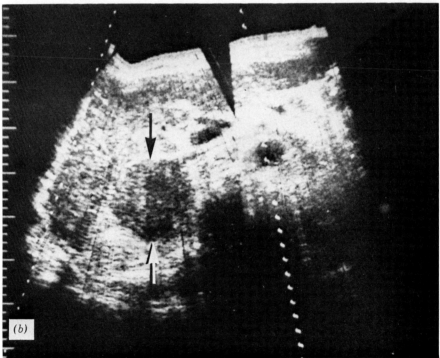

Figure 10-7 Supine longitudinal (*a*) and transverse (*b*) ultrasonograms demonstrate a typically solid suprarenal mass (arrows) that is well defined and separate from the kidney (K). This proved to be a benign cortical adenoma.

402

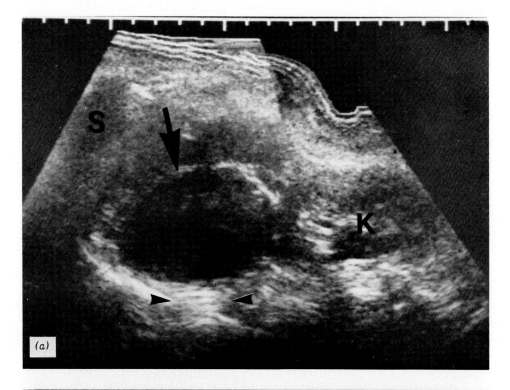

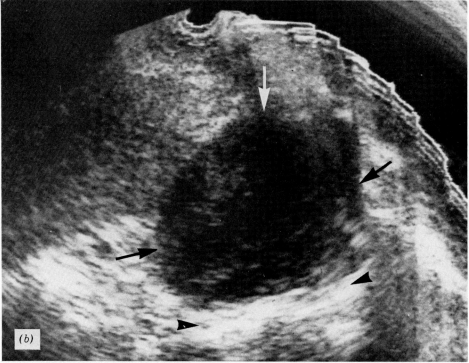

Figure 10-8 Coronal longitudinal (*a*) and transverse (*b*) ultrasonograms show a complex suprarenal mass (arrows) with a well-defined capsule and weak internal echoes, located between the spleen (S) and kidney (K). Note strong distal wall echoes (arrowheads).

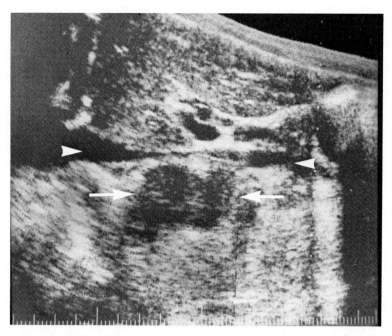

Figure 10-9 Supine longitudinal ultrasonogram shows evidence of an irregular complex mass (arrows) located posterior to the inferior vena cava (arrowheads) that is being slightly elevated and compressed. This proved to be a metastatic tumor to the right adrenal gland.

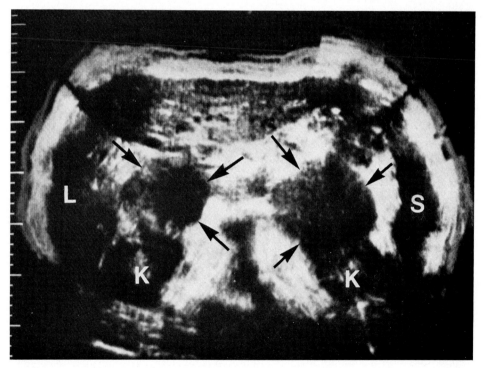

Figure 10-10 Supine transverse ultrasonogram shows evidence of bilateral complex masses (arrows) located anteromedial to the kidneys (K). This represented bilateral adrenal metastases. S = spleen; L = liver.

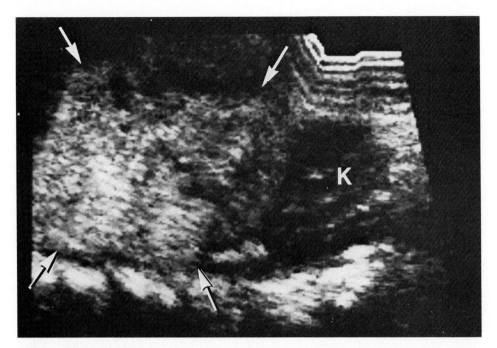

Figure 10-11 Ultrasonogram reveals an adrenal neuroblastoma (arrows), echogenic in nature, most likely due to calcification within it. K = kidney. (Courtesy of Henrietta Rosenberg, M.D. Director, Subdivision of Ultrasound, Children's Hospital of Philadelphia).

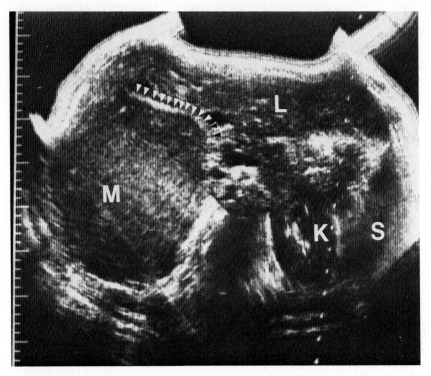

Figure 10-12 Ultrasonogram reveals displacement of the subhepatic fat (arrowheads) by an adrenal mass (M). L = liver; K = kidney; S = spleen.

CT.[8] This is not a unanimous opinion, however. Sample and Sarti reported identical accuracies for both CT and ultrasound in the diagnosis of adrenal lesions (90 percent accuracy), and Yeh reported only 3 percent false-negatives results among 34 patients with adrenal masses of various types.[12,5]

PERINEPHRIC AND PARANEPHRIC COLLECTIONS

The retroperitoneal space in the renal area is divided into two anatomic subdivisions. The space immediately surrounding the kidney is known as the perinephric space and has at its peripheral boundary the renal fascia (fascia of Gerota). (Fig. 10-13). Surrounding the renal fascia is another compartment known as the paranephric space, which, in effect, includes the remainder of the retroperitoneal space (Fig. 10-14). The paranephric space is further broken down into anterior and posterior divisions. The perinephric space is closed superiorly but open inferiorly and therefore allows fluid collections to spread caudally. Fluid accumulations occurring in these compartments consist of hematomas, abscesses, urinomas, and lymphoceles.[13–15]

Generally speaking, precise localization of fluid collections to either of the anatomic subcompartments of the retroperitoneum cannot be accomplished by ultrasound, but localization adequate to guide the surgeon in planning a proper

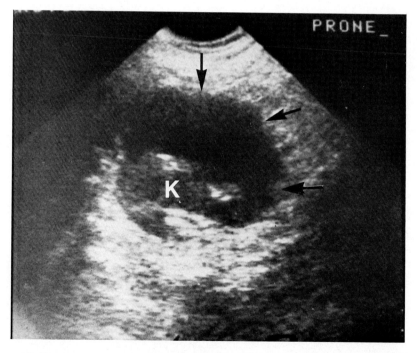

Figure 10-13 Prone transverse ultrasonogram shows the presence of a perinephric collection that has as its peripheral boundary the renal facia (arrows). This proved to be an abscess. K = kidney.

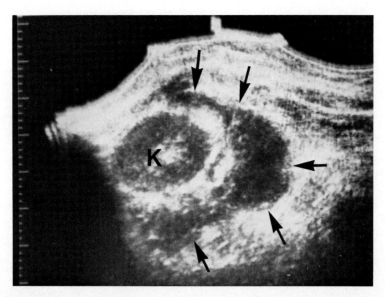

Figure 10-14 Transverse supine ultrasonogram demonstrates a paranephric collection (arrows) separated from the right kidney (K) by the more brightly reflective perinephric fat. This proved to be a hematoma.

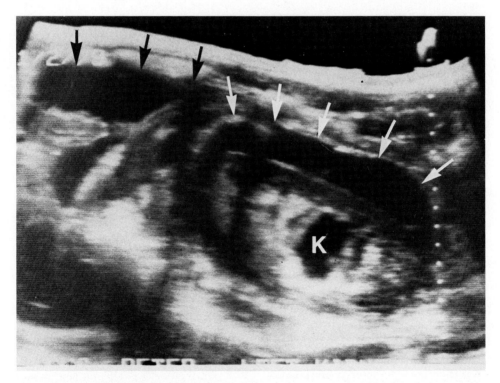

Figure 10-15 Prone longitudinal ultrasonogram shows evidence of predominantly cystic collections (arrows) superior and posterior to the kidney (K). This represented a urinoma.

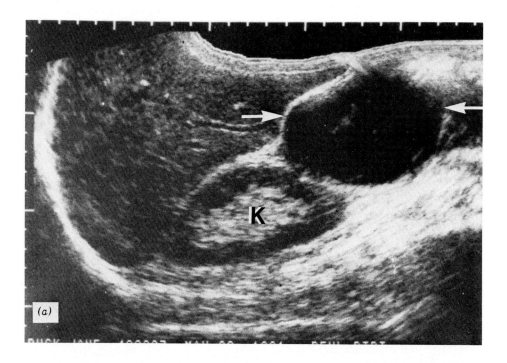

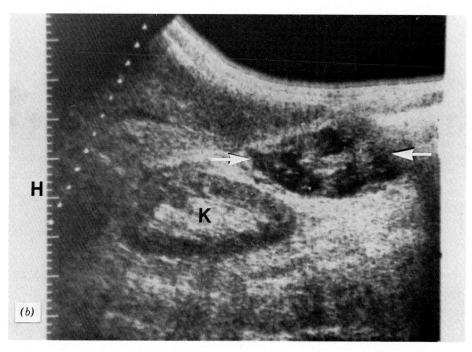

Figure 10-16 (*a*) Supine longitudinal ultrasonogram shows a predominantly cystic collection (arrows) anterior and inferior to the right kidney (K). This proved to be a hematoma the result of renal biopsy and is located in the anterior paranephric space. (*b*) A follow-up examination of the same area shows the collection (arrows) to be smaller in size with multiple internal echoes representing clot formation.

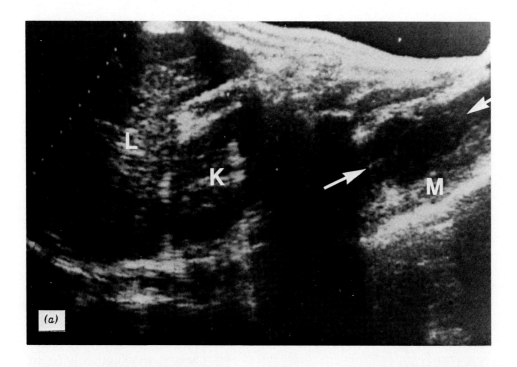

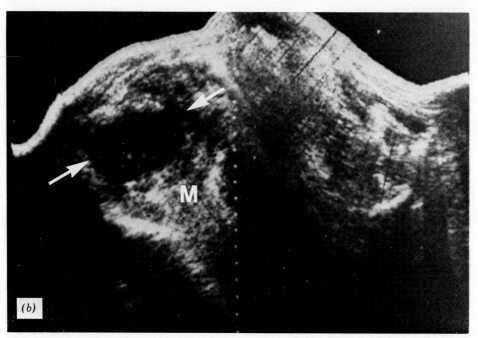

Figure 10-17 Supine longitudinal (*a*) and transverse (*b*) ultrasonograms show evidence of a complex area (arrows) located within the iliopsoas muscle (M) inferior to the kidney (K). This proved to be an abscess. L = liver.

operative approach is easily provided. While it is difficult or even at times impossible to distinguish one type of effusion from another with certainty, certain basic principles regarding fluid accumulations complicating renal transplantation apply. Thus, uninfected urinomas usually show a typical cystic pattern on sonography (Fig. 10-15). Hematomas may do likewise, but this finding is variable and is dependent on their degree of liquefaction and stage of clot dissolution (Fig. 10-16). It is not uncommon, therefore to see small particulate reflecting interfaces within hematomas. With infection, the pattern seen is usually a complex one as, for example, with perinephric abscesses. But cystic patterns, too, may be seen (Fig. 10-13).[16]

Various approaches may be needed in order to obtain maximum visualization of retroperitoneal effusions. Perinephric abscesses classically gravitate dorsal to the kidney and, therefore, usually lend themselves well to imaging in the prone position (Fig. 10-13). Other collections, however, may require varied and empirical approaches until maximum visualization is achieved. In some patients, particularly those with pelvic collections, the supine position proves to be very helpful (Fig. 10-17). Psoas abscesses may point into the groin and perinephric abscesses to the flank.

It has been mentioned that one of the main benefits of ultrasonic evaluation of retroperitoneal fluid collections is the ability to aid the surgeon in determining the optimum operative approach for these sometimes elusive masses. It should be pointed out, however, that sometimes percutaneous drainage rather than

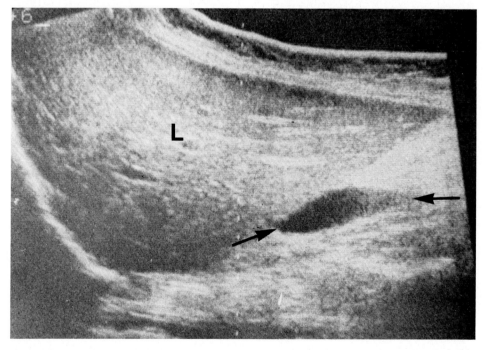

Figure 10-18 Supine longitudinal ultrasonogram delineates a fusiform type collection (arrows) located in the bed of a previously resected right kidney. This proved to be an abscess. L = liver.

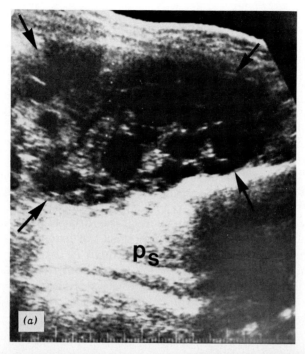

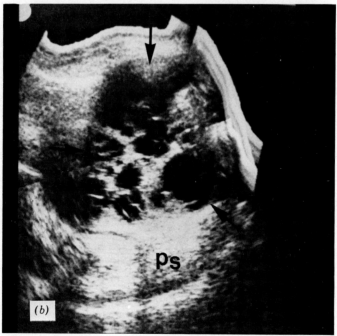

Figure 10-19 Left coronal longitudinal (*a*) and transverse (*b*) ultrasonograms show a multiloculated complex mass (arrows) having the typical pattern of cysts within a cyst described with hydatid disease. This was proven at surgery and confirmed to be located in the retroperitoneal region just lateral to the psoas muscle (PS). (Courtesy of Ruth Shilo, M.D. Tel Aviv Medical Center, Israel).

open surgical drainage is the treatment of choice, and in these instances, ultrasound also can be used to provide guidance for inserting the needle, the guide wire, and the drainage tube.[17,18] This technique is covered in more detail in Chapter 12.

Ultrasound may also be used to determine the adequacy of drainage as well as to provide a ready means of evaluating the satisfactory resolution of the collection or its potential recurrence. Of particular importance in this regard is the use of ultrasound to examine for hematoma formation following renal trauma, including needle biopsy of the kidney (Fig. 10-16). It has also been very helpful in following postoperative or posttraumatic urinomas (Fig. 10-15), and in excluding abscesses in those patients who, following renal or ureteral surgery, develop unexplained fever (Fig. 10-18). More unusual collections can also occur in the retroperitoneal area such as hydatid cysts (Fig. 10-19).

At times the quadratus lumborum muscle can appear markedly hypoechoic and can simulate a pathologic retroperitoneal collection process such as an abscess or hematoma. These potential pitfalls may be avoided if the examiner keeps in mind that the enhanced sound transmission characteristically seen with fluid collections does not occur in muscle and that this normal variant is usually bilateral. The quadratus lumborum muscle is seen most prominently when scanning is done in the prone position.[19]

RETROPERITONEAL SPACE

The retroperitoneal space contains abundant soft tissues that are not organized into well-defined organs. The space contains, for example, much loose fibroareolar tissue, fat, neurogenic elements, lymphatics, and other structures mainly of mesenchymal origin. The great vessels and their branches and the major abdominal lymph node aggregates are also found there, but, since specific chapters in this book have been allotted to them, they will not be discussed further at this time. Masses occur in the retroperitoneum that are not derived from any organ but instead appear to originate directly from the mesenchymal soft tissues. These are not to be confused with masses arising from organs that are partially or completely retroperitoneal such as the pancreas, kidneys, and adrenals or with masses primarily or secondarily involving bone and spinal cord.

Primary retroperitoneal masses may be neoplastic or nonneoplastic, and either cystic, complex, or solid. The majority of such lesions are neoplasms, however, and of these most are malignant.[20] The major nonneoplastic lesions previously described, aside from hematomas and psoas abscesses consist of retroperitoneal cysts. These cysts which in conjunction with benign neurogenic, smooth muscle and fatty tumors constitute the vast majority of benign masses. Excluding primary and secondary lymph node tumors, liposcarcoma, leiomyosarcoma, and hemangiopericytoma comprise the bulk of the malignant tumors.

The sonographic patterns of these masses depend on their physical composition. Retroperitoneal cysts, like cysts elsewhere, demonstrate a cystic ultrasonic pattern. Solid tumors, too, behave like their counterparts in other areas and produce either solid or complex ultrasonic patterns depending on the presence

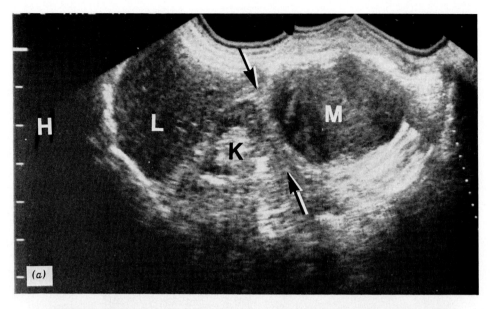

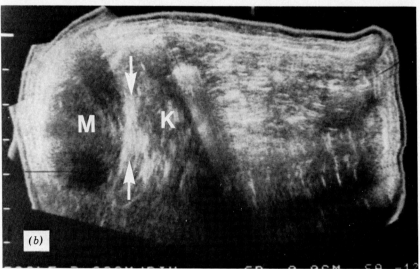

Figure 10-20 (*a*) Supine longitudinal and (*b*) transverse ultrasonograms demonstrate a large solid smooth-walled retroperitoneal mass (M) displacing the kidney (K) both medially and cephalad. Note the separation between kidney and mass delineated by intervening fat (arrows). This proved to be a fibrosing liposarcoma.

or absence of hemorrhage, necrosis, or cystic degeneration within the tumor. Karp et al. examined nine patients with retroperitoneal sarcoma of various types and found eight to have a similar ultrasonographic appearance. In these patients, the masses had regular, well-defined, smooth margins, and the tumors were solid in all cases (Fig. 10-20). Eight of nine tumors had a rich central echo pattern and usually a sonolucent periphery or a periphery with few echoes. An important ancillary observation in their series was that, in some cases, ultrasonography demonstrated displacement of the kidney and/or compression of the aorta and inferior vena cava.[21] Liposarcoma often appears as a homogeneously densely hyperechoic mass or as a hyperechoic mass intermixed with hypo- or anechoic areas (Fig. 10-21). The hyperechoic component of the mass corresponds to the fatty part of the tumor.[22]

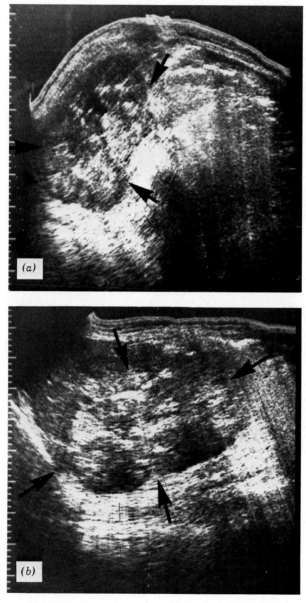

Figure 10-21 (*a* and *b*) Mixed ultrasonic pattern is seen from this large retroperitoneal tumor (arrows) having both hyper- and hypoechogenic areas. This proved to be a liposarcoma.

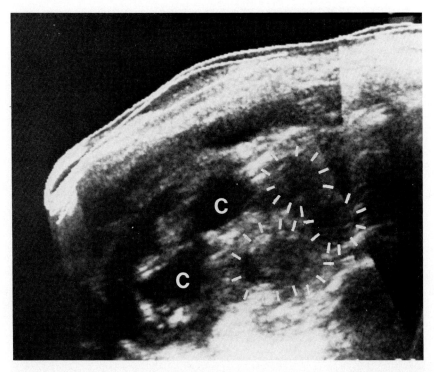

Figure 10-22 Transverse supine ultrasonogram shows evidence of retroperitoneal lymph nodes (dotted lines) that were obstructing the proximal ureter producing hydronephrosis of the right kidney. C = dilated calyces.

Cystic teratomas of the retroperitoneum also produce a mixed appearance on ultrasonography. Portions of these lesions contain fluid and have a cystic or complex appearance, while other portions contain fat and/or bone and calcium, giving hyperechoic or bright reflective zones, respectively. Masses that contain such multiple tissue components strongly suggest the diagnosis of cystic dermoid or teratoma, even though these lesions are much less common than smooth muscle and fatty sarcomas in the retroperitoneum.[23,24] With ultrasound, it is often possible to differentiate a paranephric retroperitoneal tumor from a primary renal tumor even when this distinction is not possible by urography.[19] The sonographic image of the mass and its surrounding retroperitoneal fat planes may delineate clearly a separation between the two structures even though they may appear to be indistinguishable roentgenographically (Fig. 10-20). Some retroperitoneal tumors, however, may actually invade the kidney making it all but impossible to determine their true origin. Because these lesions so often affect the ureters—usually by extrinsic compression, but occasionally by invasion as well—hydronephrosis frequently accompanies retroperitoneal masses of all types (Fig. 10-22). Retroperitoneal tumors may infiltrate and/or displace other structures. They can invade behind the aorta and vena cava, elevating or displacing them, and can even be associated with tumor invasion of the inferior vena cava (Fig. 10-9).[25,26]

Retroperitoneal fibrosis is a disease of unknown origin characterized by the

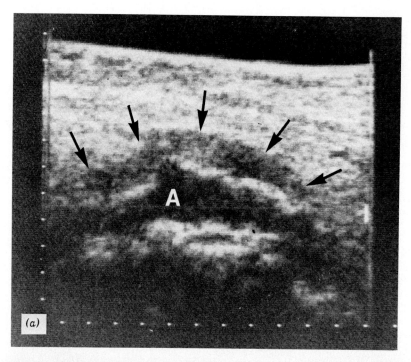

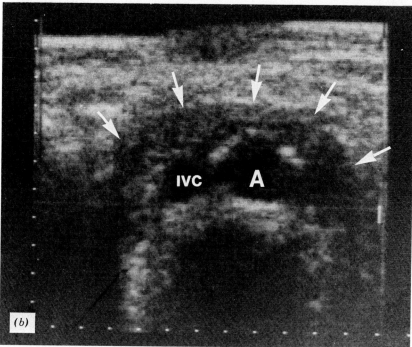

Figure 10-23 (*a*) Supine longitudinal and (*b*) transverse ultrasonograms delineate a weakly echogenic smooth-walled mass (arrows) anterior to the aorta (A) and inferior vena cava (IVC). This proved to be retroperitoneal fibrosis. Note that there is slight dilatation of the abdominal aorta.

416

presence of thick sheets of fibrous tissue in the retroperitoneal space. In many cases, it is possible to demonstrate such thick fibrous deposits by ultrasonography (Fig. 10-23).[27] Scans carried out in the supine position are usually more informative than those in the prone or other positions. There is a tendency for the mass to envelop and not displace adjacent hollow structures such as the aorta, vena cava, and ureters. The anterior margin of the lesion that conforms to and does not extend anterior to the peritoneal reflection is clearly delineated. The posterior margin, however, is poorly defined and not easily separated from adjacent structures. The lesion is minimally echogenic at low or moderate intensity settings.[27,28] The mass of fibrous tissue is often seen lying lateral to the great vessels and—if the dilated ureters can be visualized—they may be seen surmounting the ventral extent of the fibrous plaque. The fibrous tissue rarely extends above the level of L2 or below the inferior extent of the sacroiliac joints. The surgical approach to patients requiring intervention for this disease— usually because of obstructive uropathy—may be facilitated by preoperative ultrasonic demonstration of the extent of the disease. Medical treatment, if elected (i.e., steroids), may be followed by periodic ultrasound assessment.

Hypertrophy of the psoas muscle is a physiologic phenomenon seen in some muscularly well-developed individuals, and while ordinarily of no importance, it can be associated with deviation of the ureters. Visualization of an unusually thick iliopsoas muscle mass by ultrasound allows confirmation of this diagnosis, which is usually first suggested by urography.[29] Thick iliopsoas muscles may also be caused by intramuscular hemorrhage. This is not an uncommon finding in hemophiliacs or patients with other bleeding tendencies, especially those on anticoagulants who have sustained trauma.[30,31] The ultrasonic appearance of iliopsoas hematoma consists of a generalized smooth uniform enlargement of the involved muscle compared with the normal opposite side. The hematoma within the muscle is inseparable from the muscle mass itself and, in general, is characterized by a sonolucent appearance. On longitudinal sections, the enlarged muscle is spindle shaped, while on transverse sections, it has an avoid appearance. These hematomas generally absorb spontaneously allowing the muscle to eventually return to a normal appearance. The resolution of the hematoma can be monitored effectively by sonography. Abscesses may also involve the iliopsoas muscle or they may lie directly on it. Such abscesses may localize and point posteriorly in the flank or even in the groin.

URETER

While the normal ureter is rarely visualized ultrasonically because of its small diameter, variable course, and intermittent filling, the dilated ureter may be imaged with clarity (Fig. 10-24). Ureteral scanning is best performed with real-time imaging, which may allow visual observation of peristalsis and vesicoureteral reflux.[32] Reflux may be detected in some patients by sonographically observing the retrograde movement of micro air bubbles.[33] The axillary view is usually the best approach for the upper ureter, while an oblique longitudinal approach is best for the distal ureters, since this path follows the course of the ureter as it enters the bladder trigone. Other tubular structures that can be seen in this

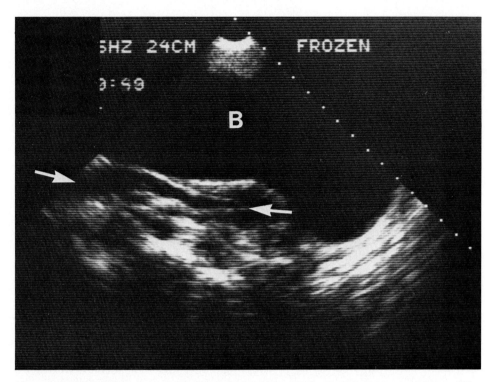

Figure 10-24 Oblique longitudinal ultrasonogram of the pelvis shows a portion of a relatively normal ureter (arrows) as it enters the bladder trigone just beneath the urine-filled bladder (B).

region are the major pelvic vessels. Confusion with the ureters is avoided by the use of real time, which demonstrates lack of pulsation in dilated ureters. Visualization of the pelvic ureter is enhanced by the presence of a full bladder, which serves as an acoustic window.

Whenever hydronephrosis is encountered, a search for ureteral dilatation should be made, and if discovered, the unilaterality or bilaterality of the dilatation should be established (Fig. 10-25). Occasionally, the ureters may be visualized as hugely dilated structures, as for example, in agenesis of the anterior abdominal wall (prune belly syndrome). Ultrasonographic visualization of the dilated ureter is particularly helpful when renal function is inadequate to produce satisfactory opacification by urography and, in addition, may be quite useful in following changes in ureteral caliber (or renal pelvic diameter) after treatment for relief of obstruction or reflux has been instituted.[34] Brandt et al. have reported ultrasonography of the urinary tract as a satisfactory alternative to excretory urography in the initial evaluation of patients with spinal cord injury. They were able to visualize dilated ureters in 43 percent of patients with ureterectasis and, using real time, could see vesicoureteral reflux in approximately one-quarter of the patients in which it existed.[32] Kessler and Altman reported ultrasonography to be 87 percent accurate in detecting reflux in children (Fig. 10-26).[33]

At times it is possible not only to demonstrate an obstructed ureter but also

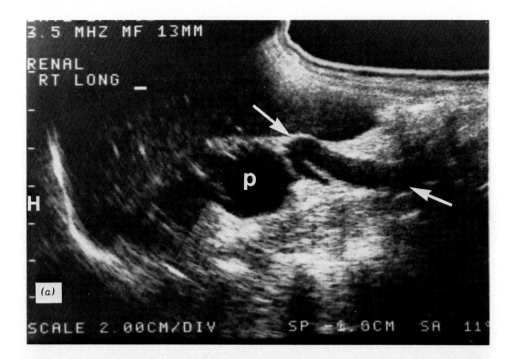

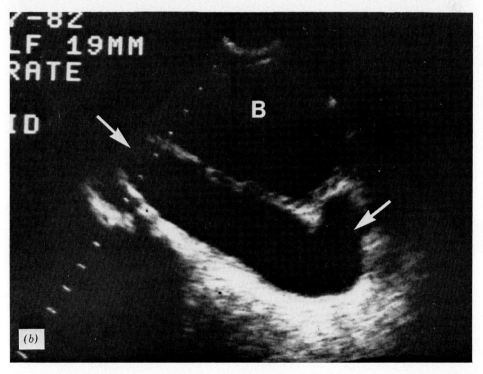

Figure 10-25 (*a*) Supine longitudinal ultrasonogram demonstrates a hydronephrotic right kidney with moderate dilatation of the pelvis (P). Just inferiorly, note a torturous dilated ureter (arrows). (*b*) Oblique longitudinal scan of the pelvic area shows the markedly dilated distal ureter (arrows) as it enters the bladder (B). (*c*) Transverse pelvic image confirmed that the obstruction was bilateral by demonstration of dilated ureters (arrows) seen posterior to the bladder (B).

419

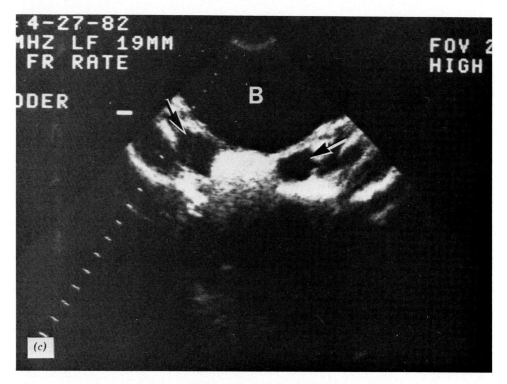

Figure 10-25 (*continued*)

to determine the cause of the obstruction. Enlarged lymph nodes, for example, may produce obstruction of the ureter resulting in hydronephrosis and/or ureterectasis (Fig. 10-22). Such enlarged lymph nodes may be easily recognized ultrasonically. Calculi in the renal pelvis and calyces have been clearly demonstrated ultrasonically,[35] and there is reason to believe that if a ureteral calculus is large enough it too may be detectable (Fig. 10-27). Small stones, of course, cannot be imaged with current state of the art ultrasonographic equipment. If a nondilated ureter can be rendered echo-producing by for example, inserting a ureteral catheter in it, its position can then be recorded ultrasonically. This technique can be employed in cases of suspected retrocaval ureter (Fig. 10-28).

A highly suggestive, if not pathognomonic, ultrasonographic appearance occurs with ectopic ureteroceles. In this condition, usually encountered in children, the dilated ureter can usually be demonstrated originating from a dilated upper portion of a duplex kidney and extending posteriorly to a region corresponding to the bladder trigone. Within the bladder, the ureterocele may be seen as a typical fluid-filled globular structure giving the appearance—when the bladder is also filled—of a "cyst within a cyst."[36] Nonectopic ureteroceles, which usually occur in adults, may also be visualized. These ureteroceles at times contain calculi that may also be demonstrated ultrasonically.

The normal jets of urine by which the ureters discharge their contents into the urinary bladder have been imaged with real time and pulsed Doppler

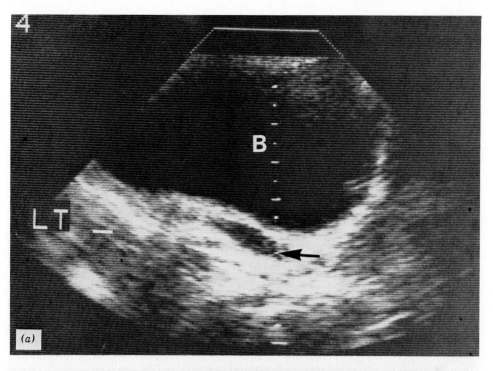

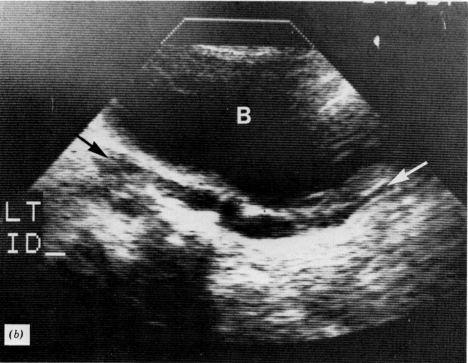

Figure 10-26 (*a*) Supine longitudinal oblique ultrasonogram of the pelvis shows evidence of a slightly prominent ureter (arrows) located just behind the bladder (B). (*b*) After partial voiding the ureter is seen to be more distended. Under real-time the progressive dilitation of the ureter due to reflux could be easily visualized.

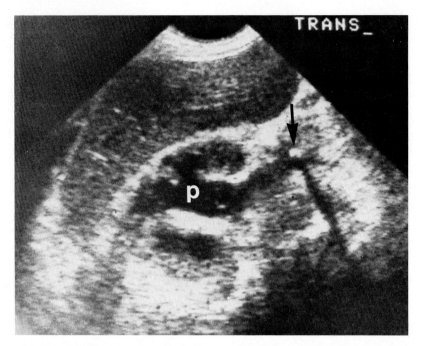

Figure 10-27 Transverse supine ultrasonogram shows evidence of dilated renal pelvis (P). The proximal ureter is visualized, and a small brightly echogenic area (arrow) with associated distal acoustic shadowing is seen. This proved to be a ureteral stone on retrograde pyelography.

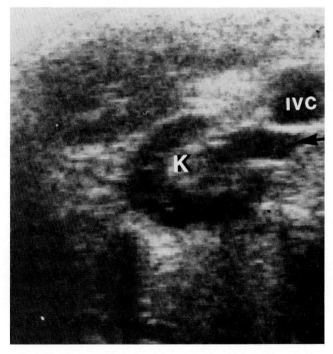

Figure 10-28 Transverse supine ultrasonogram demonstrates the presence of a dilated proximal ureter (arrow) extending behind the inferior vena cava (IVC). K = kidney. Catheterization confirmed the presence of a retrocaval ureter.

ultrasound. While the jets themselves may be clearly demonstrated, the mechanism of their ultrasonographic visualization is unclear. Theories advanced to account for the demonstration of the ureteral jets include a difference in specific gravity between ureteral and bladder urine[37] and the turbulence of the urine entering the urinary bladder.[38]

REFERENCES

1. Goldberg BB: The Retroperitoneum, in Watanabe H, Holmes JH, Holm HH, Goldberg BB (eds): *Diagnostic Ultrasound in Urology and Nephrology.* Tokyo, New York, Igaku-Shoin, 1981, p 67.

2. Sample WF: A new technique for the evaluation of the adrenal gland with gray scale ultrasonography. *Radiology* 124:463, 1977.

3. Sample WF: Adrenal ultrasonography. *Radiology* 127:461, 1978.

4. Mitty HA, Yeh HC: Radiology of the adrenals. Philadelphia, WB Saunders Co., 1982.

5. Yeh HC: Ultrasonography of normal adrenal glands and small adrenal masses. *AJR* 135:1,167, 1980.

6. Pery M, Kaftori JK, Bar-Maor JA; Sonography for diagnosis and follow-up of neonatal adrenal hemorrhage. *J Clin Ultrasound* 9:397–401, 1981.

7. Bowerman RA, Silver TM, Jaffe MH, et al: Sonography of adrenal pheochromocytomas. *AJR* 137:1,227–1,231, 1981.

8. Abrams HL, Siegelman SS, Adams DF, et al: Computed tomography versus ultrasound of the adrenal gland: A prospective study. *Radiology* 143:121–128, 1982.

9. Berger PE, Kuhn JP, Munschauer RW: Computed tomography and ultrasound in the diagnosis and management of neuroblastoma. *Radiology* 128:663–667, 1978.

10. Hartman DS, Sanders R: Wilms' tumor versus neuroblastoma: Usefulness of ultrasound in differentiation. *J Ultrasound Med* 1:117–122, 1982.

11. Gore RM, Callen PW, Filly RA: Displaced retroperitoneal fat: Sonographic guide to right upper quadrant mass localization. *Radiology* 142:701–705, 1982.

12. Sample WF, Sarti DA: Computed tomography and gray scale ultrasonography of the adrenal gland: A comparative study. *Radiology* 128:377, 1978.

13. McCullough DL, Leopold GR: Diagnosis of retroperitoneal fluid collections by ultrasonography: Series of surgically proved cases. *J Urol* 115:656, 1976.

14. Laing FC, Jacops RP: Value of ultrasonography in the detection of retroperitoneal inflammatory masses. *Radiology* 123:169–172, 1977.

15. Fried AM, Williams CB, Litvak AS: High retroperitoneal lymphocele: Unusual clinical presentation and diagnosis by ultrasonography. *J Urol* 123:583–584, 1980.

16. Kressel HY, Filly RA: Ultrasonographic appearance of gas-containing abscesses in the abdomen. *AJR* 130:71, 1978.

17. Elyaderani MK, Subramanian VP, Burgess JE; Diagnosis and percutaneous drainage of a perinephric abscess by ultrasound and fluoroscopy. *J Urol* 125:405–407, 1981.

18. Gerzof SG, Gale ME: Computed tomography and ultrasonography for diagnosis and treatment of renal and retroperitoneal abscesses. *Urol Clin North Am* 9:185–193, 1982.

19. Callen PW, Filly RA, Marks WM: The quadratus lymborum muscle: A possible source of confusion in sonographic evaluation of the retroperitoneum. *J Clin Ultrasound* 7:349–352, 1979.

20. Ackerman LV: Tumors of the retriperitoneum, mesentery and peritoneum in *Atlas of Tumor Pathology*, sec 6. Washington, D.C., 1954.

21. Karp W, Hafstrom LO, Jonsson PE: Retroperitoneal sarcoma: Ultrasonographic and angiographic evaluation. *Br J Radiol* 53:525–531, 1980.

22. Yiu-Chiu V, Chiu L: Ultrasonography and computed tomography of retroperitoneal liposarcoma. *CT: J Comput Tomogr* 5:98–110, 1981.

23. Weinstein BJ, Lenkey JL, Williams S: Ultrasound and CT demonstration of a benign cystic teratoma arising from the retroperitoneum. *AJR* 133:936–938, 1979.

24. Aston JK: Ultrasound demonstration of retroperitoneal teratoma. *J Clin Ultrasound* 7:377–378, 1979.

25. Kurtz AB, Rubin C, Goldberg BB: Ultrasound diagnosis of masses elevating the inferior vena cava. *AJR* 132:401–406, 1976.

26. Pussell SJ, Cosgrove DO: Ultrasound features of tumor thrombus in the IVC in retroperitoneal tumors. *Br J Radiol* 54:866–869, 1981.

27. Fagan CJ, Larrieu AJ, Amparo EG: Retroperitoneal fibrosis: Ultrasound and CT features. *AJR* 133:239–243, 1979.

28. Center S, Schwab R, Goldberg BB: The value of ultrasonography as an aid in the treatment of idiopathic retroperitoneal fibrosis. *J Ultrasound Med* 1:87–89, 1982.

29. Bree RL, Green B, Keiler DL, Genet EF: Medial dexiation of the ureters secondary to psoas muscle hypertrophy. *Radiology* 118:691, 1976.

30. Kumari S, Fulco JD, Karayalcin G, Lipton R: Gray scale ultrasound: Evaluation of ileopsoas hematomas in hemophiliacs. *AJR* 133:103–106, 1979.

31. Wiggers RH, Rosekrans P: Ultrasonographic diagnosis of psoas hematoma. *Diagn Imaging* 49:98–105, 1980.

32. Brandt TD, Neiman HL, Calenoff L, et al: Ultrasound evaluation of the urinary system in spinal-cord-injury patients. *Radiology* 141:473–477, 1981.

33. Kessler RM, Altman DH; Real-time sonographic detection of vesicoureteral reflux in children. *AJR* 138:1,033–1,036, 1962.

34. Forsberg L, Malmfors G, Mortensson W, White T: Ultrasound examination of the kidney after Politano-Leadbetter ureteroneocystostomy. *Acta Radiol Diagn* 22:349–351, 1981.

35. Pollack HM, Arger PH, Goldberg BB, Mulholland SG: Ultrasonic detection of non-opaque renal calculi. *Radiology* 127:233–237, 1978.

36. Morgan CL, Grossman H, Trought WS, Oddson TA; Ultrasonic diagnosis of obstructed renal duplication and ureterocele. *South Med J* 73:1,016–1,019, 1980.

37. Kremer H, Dobrinski W, Mikyska M, et al: Ultrasonic in vivo and in vitro studies on the nature of the ureteral jet phenomenon. *Radiology* 142:175–177, 1982.

38. Dubbins P, Kurtz AB, Darby J, Goldberg BB: Ureteric jet effect: The echographic appearance of urine entering the bladder. *Radiology* 140:513–515, 1981.

11

Lower Urinary Tract and Testes

Matthew D. Rifkin
Barry B. Goldberg

INTRODUCTION

Ultrasound is an important diagnostic imaging modality for evaluating the urinary tract. Initially used for differentiating cystic from solid masses in the kidneys, the urinary bladder and the remainder of the lower urinary system are now frequently examined. The bladder can be evaluated when distended with urine, and it also serves as an acoustic window to study the remainder of the pelvis. The prostate and the scrotum can also now be analyzed using ultrasound, the result of recent developments of high-resolution specialized equipment during the past few years.

THE URINARY BLADDER

The urinary bladder, the largest potential space in the pelvis, is most often imaged when it is used as an acoustic window to evaluate the adjacent pelvic structures. The bladder must be distended with at least one liter of fluid (i.e., urine or other material).

Anatomy

The bladder wall is composed of four layers: (*1*) the mucosa, a thin layer of transitional cell epithelium; (*2*) the submucosa, consisting of areolar tissue that connects the muscular layer with the mucosa; (*3*) the muscularis, consisting of three layers of smooth muscle; and (*4*) the serosa, the outer most layer derived from the peritoneum and only present on the superior portion of the bladder.[1]

With the urinary bladder distended, the peritoneum forms two potential spaces in the pelvis, the anterior paravesical space and posteriorly, the cul-de-sac. Inferior to the anterior peritoneal reflection, the urinary bladder is in direct contact with the pubic bones. In men, the posterior bladder wall is adjacent to the seminal vesicles, the vas deferens, and more inferiorly at the

425

bladder base, the prostate. The uterus and adnexal structures are the posterior borders in women, and because of the various normal anatomic placements, their position is inconsistent. The ureters insert at the trigones that are bilaterally symmetrically situated at posterior lateral aspects of the bladder.

When the bladder is distended, its lateral caudad margins are bordered by the acetabulum, constricting its shape to appear square (Fig. 11-1a). As the bladder extends cephalically, the lack of bony margins allows it to assume a more rounded shape (Fig. 11-1b).[2] Ultrasonically, the bladder walls are sharply defined posteriorly and laterally. The anatomic layers of the bladder are not clearly demarcated on the sonogram.

The ureteral insertion may be defined, when, during real-time examination, bright echoes are noted in the bladder as urine flows from the ureter in the region of the trigone. This sporadic disruption of the anechoic fluid in the bladder caused by flow differences is known as the "jet effect" (Fig. 11-2).[3,4]

Technique

There are numerous approaches available to evaluate the bladder. The suprapubic-abdominal approach is the simplest to use.[5] Recently, specialized sonoendoscopic probes have been developed that allow examination with transurethrally or transrectally placed ultrasound transducers.[6-8]

B-scan contact images can be obtained in both transverse and longitudinal projections at 0.5 to 1.0 cm intervals by placing the transducer on the abdomen immediately superior to the pubic bone and angling it in a slightly caudad direction. Sector and linear array real-time evaluation can also be used with excellent results.[5] The gain controls should be adjusted so that the inner contents of the bladder are anechoic. Minimal reverberation echoes at the anterior portion are acceptable.

The specialized transurethral sonoendoscopes with the transducers placed in the tip of the probe requires the patient to be cystoscoped.[6,7] The male patient requires general or spinal anaesthesia, and the study is usually performed in the operating room. Women may be studied with mild sedation as out-patients. The technique using B-scan equipment, known as radial scanning, produces images in transverse orientation, known as radial scanning. Following urethral catheterization with the rigid endoscope, images of the urinary bladder are recorded at 0.5 cm intervals from the caudad portion at the origin of the urethra to the fundus (the most superior aspect of the urinary bladder). The bladder, which must be distended for this examination, may be filled during the procedure via the sonoendoscope, which has specifically designed channels for this purpose.

Sonoendoscopes with special transducers have also been manufactured for transrectal placement. These are used for the evaluation of both the urinary bladder and prostate and produce images in transverse or longitudinal planes depending on the unit.[8,9]

Ultrasonic Diagnosis

Both intrinsic and extrinsic abnormalities can be seen during routine ultrasonic evaluation. Filling defects, bladder wall irregularities and foreign material can

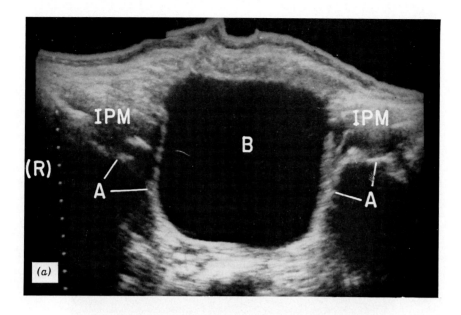

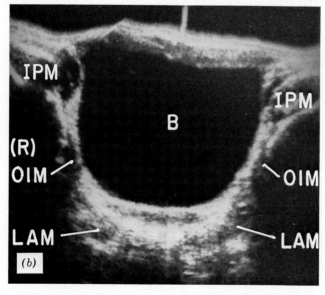

Figure 11-1 (*a*) Transverse image of fluid-filled bladder at its caudad margin. The bladder demonstrates a squared-off appearance as it is visualized in its most caudad portion. The acetabula (A) and the iliopsoas muscles (IPM) anteriorly are the constricting lateral borders to the bladder. (R) = patient's right side. (*b*) Transverse image of the fluid-filled urinary bladder in its cephalad portion. The rounded urinary bladder is noted bordered by the iliopsoas muscles (IPM) anterolaterally, the obturator internus muscles (OIM) laterally, the levator ani muscles (LAM) posteriorly. B = bladder; (R) = patient's right side.

427

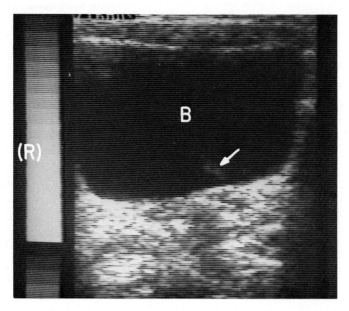

Figure 11-2 Ureteral jet phenomena. A real-time image demonstrates the fluid-filled urinary bladder (B) with an echogenic area extending from the posterolateral margin on the left side (arrow), which is caused by the turbulence produced by the urine being expelled from the distal ureter into the bladder. (R) = patient's right side.

be noted with great accuracy.[5] Transitional cell carcinoma is usually denoted as a focal area of wall thickening. These echogenic masses may be small (Fig. 11-3) or quite extensive (Fig. 11-4) and can often be seen extending beyond the wall. Fungating, polypoid cancers (Fig. 11-5) may be acoustically difficult to differentiate from some benign lesions, such as, consolidated blood clot or nonshadowing calculi.[5]

The accurate staging of cancers is useful prognostically (the highest grade having the worst prognosis) and as a guide in planning appropriate therapy. The clinical grading system, applicable to ultrasound classifies malignancy into four categories:[10]

1. Limited to the mucosa
2. Invading the submucosa
3. Invading the bladder wall musculature
4. Extending beyond the muscle layer

Staging of these cancers can be performed with the currently available ultrasound modalities. The abdominal approach appears as accurate as computed tomography and more accurate than clinical staging by bimanual examination and cystoscopy.[11] The most sensitive method appears to be by transurethral endosonoscopic evaluation where highly significant correlation to histologic specimens are obtained (Fig. 11-6).[6,7]

The Stage I lesions, which are as small as a few millimeters, are the most difficult to detect ultrasonically, often seen only with the transurethral sonoendoscope. The larger, more invasive lesions can be accurately staged by all methods.[12-14]

The transurethral endoscope demonstrates both small and large masses. Varying the distension of the bladder with fluid permits evaluation of vesical wall pliability, which can be caused by neoplastic infiltration. The presence of these changes may alter treatment planning.[7]

Inflammatory reactions of the bladder, cystitis, are usually diffuse processes (Fig. 11-7). Sonographically, the bladder appears thickened and echogenic. Acoustically, the mixed lesions may represent massive edema that is seen with bullous cystitis.[5]

Recently, cases of focal cystitis have been demonstrated that have focal hyperechoic areas of thickening with the remainder of the bladder wall appearing normal (Fig. 11-8). This has been seen in primary cystitis and secondary inflammation from an extrinsic cause, diverticulitis. Both the histologic and ultrasonic findings were confined to a small area of mucosa in the urinary bladder. These focal abnormalities must be differentiated from the more common diffuse cystitis with an additional larger focally edematous area, and with focal malignancy.[15]

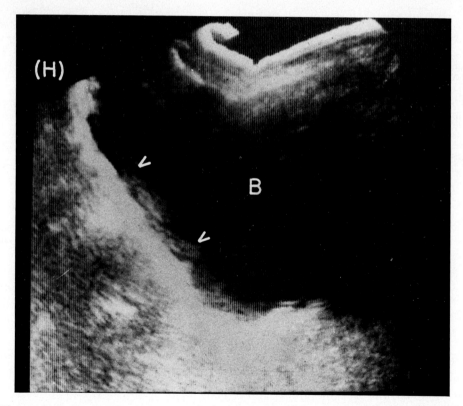

Figure 11-3 Grade II transitional cell bladder carcinoma. A grade II transitional cell carcinoma of the urinary bladder is noted involving the posterior aspect of the bladder wall (arrowheads). The irregular margination is involving the mucosa and portions of the submucosa. B = bladder; (H) = toward patient's head.

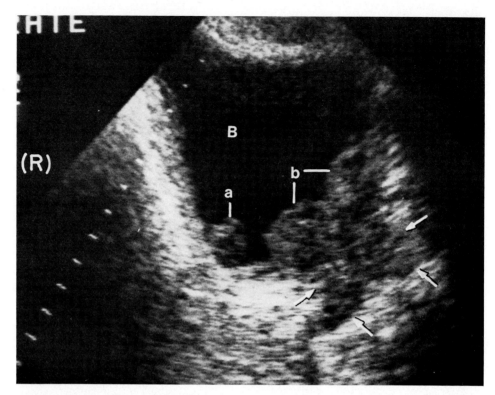

Figure 11-4 Grade IV invasive transitional cell carcinoma of the bladder. Transverse image of the urinary bladder (B) demonstrates multiple lobulated masses (a and b). Lesion "a" appears to be involving only the mucosa and submucosa equivalent to a stage II lesion, whereas lesion "b" is infiltrating through the bladder wall into the pelvic sidewalls (arrows), a stage IV lesion. (R) = toward patient's right side.

Ureteroceles, invaginations of the ureteral orifice into the bladder are smooth, well-defined cystic areas suggesting masses within or near the wall of the bladder (Fig. 11-9).[16,17] A diagnostic clue to the proper diagnosis is the visualization of the "jet" phenomenon. If this is not seen, the diagnosis may also be suggested by the mass' position at the trigone.

A Foley catheter in the bladder is detected by visualization of the balloon distended with fluid, which is also secured by the catheter at the bladder base. Bright linear reflections from the walls of the foley as it extends from the urethra into the bladder are also seen (Fig. 11-10).

Calculi are detected as hyperechoic focal echoes that cause shadowing (Fig. 11-11). These stones may be single or multiple and should move with a change in the patient's position, that is, from supine to decubitus views. However, with acute or chronic inflammation, some calculi may adhere to the bladder wall, mimicking carcinoma. In these cases, enhancement of the acoustic shadowing from the stone may be noted by decreasing the gain. These brightly reflective echoes and shadows are not always due to calcium within the stone. They are dependent on compactness and molecular density of the calculus and are seen with stones other than calcium, such as magnesium and uric acid.[5]

Blood clots may be noted as intravesical masses of varying echogenicity. The acoustic reflectivity of the hematomas changes as the amount of fibrin and other components vary. The lesions may be focal or diffuse, occasionally fixed to the wall, but more often freely movable (Fig. 11-12).[5]

Occasionally, fluid levels may be noted when two liquid substances of varying density are present (Fig. 11-13). By repositioning the patient, the fluid levels also change. Phosphate and cholesterol deposits in the urine have been seen to cause this effect.

Diverticulum appear as fluid-filled masses of varying size extending from the wall of the urinary bladder (Fig. 11-14).[5,18] The diagnosis is often not difficult, but if not clear, a postvoid study may show emptying of the urinary bladder with either no change or enlargement in the size of the diverticulum, although it may also empty.

Less common perivesical abnormalities have also been described. Abscesses and other fluid collections, including rectus sheath hematomas and anterior paravesical fluid collections appear as anechoic, hypoechoic, or rarely acousti-

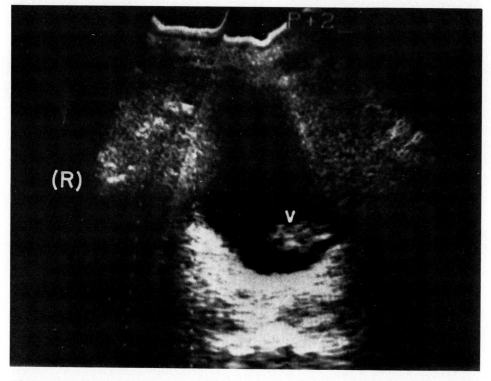

Figure 11-5 Fungating bladder carcinoma. Transverse image demonstrates an intravesical polypoid-type fungating irregular echogenic mass (arrowhead) caused by transitional cell carcinoma. (R) = toward patient's right side.

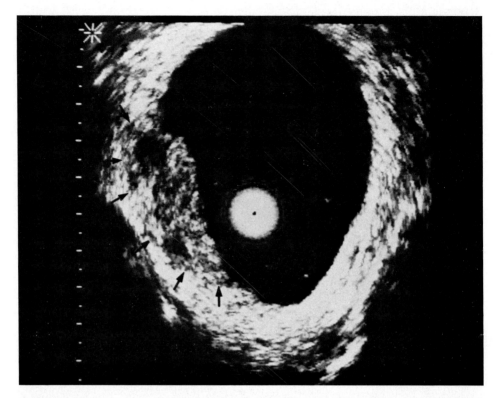

Figure 11-6 Transurethral ultrasound of grade III carcinoma. A transurethral ultrasound scan of the urinary bladder demonstrates the probe in the midportion of the fluid-filled bladder. An acoustically mixed lesion extending into the lumen of the bladder and involving the muscularis portion of the bladder is noted (arrows). No demonstrable extension into the pelvic sidewall is present. (Courtesy of Hans Holm, M.D., Copenhagen, Denmark.)

cally complex lesions (Fig. 11-15).[5,18] They are usually distinctly separate from the urinary bladder, and in cases involving abscesses or hematomas, may appear as mildly echogenic areas depending on the maturity of the collection. These lesions are more accurately defined by the suprapubic approach. It is essential that the pathologic area be studied both with a full bladder and again after voiding. Urinomas and lymphoceles in the pelvis have also been detected and are more common in patients who have undergone previous renal transplant.[18] Endometriosis, involving both the bladder wall and the perivesical spaces, have been reported both as cystic and solid masses.[19] Other uncommon lesions, including metastatic disease, leiomyomas, and arteriovenous malformations have also been demonstrated as rare causes of bladder wall masses.[21]

Pelvic lipomatosis has been reported as a rare entity that can be suggested by ultrasound. The bilateral pelvic fat deposits are seen as echogenic masses compressing the fluid-filled urinary bladder. Other imaging modalities (CT and cystography) will be confirmatory.[5,22]

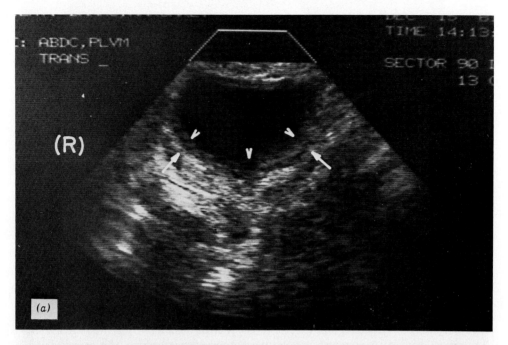

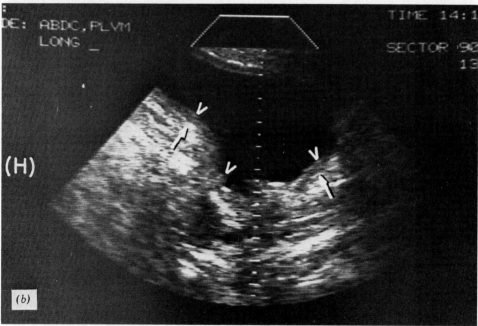

Figure 11-7 Cystitis. Transverse (*a*) and longitudinal (*b*) images demonstrate diffuse inflammatory change of the urinary bladder with thickening of the bladder wall (arrowheads). The muscularis (arrows) is not involved in this patient with diffuse inflammation. (R) = toward patient's right side; (H) = toward patient's head.

433

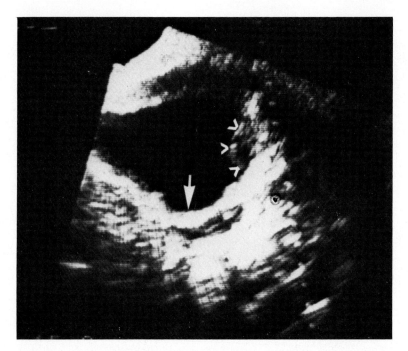

Figure 11-8 Focal inflammatory change of the urinary bladder. Focal inflammation of the urinary bladder is demonstrated on the left side (arrowheads). The remainder of the urinary bladder wall demonstrates no acoustic abnormality (arrow). This focal abnormality was secondary to diverticulitis. (R) = toward patient's right side.

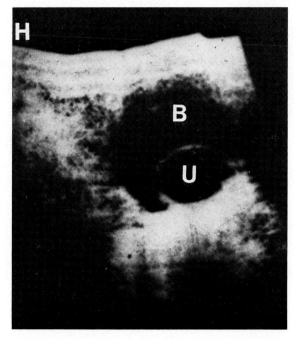

Figure 11-9 Ureterocele. Longitudinal image demonstrates a fluid-fluid, anechoic mass (U), a ureterocele, impinging on the posterolateral aspect of the bladder (B). (H) = toward patient's head.

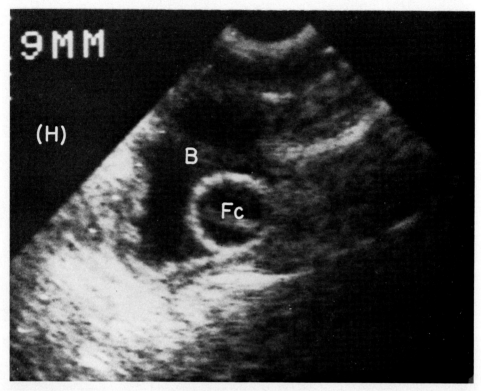

Figure 11-10 Foley catheter. Longitudinal image of the urinary bladder (B) demonstrates a circular filling defect (FC) with bright echogenic margins and a linear echogenic foci representing the Foley catheter with its balloon in the urinary bladder. The bladder walls appear thickened and irregular because the bladder is partially collapsed. (H) = toward patient's head.

Urine volume and residual urine measurements have been accurately estimated using ultrasound. The simplest and most accurate technique uses the abdominal approach. The urinary bladder is examined with a full bladder, and after voiding, repeat measurements are taken. Formulas have been devised to calculate the change in the urine and residual volumes.[23-25] This technique is most useful for the diagnosis of bladder contractility, neurogenic bladder, and bladder outlet obstruction, particularly when catheterization is contraindicated.

Suprapubic Bladder Aspiration

The use of ultrasound, as described in the aspiration biopsy chapter, allows safe, accurate suprapubic aspiration of urine. This technique is most useful in the neonate, newborn, and young pediatric age group where voiding on demand and the ability to obtain a clean-catch urine for bacteriologic studies may be difficult. The use of ultrasound permits evaluation of bladder distension and guides placement of the needle for aspiration decreasing the risk of complications. Suprapubic puncture has also been used to deflate Foley catheters when the urethral channel has occluded and will not empty in a normal fashion.[26]

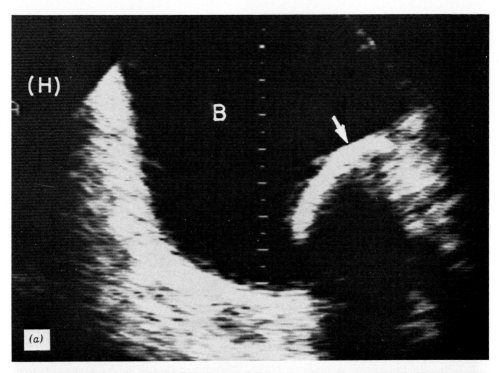

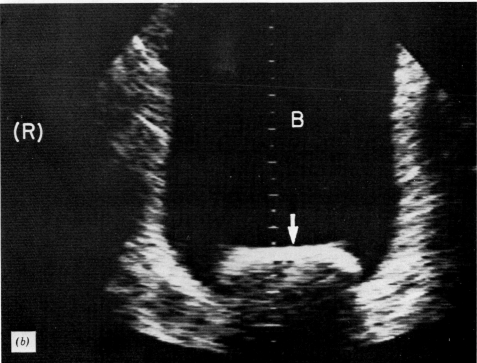

Figure 11-11 Bladder calculus. Longitudinal (*a*) and transverse (*b*) images of the urinary bladder demonstrate a brightly echogenic defect (arrow) within the urinary bladder (B). Acoustic shadowing is noted from this large bladder calculus. (R) = toward patient's right side; (H) = toward patient's head.

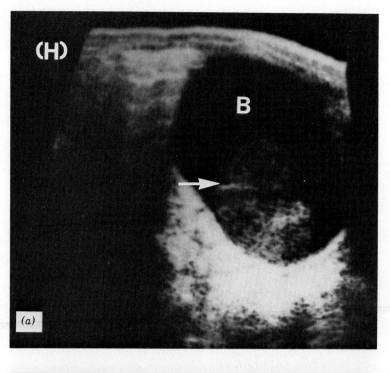

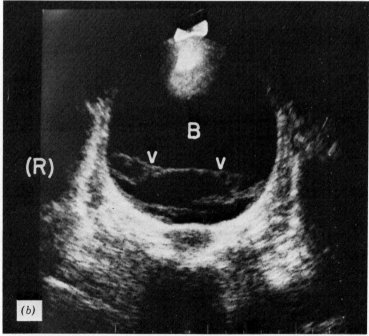

Figure 11-12 Hematoma. (*a*) Longitudinal image demonstrates an echogenic area (arrow) within the bladder. The mass, a large clotted hematoma, has varying echogenic areas. (H) = toward patient's head. (*b*) Poorly defined fluid levels are noted with bright linear echoes (arrowheads) in the urinary bladder (B). The echogenic defects are secondary to a resolving hemorrhage. (R) = toward patient's right side.

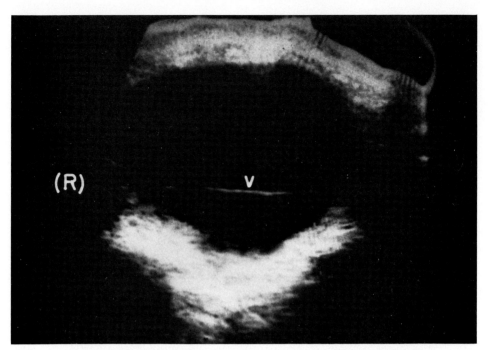

Figure 11-13 Phosphates in the bladder. A transverse image of the urinary bladder demonstrates a fluid-fluid level (arrowheads) due to phosphate accumulation in the urine. The demarcation of the two levels is clearly defined. (R) = toward patient's right.

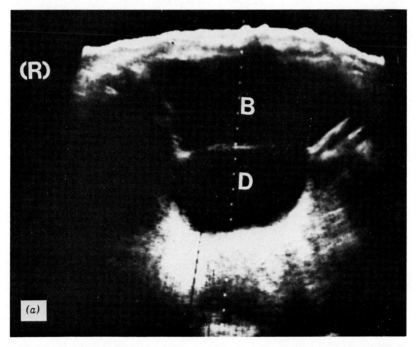

Figure 11-14 Bladder diverticulum. Transverse images demonstrate fluid-filled masses (D) representing a bladder diverticulum posterior to the bladder (B). The connection of the bladder and diverticulum may not be seen (*a*), but by careful angling of the transducer, it can often be demonstrated (*b*). (R) = patient's right side.

438

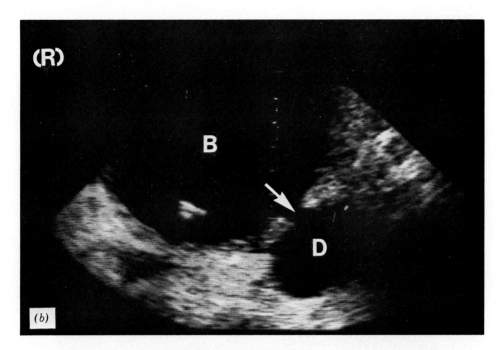

Figure 11-14 (*continued*)

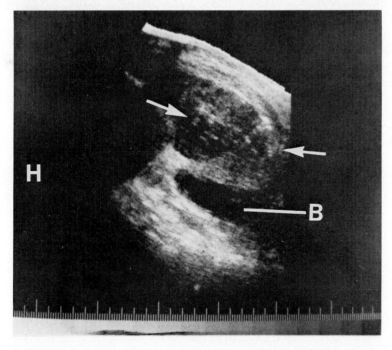

Figure 11-15 Anterior paravesical space hematoma. Longitudinal examination demonstrates (B) complex mass (arrows) extending from the anterior abdominal wall compressing the antero-superior aspect of the urinary bladder (B). (H) = toward patient's head.

439

URETER

The distal ureters can often be detected by abdominal sonography, particularly when the urinary bladder is adequately distended (Fig. 11-16). However, ultrasonic diagnosis of ureteral abnormalities except for the visualization of marked ureteral dilatation is limited (Fig. 11-17).

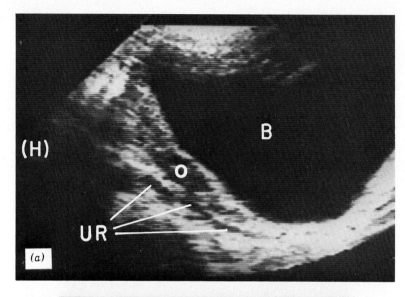

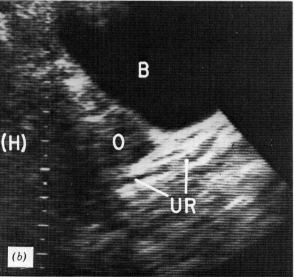

Figure 11-16 Normal ureter. The normal ureter (Ur) is visualized in longitudinal axis (*a* and *b*) posterior to the ovary (O). In transverse projection (*c*), the ureter (Ur) is noted proximal to insertion into the trigone. (H) = toward patient's head; (R) = toward patient's right; UR = ureter; IPM = iliopsoas muscle; B = bladder; U = ureter; O = ovary.

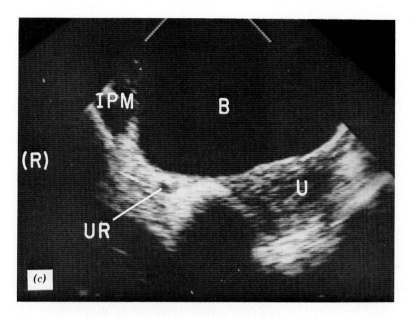

Figure 11-16 (*continued*)

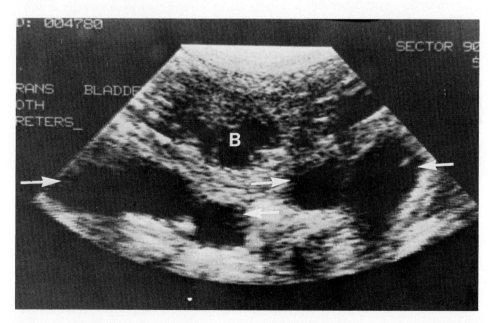

Figure 11-17 Hydroureter secondary to posterior urethral valves. A transverse image demonstrates a partially filled urinary bladder (B) anterior in the midline. Posterior to the bladder are bilateral markedly dilated ureters (arrows) due to chronic hydronephrosis.

441

URETHRA

The benefits of the ultrasonic evaluation of the urethra in both men and women are limited. Detection of diverticulum of the female urethra has been reported, but is a rare entity.[27] Studies have attempted to evaluate the female patient for stress incontinence using real-time ultrasonography of the female urethra. The standard suprapubic approach is used with the transducer placed on the abdomen and angled caudally. The relationship of the urethra to the bladder neck in the fluid-filled bladder can then be ascertained. Abnormalities in this normal angle, flatness of the bladder base, and abnormal mobility and funnelling of the urethrovesical junction is evidence of incontinence.[28]

ULTRASOUND OF THE PROSTATE GLAND

Anatomy

The prostate measures approximately $3 \times 3 \times 2.5$ cm and is situated in the perineum with the inferior portion (the apex) abutting the urogenital diaphragm. The posterior margin, a portion of the posterior lobe, is adjacent to the rectum, and the anterior margin apposes the anterior prostatic fascia, a collection of vascular structures and fatty material. The symphysis pubis is directly ventral to this fascia. Laterally, the levator ani and obturator internus muscles border the gland. The urinary bladder is positioned at the gland's superior border, termed the *base* of the prostate. The seminal vesicles are situated at the superior posterior aspect of the prostate, posterior to the urinary bladder, and anterior to the rectum.[1]

The normal prostate weighs approximately 20 g,[29] and in the adult, is divided into five major lobes. The anterior lobe is situated from the anterior margin of the prostate to the prostatic urethra, which traverses the middle of the gland in longitudinal plane. The median lobe is situated between the prostatic urethra and the ejaculatory ducts, which course from the insertion of the vas deferens and ejaculatory ducts just lateral to the midline. The duct joins the prostatic urethra at its caudad portion within the prostate. The posterior lobe lies between the ejaculatory ducts and the posterior margins of the gland. The two lateral lobes, which comprise the bulk of the gland, are also situated posteriorly and laterally abutting both the middle and posterior lobes.[1] The different lobes are ultrasonically indistinguishable.

Before the advent of ultrasound, imaging of the prostate was limited to plain films of the pelvis, excretory urography, and computed tomography. Diagnostic capabilities were minimal. The plain films may demonstrate calcifications, suggestive of either chronic prostatitis or healed necrosis. The excretory urogram can define elevation of or impingement on the bladder floor, evidence of gland enlargement. Irregular indentation could suggest malignancy, but is not conclusive. Computed axial tomography defines enlargement of the gland. The differentiation of benign and malignant processes can only be made when neoplastic extension outside the capsule into the seminal vesicles, the pelvic sidewalls, or other adjacent structures occurs. This is diagnostic of carcinoma. Lesions that are isolated to the prostate cannot be diagnosed.[30]

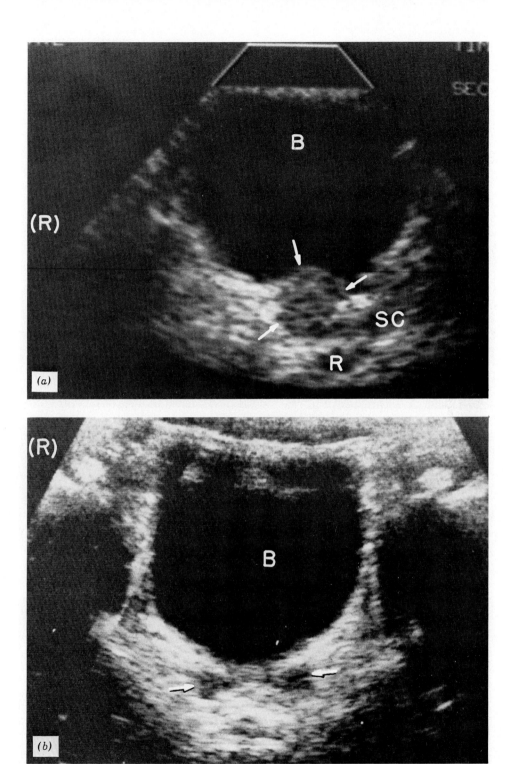

Figure 11-18 Normal prostate and seminal vesicles. (*a*) The normal prostate (arrows) is seen in transverse orientation in the midline and posterior to the bladder (B) bordered posteriorly and laterally by the rectum (R) and the sigmoid colon (SC). (*b*) The seminal vesicles are noted in their classic bow tie shape (arrows) in the midline posterior to the bladder. (R) = toward patient's right.

443

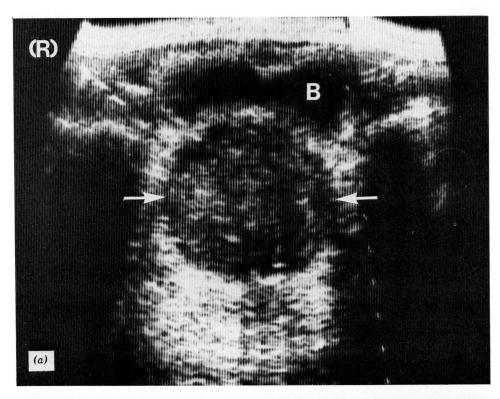

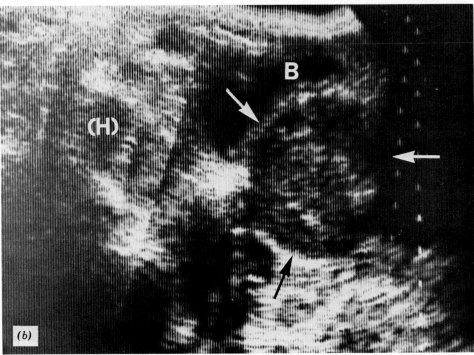

Figure 11-19 Prostatic enlargement. Transverse (*a*) and longitudinal (*b*) images demonstrate a markedly enlarged prostate (arrows) impinging on the urinary bladder (B). Echogenic changes representing diffuse benign prostatic hypertrophy are noted throughout the gland. (H) = toward patient's head; (R) = toward patient's right.

Evaluation of Size

The use of ultrasound to evaluate the gland was initially limited to the suprapubic, abdominal approach. This modality, using standard ultrasound equipment, either B-scan contact or real-time (linear array or sector scanner) machinery yields extensive information.[31,32] With the urinary bladder adequately distended, the transducer is placed on the anterior abdominal wall immediately superior to the symphysis pubis and angled caudally. The prostate can usually be visualized (Fig. 11-18), particularly if enlarged (Fig. 11-19). Early studies were able to accurately define prostatic size and correlate this with its weight.[33–35] The preoperative determination of the gland's size is of marked importance for appropriate surgical treatment of benign hypertrophy. For technical reasons, glands larger than 60 g are often excised by a suprapubic or retropubic open prostatectomy, whereas those smaller than 60 g are more appropriately removed by transurethral resection.[36]

Two methods have been devised that yield adequate results. The simplest measures the largest diameters of the anteroposterior and the lateral dimensions (Fig. 11-20) obtained in a single transverse scan of the prostate and compares their average to a chart (Table 11-1).[34] A second method measures the three largest diameters of the lateral anteroposterior and cephalocaudad dimensions. This requires both a transverse and longitudinal scan. The size is then obtained

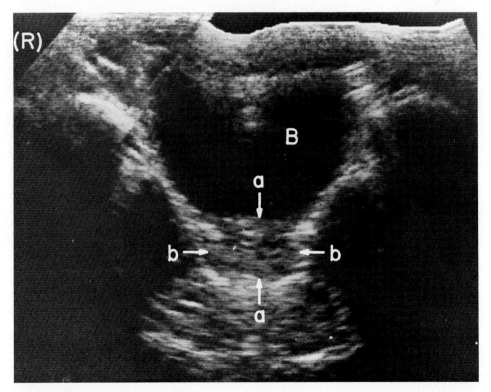

Figure 11-20 Calculations for prostate size. The oval-shaped prostate (arrows) is slightly enlarged in this transverse image. The anterior-posterior dimensions a/a and the lateral dimensions b/b can be measured. B = bladder; (R) = toward patient's right.

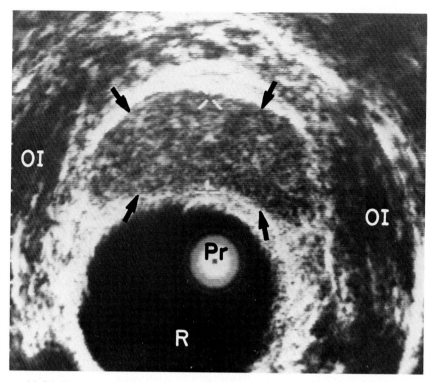

Figure 11-21 Transrectal ultrasound of the normal prostate. The probe (Pr) is placed in the rectum (R). The prostate is oriented in transverse axis on this radial scan (arrows). It is bordered by the rectum posteriorly, the anterior prostatic fascia anteriorly, and the obturator internus muscles (OI) laterally. The normal low-level homogeneous acoustic texture of the gland is demonstrated. (In: *Ultrasound Annual 1983*, edited by RC Sanders and M Hill. Raven Press, N.Y.)

using the formula for a sphere, $\frac{4}{3} \pi r^3$.[33] The resulting value expressed in cubic centimeters is approximately equivalent to the weight in grams. The specific gravity of prostatic tissue is 1.05 g per cubic centimeter. Thus, the area $(\text{cc}^3) \in 1.05 \text{ g/cc}^3 = $ weight.

Sonoendoscopy

Recently, both experimental and commercially available specialized endosonoscopic probes have been developed for transurethral[37-39] and transrectal examinations.[39-47] The initial equipment used static radial scans, which like the urinary bladder studies presented the image in a transverse orientation. The sonoendoscope used for bladder evaluation can also be used to study the prostate. The transrectal approach is simpler to use, has less complications, and currently is more acceptable for prostatic evaluation. Linear array real-time rectal probes have been developed recently.[44,47] This device not only uses constant imaging by a real-time system, but also presents the scan in longitudinal fashion. The equipment is as easy to use as those employing the radial scan.

The normal prostate, as seen on the transrectal examination, has well-defined margins, with the capsule intact (Fig. 11-21 and 11-22). The gland demonstrates low to moderate level homogeneous echogenicity without evidence of focal change. In the longitudinal linear array examination, the collapsed prostatic urethra may be defined as linear reflections off the apposed walls of the tubular structure (Fig. 11-22*a*) or partially fluid-filled (Fig. 11-22*b*). Patients who have previously undergone transurethal resection show a typical defect in the cephalad margin of the prostatic urethra (Fig. 11-23). The longitudinal scan may define the ejaculatory ducts as parallel echogenic lines off the apposed walls in its the proximal portion just posterior to the porstatic urethra (Fig. 11-22*b*).

The seminal vesicles may be seen with the abdominal approach (Fig. 11-18) or the radial scan (Fig. 11-24) as distinctly separate from and superior to the prostate. The echogenic texture is also homogeneous, but of lower reflectivity

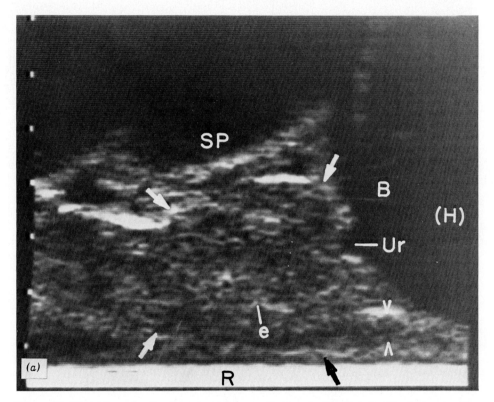

Figure 11-22 (*a*) Longitudinally oriented normal prostate. The longitudinal examination of the prostate with the probe placed in the rectum (R) demonstrates the gland (arrows) to be homogeneously echogenic. The prostatic urethra is seen at its proximal portion (Ur) exiting from the bladder (B). The apposed walls of the ejaculatory duct (e) are seen transiently in the posterior portion of the gland. The seminal vesicles are defined (arrowheads) just superior to the prostate. (H) = toward patient's head; SP = symphysis pubis. (In: *Ultrasound Annual 1983*, edited by RC Sanders and M Hill. Raven Press, N.Y.) (*b*) Longitudinal transrectal ultrasound of the normal prostate. The prostatic urethra (Ur) is noted in a distended state traversing from the bladder (B) toward the membranous portion of the urethra. The ejaculatory duct (e) is noted by its echogenic reflections from its apposed walls. Arrows = prostatic margins; (H) = toward patient's head.

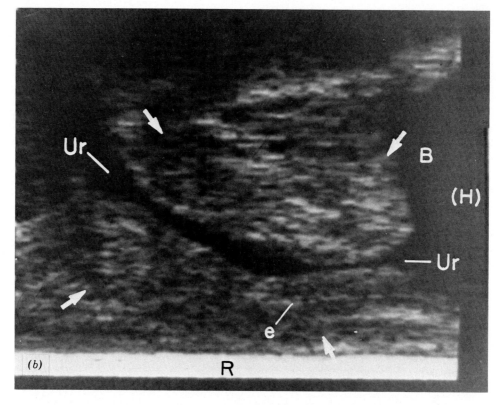

Figure 11-22 (*continued*)

than the prostate. The longitudinal sonogram may demonstrate the seminal vesicles posterior and superior to the gland (Fig. 11-22).

Hypertrophy

Until recently it had been assumed that benign prostatic hypertrophy was a diffuse process involving the entire gland (Fig. 11-25). The echogenicity would be abnormal throughout the gland, although some areas of focal abnormality could be defined. Recent evidence has demonstrated that benign prostatic hypertrophy may also have distinct areas of focal abnormality (Fig. 11-26)

Table 11-1 Suprapubic Abdominal Examination: Correlation of Prostate Weight to Transverse Average Diameter of the Prostate[34]

Degree of Size	Diameter (cm)	Weight (cm)
I	3.0–3.8	30
II	3.8–4.5	30–50
III	4.5–5.5	50–80
IV	5.5	85

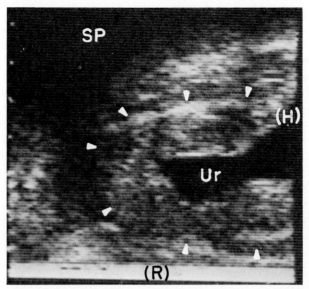

Figure 11-23 Prostatic resection defect. Longitudinally oriented transrectal sonogram of the prostate (arrowheads) demonstrates defect of the proximal prostatic urethra (Ur) due to previous transurethral resection. R = rectum; (H) = toward patient's head; SP = symphysis pubis.

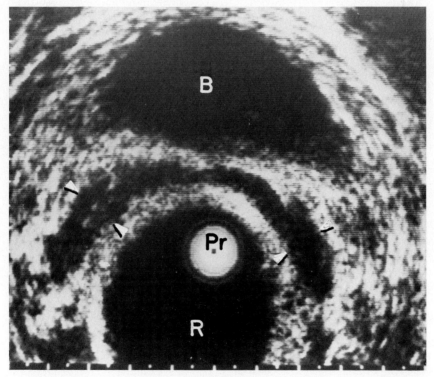

Figure 11-24 Transrectal scan of the seminal vesicles. A static radial scan of the seminal vesicles (arrowheads) demonstrates the bow tie-shaped hypoechoic but homogeneous echogenic structures between the rectum (R) and the bladder (B). The transrectally oriented image is obtained by the probe (Pr) placed in the rectum. (In: *Ultrasound Annual 1983*, edited by RC Sanders and M Hill. Raven Press, N.Y.)

449

occurring in up to 75 percent of patients.[47] These foci are often hyperechoic, but may be purely hypoechoic or of mixed acoustic reflectivity.

Approximately 75 percent of these focal lesions are more than 3 to 4 mm thick and sonographically more reflective than the prostatic capsule (Fig. 11-26). The remaining 25 percent of the hyperechoic foci are thin and only slightly more echogenic than the normal prostate. Only about 30 percent of these lesions demonstrate acoustic shadowing. Pathologic studies have demonstrated that only those foci that shadow are indeed calcification (Fig. 11-27). The remainder of these focal areas of benign prostatic tissue do not have calcium.[47]

Diffuse prostatitis may not be differentiable from some examples of diffuse benign prostatic enlargement. The echogenic characteristics are similar, having increased, decreased, or diffusely mixed echogenicity throughout the entire gland.[47] The gland in prostatitis is often normal sized.

Malignancy

Carcinoma of the prostate is usually a focal process. Alterations in acoustic texture should be localized, although invasion of the capsule may be present.

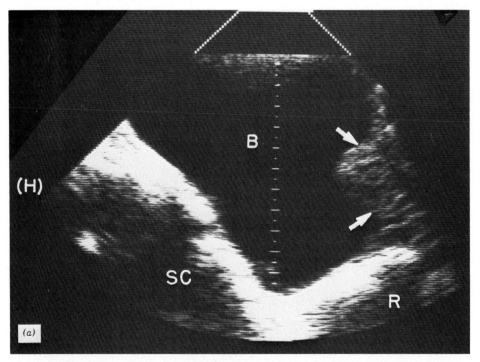

Figure 11-25 Prostatic hypertrophy. The enlarged prostate (arrows) is seen impinging on the bladder in the longitudinal image obtained by a suprapubic abdominal approach (*a*). The longitudinal transrectal linear array real-time examination (*b*) also demonstrates an enlarged gland (arrows) with subtle diffuse increase in echogenicity. When prostatic enlargement (arrows) extends intravesically, it can also be demonstrated on the transrectal approach impinging on the urinary bladder (*c*). (H) = toward patient's head; R = rectum; SC = sigmoid colon; B = bladder; SP = symphysis pubis.

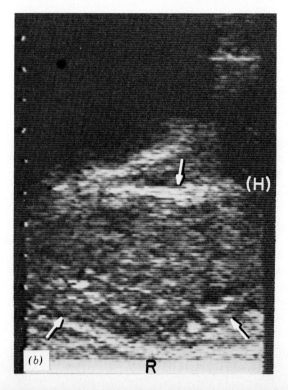

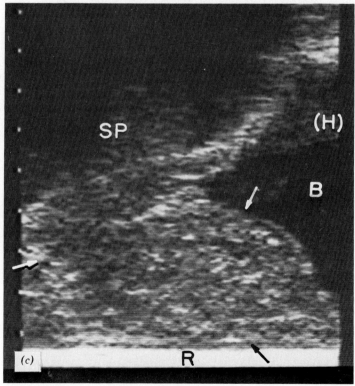

Figure 11-25 (*continued*)

451

The echogenicity may be hyperechoic or of mixed echogenicity, but is rarely, if ever, purely hypoechoic.[47] Evidence suggests that the malignant changes within foci are usually of low-level reflectivity measuring slightly greater than the gland itself and of minimal thickness measuring approximately 2 to 3 mm (Fig. 11-28). Many studies have demonstrated the ability to detect focal abnormalities of the prostate that, on surgical resection, were proven to be cancer in approximately 95 percent of all malignant lesions.[43,46,48] However, because there is a significant overlap between cancer and benign disease, many benign lesions that mimic carcinoma cannot be differentiated ultrasonically without tissue diagnosis.

Findings that suggest benign as opposed to malignant disease include: (1) brightly echogenic foci, (2) thickly echogenic foci, (3) shadowing that should not be seen with carcinoma, and (4) purely hypoechoic focal lesions.[47]

Invasion of the prostatic capsule, the seminal vesicle, or the pelvic sidewalls are highly suspicious for malignancy (Fig. 11-29). Focal lesions within normal-sized glands may represent a benign process and cannot be considered malignant unless they have the acoustic criteria for cancer. Biopsy is often needed for definitive diagnosis.

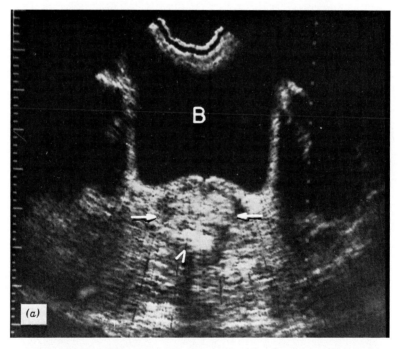

Figure 11-26 Echogenic foci benign prostatic hypertrophy. Benign prostatic hypertrophy can demonstrate focal increased echoes in a specific portion of the gland. When the foci are brightly echogenic they can be demonstrated in the transabdominal approach (*a*). The acoustic shadowing (arrowhead) is from a calcified focus. The radial scan (*b*) of a second patient demonstrates echogenic foci (arrowhead) in the posterior portion of the gland, and a third patient studied with the longitudinal linear array equipment (*c*) shows clearly demarcated echoes in the caudad area of the prostate (H) = toward patient's head; B = bladder; APF = anterior prostatic fascia; Arrows = prostatic margins. (Part *b* courtesy of Dr. Bruno Squassabia).

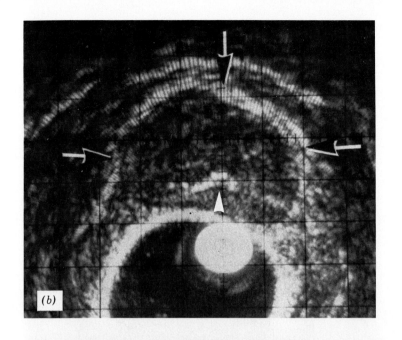

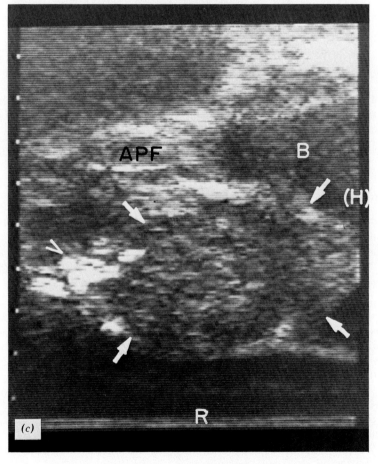

Figure 11-26 (*continued*)

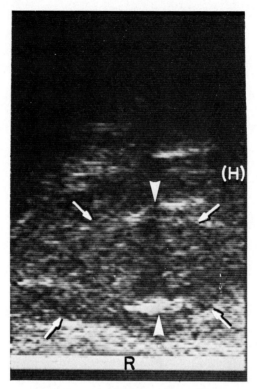

Figure 11-27 Prostatic calcification. Longitudinal linear array examination of the prostate demonstrates a slightly enlarged gland (arrows) with a brightly echogenic focus in the posterior portion of the prostate with shadowing (arrowhead). The sound originates in the rectum, extending anteriorly, so shadowing is also in a direction away from the rectally placed transducer. R = rectum; (H) = toward patient's head.

Biopsy

Despite the suggestions for differentiating the various disease processes by ultrasound, histologic diagnosis is usually required. Because of this, techniques have been developed to guide biopsy needles into the acoustically abnormal areas. This is of particular importance for patients who exhibit ultrasonically focal lesions that are not palpable on digital rectal examination.

Figure 11-28 Prostatic carcinoma. The areas of prostatic carcinoma are denoted by scattered echogenic foci. (*a*) A radial scan, demonstrates the prostate (arrowheads) to be oriented slightly laterally. The carcinoma is demonstrated by brightly echogenic foci (arrows) with apparent extension into the right pelvic sidewall. Two other patients had less defined areas of carcinoma, seen on the longitudinal linear array examination (*b* and *c*). Part *b* demonstrates scattered, slightly echogenic punctate foci throughout the midportion of the gland (arrowheads) in a normal-sized prostate (arrows). A relatively large echo (arrowhead) is demonstrated without acoustic shadowing (*c*) demonstrating carcinoma in a normal-sized gland (arrowheads) in a third patient. SP = symphysis pubis; R = rectum; APF = anterior prostatic fascia; X = water in distended rectum. (Part *a* courtesy of Dr. Bruno Squassabia).

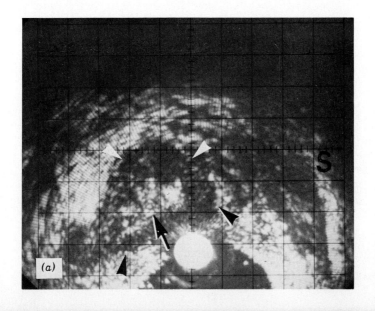

(a)

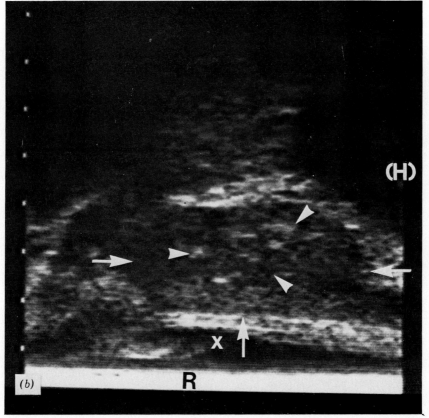

(b)

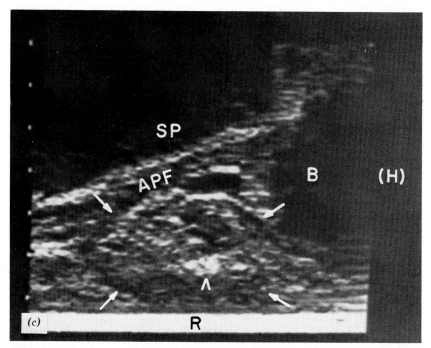

Figure 11-28 (*continued*)

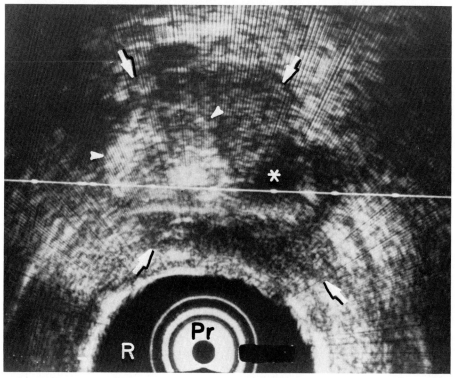

Figure 11-29 Invasive prostatic carcinoma. A transrectal radial scan of the prostate demonstrates an invasive carcinoma (arrowheads) of the prostate (arrows) invading the right lateral margins of the gland and deviating the ureter (*) to the left. R = rectum; Pr = probe. (In: *Ultrasound Annual 1983*, edited by RC Sanders and M Hill. Raven Press, N.Y.)

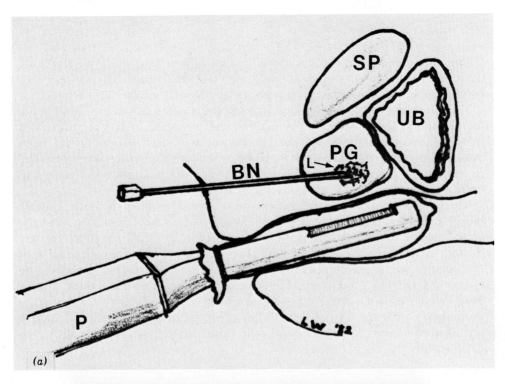

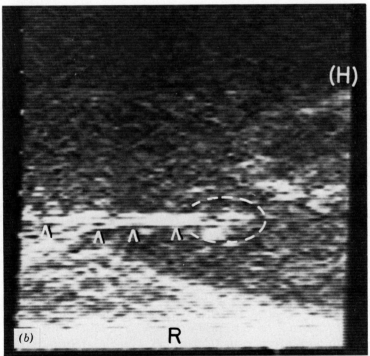

Figure 11-30 Transrectally ultrasonically guided transperineal biopsy. (*a*) Schematic drawing of the biopsy procedure demonstrates a probe (P) placed in the rectum. The biopsy needle (BN) is placed into a lesion (L) in the prostate (PG). SP = symphysis pubis; UB = urinary bladder. (*b*) A longitudinally oriented image demonstrates the biopsy needle (arrowheads) placed into the lesion (circled). R = rectum; (H) = toward patient's head. (Part *b* in: *Ultrasound Annual 1983*, edited by RC Sanders and M Hill. Raven Press, N.Y.)

The abdominal approach has limited value in detecting subtle focal abnormalities. For this reason, guidance to these focal areas, particularly in normal-sized glands, which are poorly seen on the suprapubic approach, is limited.[47]

Techniques have been developed that use the transrectal radial scan to guide the percutaneous transperineal biopsy.[49,50] Because static images are presented in transverse orientation, the needle cannot be visualized until it has been inserted into the area of the prostate being examined. Therefore, it is impossible to alter the course of the needle at will during biopsy, limiting the benefit to be realized from this type of ultrasonic guidance.

The longitudinal linear array examination appears to allow the most accurate biopsy guidance. The image is presented in longitudinal orientation, and the biopsy needle once placed into the perineum, can be visualized in its entirety during its insertion into the prostate (Fig. 11-30).[51,52] Altering the course of the needle can be accomplished as required during the biopsy procedure to ensure its proper placement. The biopsies using these techniques can be performed with a large bore needle to obtain a core of tissue for histologic evaluation[51] or a small-gauge needle for cytologic diagnosis.[52] This technique has allowed biopsy diagnosis of clinically unsuspected but ultrasonically suspicious lesions.[53]

SCROTUM

Evaluation of the scrotum before the development of ultrasound was limited to physical palpation alone. With the advent of the earliest ultrasound equipment, the delineation of some of the scrotal contents could be made. However, with the availability of high-resolution equipment, particularly dedicated small parts scanners, the full impact of the diagnostic capabilities of ultrasound can now be demonstrated.

Technique

Currently, there are multiple modalities that may be used to study the scrotum. Contact B-scan images should be performed using a high-resolution transducer, preferably 7.5 or 10 MHz, although a 5-MHz transducer can be used. Direct contact of the transducer on the scrotum yields exquisite detail.[54,55] A water bath placed between the transducer and the scrotum can be used with similar accuracy.[56] Small parts high-resolution real-time equipment, both with sector scan transducers and linear array machinery also yields excellent results.[57] Both longitudinal and transverse orientation should be studied with either contact or real-time studies. The use of real time permits rapid evaluation and is also simpler to use requiring less technical expertise to produce satisfactory images.

Dedicated automated water-path machines with the transducers situated in the water have also been used. This technique requires the scrotal sac to be submersed into the warmed water bath. The automated equipment then obtains images of the scrotum and its contents at prescribed intervals.[58] The major limiting factors of this equipment are the lesser resolution of the machinery and the small size of the images, which may be unable to detect small or subtle lesions.

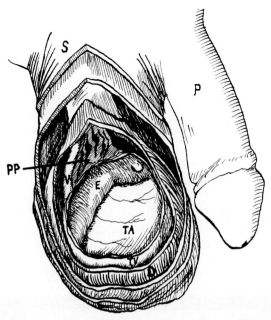

Figure 11-31 Anatomic drawings of the prostate. A sagittal image of a schematic drawing of the scrotum shows the tunica albuginea (TA) tightly adherent to the testes. The epididymis (E) is situated posterior to the testicle, and both are covered by the tunica vaginalis (TV) and Dartos fascia (D). The vas deferens (V) and the pampiniform plexus (PP) are noted ascending in the spermatic cord. S = scrotal sac; P = penis.

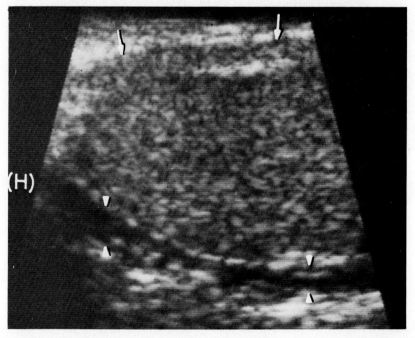

Figure 11-32 High-resolution examination of the normal testicle. Longitudinal examination of the normal testicle demonstrates its anterior margin (arrows) abutting the skin surface. The epididymis (arrowheads), posterior to the testis, is a hypoechoic structure compared to the homogeneous texture of the testicle itself. The bright echoes surrounding the epididymis are its fascial lining. (H) = toward patient's head.

459

During all of these procedures, the patient should be positioned to preserve maximum modesty. The scrotum can be supported by a towel placed beneath the scrotal sac and tightly tucked under the patient's thighs. The penis is then placed on the patient's lower abdomen and covered with a towel. This position allows direct contact of the transducers on the patient's scrotum without requiring direct contact by the examiner's hands.

Uses of Ultrasound

Ultrasonic evaluation yields accurate detection of multiple abnormal processes. A clinically palpable mass can be defined, and differentiation between testicular and extratesticular lesions is very accurate. Young men may have evidence of metastatic lesions within the retroperitoneum and/or the mediastinum. Evaluation of the testes for a subclinical primary tumor is often required despite a

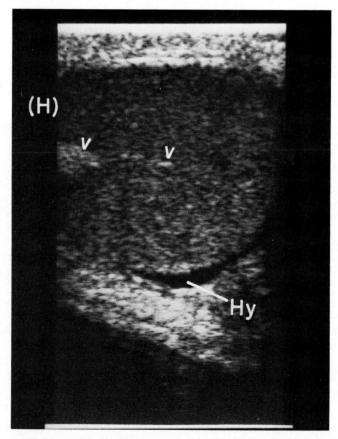

Figure 11-33 High-resolution normal testicle. Longitudinal scan of the normal testicle demonstrates the normal homogeneous echogenic texture to be disrupted by a bright echogenic band (arrowheads) from the mediastinum testis. A small amount of fluid (Hy) denoting the normal fluid between the two layers of the tunica vaginalis is noted. (H) = toward patient's head.

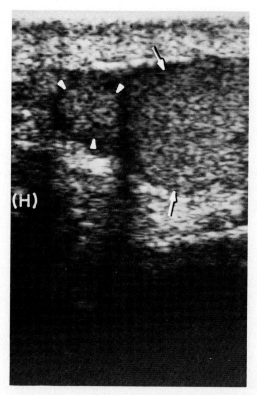

Figure 11-34 Normal head of the epididymis. A longitudinal high-resolution examination of the scrotum demonstrates a normal-sized and echogenic testicle (arrows). Superior to the testis is the head of the epididymis (arrowheads). (H) = toward patient's head.

negative physical examination. Clinically unsuspected small, subtle lesions have been detected as the primary lesion in many patients.[59]

Fluid collections can be consistently differentiated by ultrasound and solid lesions defined. Traumatic changes, including hemorrhage, testicular disruption, and occasionally torsion may be detected. Inflammatory changes, including epididymitis and orchitis, are often diagnosed with ultrasound, often differentiating these abnormalities from other more ominous lesions.

A varicocele may be present in many normal men, but may also be the only cause for male infertility. The delineation of varicoceles, even subtle, clinically indiscrete lesions has been shown to be possible with the use of diagnostic ultrasound.[60]

The Normal Scrotum

The normal testis measures approximately 3.0 × 2 × 2.5 cm and is lined by a tight fascial membrane, the tunica albuginea. A double serous membrane, the tunica vaginalis, surrounds the entire testis and embryologically originates from the peritoneum. A few cubic centimeters of fluid are normally present between the two layers. The testis has a small appendage superiorly, the appendix.

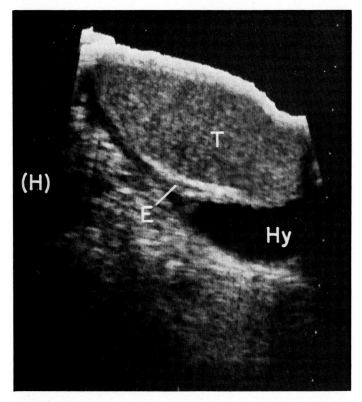

Figure 11-35 Hydrocele. Longitudinal examination of the scrotum demonstrates a normal testis (T) and epididymis (E). A small, hydrocele (Hy), is noted posterior. The normal apposition of the epididymis to the testis is not disturbed.

The epididymis is situated along the posterior margin of the testis. The largest portion, the head, is situated superior to the testicle, and the remainder of the epididymis (the body), which is about 2 to 3 mm thick, courses along the posterior margin inferiorly. A small protuberance off the head is the epididymal appendix (Fig. 11-31).

The spermatic cord, which courses through the inguinal canal to the superior margin of the testis, is composed of the vas deferens, the testicular artery, the draining veins of the scrotum, the pampiniform and cremesteric plexi, and the nerves and lymph channels.[1]

Acoustically, the testicle is very homogenous and of low-level echogenicity (Fig. 11-32). A brightly echogenic band, representing the mediastinum testis, is occasionally seen in the superior aspect (Fig. 11-33). Both testes are usually symmetrically sized and shaped, however, anatomically, the position may vary, one usually being situated more caudally than the other. The appendix of the testis may only be seen when hydroceles are present.

Sonographically, the normal epididymis is no greater than 2 to 3 mm and is of variable echogenicity, defined by two thin echogenic bands representing fascial lining (Fig. 11-32).[61]

Previous reports describe the epididymis as highly echogenic.[54] This probably

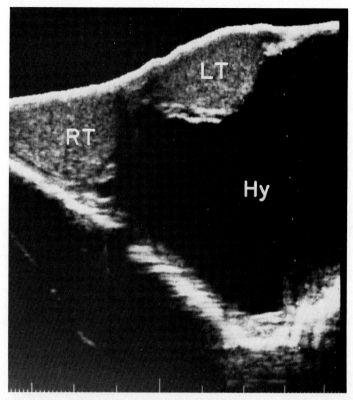

Figure 11-36 Large hydrocele. A transversely oriented B-scan of the scrotum demonstrates a normal right (RT) and left (LT) testicle. A large hydrocele (Hy) is on the left side.

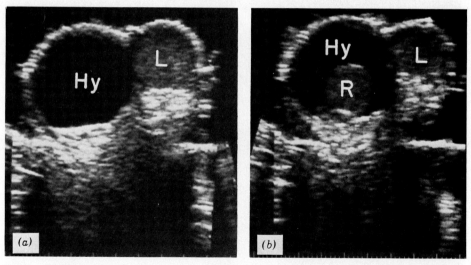

Figure 11-37 Right-sided hydrocele. Transverse images of the scrotum demonstrates normal right (R) and left (L) testes. Because the testes are situated at different cephalocaudad levels, a large hydrocele is noted superiorly involving the right side (*a*) at the level where the left testicle is visualized, but no contralateral testis is noted. (*b*) At a slightly more caudad position, the superior aspect of the right testis with the hydrocele is still present.

relates to the inability of the equipment to resolve the fascial lining from the less echogenic epididymis.

The epididymal head, larger than the body (up to 15 mm in diameter), is also slightly more echogenic, but remains homogeneous (Fig. 11-34). The appendix of the epididymis cannot be visualized with ultrasound.

The use of high-resolution machines permits identification of some normal venous channels of the pampiniform plexus. This fluid-filled structure, no greater than 1 to 2 mm in diameter, may be seen just superior to the testis.[60]

Fluid Collections

There is normally less this 5 cc of fluid within the tunica vaginalis. Three types of abnormal fluid collections occur within the scrotum: (1) hydroceles, (2) cysts, and (3) varicoceles.

Hydroceles are abnormal fluid collections between the two layers of the tunica vaginalis. They may be primary (simple hydroceles) or be secondary to a specific inciting cause. The simple hydrocele can be quite small (Fig. 11-35) or large (Figs. 11-36 and 11-37). In acute or subacute hydroceles, the walls of the scrotum are normally thin. Transillumination usually delineates these fluid collections. Light does not transmit through the solid testis, whereas it is seen

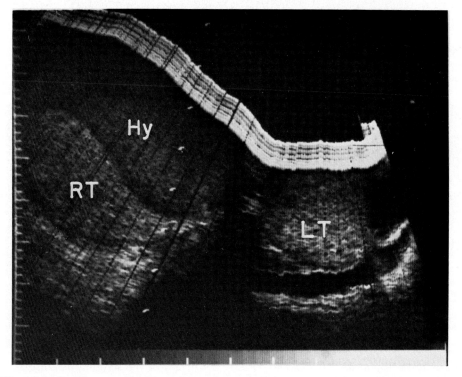

Figure 11-38 Hematocele. Transverse images of the scrotum demonstrates a normal right (RT) and left (LT) testes. A right-sided anterior hypoechoic but echogenic collection is noted (Hy). This proved to be hemorrhagic material collecting following inguinal herniorrhaphy.

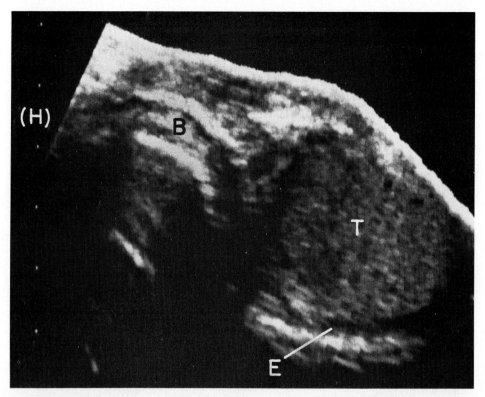

Figure 11-39 Hernia. Longitudinal examination demonstrates a normal testis (T) and epididymis (E). Superior to the testis are bright echogenic areas (B) with loss of the sound transmission (shadowing) representing air-filled bowel. (H) = toward patient's head.

with fluid collections. This is a simple test that often differentiates masses from fluid accumulation within an enlarged scrotum. However, there are cases, particularly with chronic hydroceles, where the walls of the scrotum become thickened and do not permit adequate transillumination. Differentiation between fluid and solid components is not possible in these patients.

Reactive hydroceles are due to a variety of causes. Tumors, both benign and malignant, inflammation, and trauma may cause small hydroceles.

Hydroceles, because they are fluid, are usually acoustically anechoic collections. They may occur in any region of the scrotum. When posteriorly placed, they usually do not displace the epididymis from the testis. Loculations may occur, and in cases of inflammation or hemorrhage, subtle echogenic areas may be seen scattered throughout the fluid (Fig. 11-38). Cholesterol deposits may cause a diffuse low-level echogenicity. As these processes resolve, septations may develop, which represent fibrin deposits and adhesions.[62] Hydroceles may also occur in patients with disruption of the inguinal ring and free communication of abdominal ascitic fluid.

Hematoceles are complicated hydroceles where fluid collects within the tunica vaginalis, secondary to trauma, surgery, or rarely, spontaneously in patients with bleeding diatheses.[62] They may be echogenic, acoustically mixed, or purely anechoic lesions (Fig. 11-38).

Herniation of bowel into the scrotum also occurs. Both direct and indirect hernias have been correctly identified.[63] The accurate diagnosis is simplified when the bowel is identified within the scrotum. Bowel can appear as (a) fluid-filled structures, (b) solid-filled masses, where the loops of bowel may be identified in transverse section with a solid echogenic center and a thin hypoechoic rim representing the bowel wall, (c) gas-filled (Fig. 11-39), noted as shadowing or (d) a combination of three findings (Fig. 11-40).The diagnosis is simplified when peristalsis is identified on real-time examination.[62] It may be difficult to differentiate a hernia from a primary extratesticular mass when only a small portion of omentum without bowel is present in the scrotum.

Although cystic collections of the scrotal contents are not uncommon, cysts of the testis and the tunica albuginea are distinctly unusual. Acoustically, however, they are quite characteristic being anechoic lesions with sharp back walls and enhanced through transmission (Fig. 11-41).[64]

A spermatocele is a cystic dilatation of the ducts of the epididymis filled with

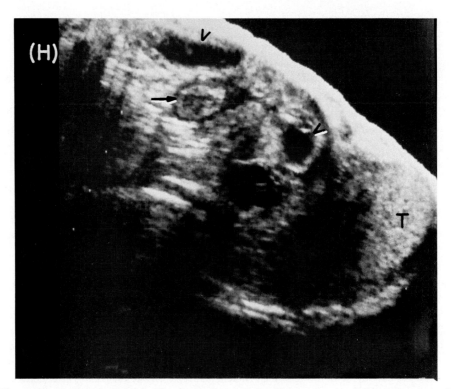

Figure 11-40 Hernia. Longitudinal examination demonstrates a small but normal portion of the testis (T). Multiple loops of bowel, some fluid-filled (arrowheads) and others distended with feces (arrow), are noted cephalad to the testicle. (H) = toward patient's head.

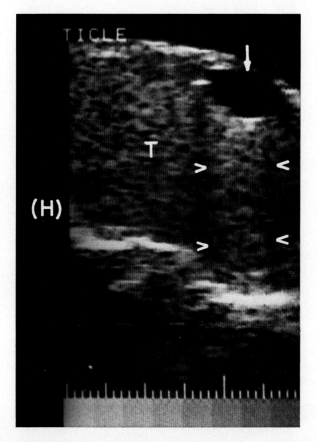

Figure 11-41 Intratesticular cyst. Longitudinal examination of the testis (T) demonstrates an anechoic fluid-filled mass (arrow) with no internal echoes, sharp margins, and acoustic sound enhancement (arrowheads). These findings are consistent with and were confirmed at surgery to be an intratesticular cyst. (H) = toward patient's head.

creamy fluid and sperm (Fig. 11-42). They are usually within the epididymal head. Epididymal cysts are also fluid-filled masses that can be quite small or massive, focal or lobulated, and may be situated any place within the epididymis (Fig. 11-43). Ultrasonically, differentiation between these two processes is not possible.

A varicocele is abnormal dilatation of the draining veins of the scrotum. The major vessels draining the testis are the pampiniform plexus, which flow into the cremasteric vein and subsequently into the internal spermatic vein. The cremasteric plexus is distinctly dorsally placed, usually draining the nontesticular contents of the scrotum; its major flow is into the cremasteric vein, but it also has anastomosing channels to the pampiniform plexus. The left internal spermatic vein drains into the left renal vein, and because of this course, backup of venous drainage and dilatation may occur. These cases of varicoceles are seen in approximately 15 to 20 percent of normal adult men. However, it has

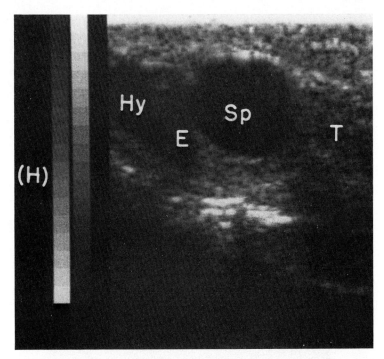

Figure 11-42 Spermatocele. Longitudinal examination demonstrates superior to the testis (T) the epididymis (E), a small hydrocele (Hy), and a well-defined fluid collection with sharp margins and sound enhancement, which was confirmed at surgery to be a spermatocele (Sp). (H) = toward patient's head.

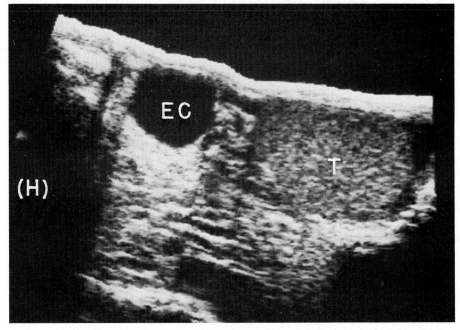

Figure 11-43 Epididymal cyst. Longitudinal examination of the scrotum demonstrates the testis (T) to be acoustically unremarkable. Superiorly, in the region of the epididymal head, is a large cystic collection (EC), an epididymal cyst. (H) = toward patient's head.

468

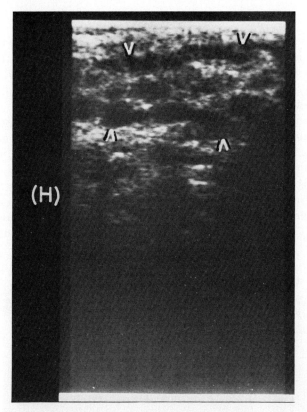

Figure 11-44 Varicocele. High-resolution examination of the spermatic cord demonstrates dilated, tortuous fluid-filled structures consistent with dilated venous plexes (arrowheads). This small but clinically evident varicocele demonstrated veins to be as large as 4 mm in diameter. (H) = toward patient's head.

also been seen in approximately 35 to 40 percent of infertile and subfertile men. The majority of these patients become fertile following correction of the varicocele. The size of the venous dilatation appears to be unrelated to the physiologic effect.

The right internal spermatic vein drains directly into the inferior vena cava. Unilateral idiopathic right-sided varicoceles are quite unusual. When seen, an underlying cause such as mass compressing the inferior vena cava or the internal spermatic vein on the right side must be excluded.

Small varicoceles may be demonstrated as multiple tubular, tortuous vessels measuring anywhere from 4 to 6 mm in diameter seen predominantly with high-resolution equipment to large lesions up to a few centimeters in diameter. All lesions should dilate with valsalva maneuver, i.e., when decreasing venous return, or when the patient assumes the erect position (Fig. 11-44). The normal veins do not dilate. Ultrasound evaluation for varicoceles is as, if not more, accurate than any other diagnostic imaging modalities.[60]

Inflammation

Epididymitis is an inflammatory reaction of the epididymis, which clinically appears as a painful enlargement of the epididymis. Acoustically, the epididymis enlarges and becomes hypoechoic compared to normal. This is a diffuse process that can be quite extensive or minimal (Figs. 11-45, 11-46, and 11-47).[65–68]Reactive small or large fluid collections may be present.

Secondary orchitis may occur with epididymitis. In these cases, the entire testis may be abnormal, demonstrating diffusely decreased echogenicity. Focal lesions occur rarely, and when present, are usually situated immediately apposed to the epididymis.[69]

Focal orchitis or abscess without primary insiting epididymitis is an unusual finding seen sonographically as hypoechoic areas infiltrating the normal testis. Occasionally they may be well defined (Fig. 11-48). These lesions cannot be sonographically differentiated from primary infiltrating neoplastic conditions.

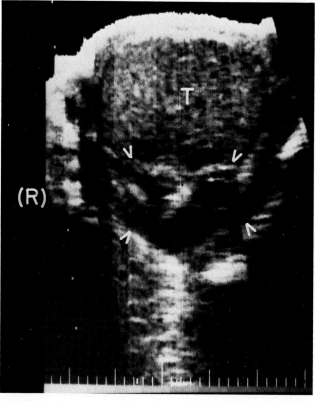

Figure 11-45 Acute epididymitis. A transverse image demonstrates the testis (T) to be acoustically unremarkable. The epididymis, situated posterior to the testis, is markedly dilated, hypoechoic, and poorly defined (arrowheads). This is an example of acute fulminant epididymitis. (R) = patient's right side.

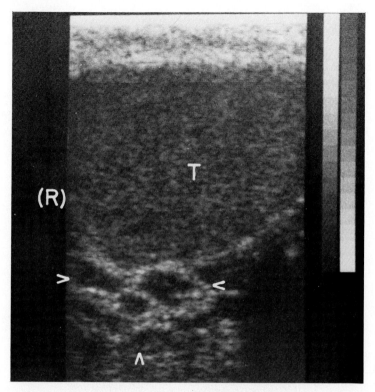

Figure 11-46 Partially healed epididymitis. Transverse image shows a normal testis (T), but the epididymis is slightly enlarged and lobulated (arrowheads). The echogenicity has returned to normal in this patient recovering from acute epididymitis. (R) = patient's right side.

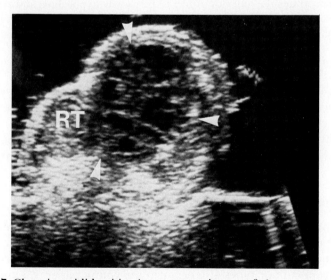

Figure 11-47 Chronic epididymitis. A transverse image of the scrotum demonstrates large, hypoechoic structure with multiple tubular and hypoechoic areas (arrowheads). This area is superior to the left testis. The findings were confirmed to be chronic inflammatory change of the left epididymis. The right testis (RT) is normal.

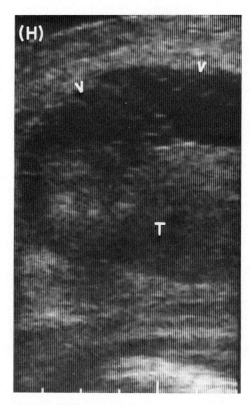

Figure 11-48 Focal orchitis. A high-resolution longitudinally oriented examination of the testis demonstrates the anterior aspect to be grossly hypoechoic and poorly defined (arrowheads) in comparison to the posterior aspect of the testis (T), which is acoustically unremarkable. (H) = toward patient's head.

Abscesses, unlike primary testicular tumors, are not isolated to the younger age group. Clinically they are quite painful, and the testis is diffusely edematous.

Diffuse orchitis has similar clinical findings as focal inflammation. Sonographically, the entire testes is acoustically abnormal, usually grossly hypoechoic (Fig. 11-49). Small reactive hydroceles are usually seen with all inflammatory processes.

Neoplasms of the Testis

Multiple neoplasms affect the testes. Seminoma, the most common primary testicular lesions, is usually seen in younger men between the ages of 18 and 40. Embryonal cell carcinoma, choriocarcinoma, and mixed germ cell lesions involving various tumor types also occur in the young patients. Lymphoma and leukemia occur in all age groups. Metastatic lesions and epididymal tumors are rare causes of focal space-occupying neoplastic lesions of the scrotum.[65–70]

All the infiltrating tumors have similar sonographic findings. Small lesions are focally hypoechoic and usually poorly defined, although some margins may be distinct (Fig. 11-50). The larger lesions may involve the entire testes often with little or no residual normal tissue (Figs. 11-51 and 11-52). Rarely, areas of increased echogenicity may be seen. This may occur with mixed cellular malignancy. Both primary and secondary lesions, such as leukemia, have similar acoustic properties. Focal, clinically nonpalpable lesions as small as 3 mm have been accurately defined.[59] When young men have mediastinal or retroperitoneal adenopathy, sonography of the scrotum can identify a testicular cause if present.

Trauma

Traumatic lesions of the testicle can include torsion, injury by foreign bodies (Fig. 11-53), and crushing injuries. Disruption of the testis with poor definition

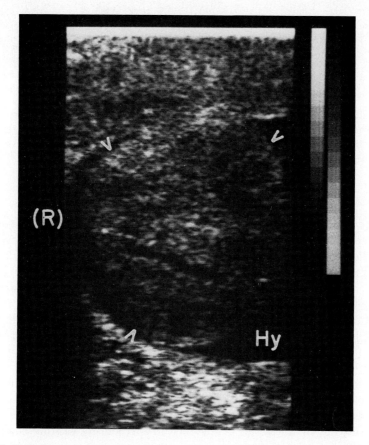

Figure 11-49 Diffuse orchitis. The testis (arrowheads) in this transverse high-resolution image is diffusely hypoechoic with areas of inhomogeneous echogenicity scattered throughout the organ. A small reactive hydrocele (Hy) is demonstrated posteriorly. (R) = patient's right side.

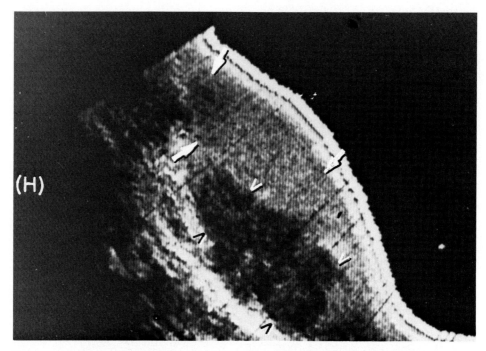

Figure 11-50 Seminoma. Longitudinal examination of the testis demonstrates the anterosuperior portion of the gland (arrows) to be of normal echogenic texture. A hypoechoic mass (arrowheads) involving the posteroinferior portion of the organ was a seminoma. (H) = toward patient's head.

and change in echogenicity is the most common sonographic finding. Testicular trauma from blunt trauma may result in rupture, where the testis cannot be differentiated from the surrounding hemorrhagic change (Fig. 11-54). If a hemorrhagic fluid collection, a hematocele, occurs, its margins are indistinguishable from the injured testicle. In these cases, hemorrhage may appear as areas of varied echogenicity, being increased or decreased.[69,72,73]

Acute torsion, where the spermatic cord twists disrupting the single arterial blood supply to the testes, is an acute surgical emergency. Restoration of blood flow is required within 7 to 8 hours to preserve testicular function. Acute torsion has no distinct acoustic characteristics. The testis may be slightly enlarged and echo-poor or normal.[71] Subacute or chronic torsion may demonstrate an enlarged testis, which may be diffusely echogenic. Hypoechoic cystic areas due to hemorrhage and necrosis have been seen. Untreated, the testis will infarct resulting in areas of increased echogenicity representing fibrotic change and reaction.

Gunshot wounds may result in the presence of a foreign body. Reactive hydroceles or hematoceles may occur, and the testes may also exhibit acoustic changes of edema (increased echogenicity) and disruption of the normal acoustic characteristics.

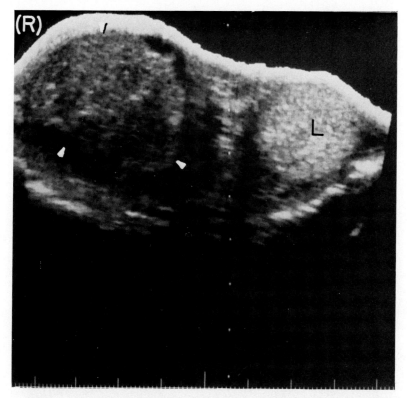

Figure 11-51 Mixed cellular malignancy. Transverse images of the scrotum demonstrate a normal left (L) testis. The right testis (arrowheads) is diffusely inhomogeneous, mostly hypoechoic. Mixed cellularity was noted histologically with portions of seminoma, choriocarcinoma, and embryonal cell carcinoma. (R) = patient's right side.

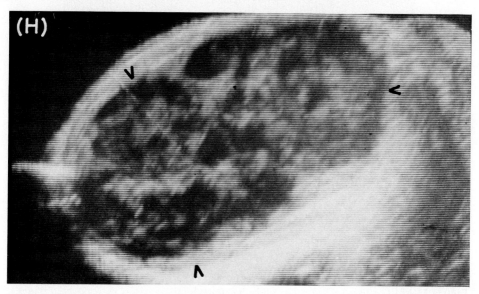

Figure 11-52 Lymphoma. A longitudinal examination of the testis demonstrates the organ to be slightly enlarged (arrowheads) and acoustically diffusely inhomogeneous. Lymphoma was proven histologically. (H) = toward patient's head.

475

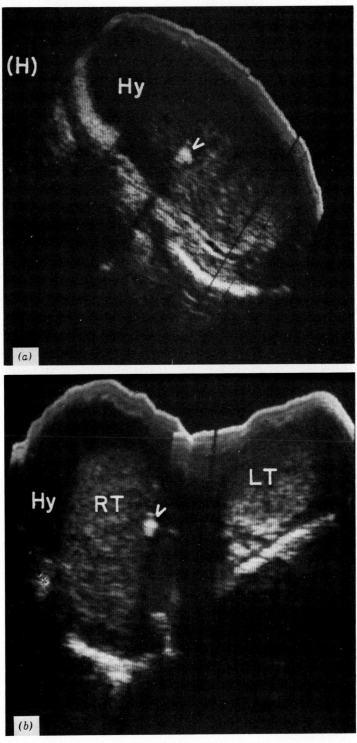

Figure 11-53 Trauma with foreign body. Longitudinal (*a*) and transverse (*b*) images of the scrotum demonstrates a normal left testis. The right testis (RT) is enlarged with an echogenic focus (arrowhead) that shadows. There is also a small hydrocele (Hy). The echogenic focus represents metallic fragments from a bullet, and the hemorrhagic hydrocele was secondary to the trauma. (H) = toward patient's head.

476

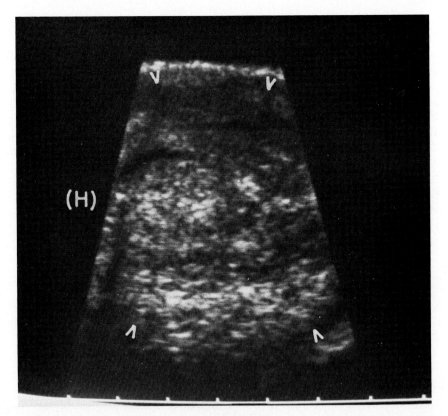

Figure 11-54 Testicular rupture. Longitudinal high-resolution examination of the testis demonstrates the organ to be poorly defined with areas of increased, and a few areas of decreased, echogenicity scattered throughout the testis (arrowheads). This patient had direct trauma to the testis with hemorrhagic changes extending through the tunica albuginea. (H) = toward patient's head.

REFERENCES

1. Gray H: *Gray's Anatomy*, ed 28, CM Goss, (ed). Philadelphia, Lea & Febiger, 1966.
2. Kurtz AB, Rifkin MD: Ultrasound of the normal female pelvis, in Callem P (ed): *Ultrasound in Obstetrics and Gynecology*, Philadelphia, W.B. Saunders Co, 1983.
3. Dubbins PA, Kurtz AB, Darby J, Goldberg BB: Ureteric jet Effect: The echographic appearance of urine entering the bladder. *Radiology* 140:513–515, 1981.
4. Kremer H, Dobrinski W, Mikyska M, et al: Ultrasonic in vivo and in vitro studies on the nature of the ureteral jet phenomenon. *Radiology* 142:175–177, 1982.
5. Bree RL, Silver TM: Nongynecologic bladder and perivesical ultrasound. *Urol Radiol* 4:135–145, 1982.
6. Nakamura S, Niijima T: Staging of bladder cancer by ultrasonography: A new technique by transurethral intravesical scanning. *J Urol* 124:341–344, 1980.
7. Schuller J, Walther, V, Schmiedt E, et al: Intravesical ultrasound tomography in staging bladder carcinoma. *J Urol* 128:264–266, 1982.
8. Watanabe H, Ohe H, Saitoh M, et al: Transrectal radial cone scanning for the

staging of urinary bladder tumors, in White D, Lyons EA (eds): *Ultrasound in Medicine*. New York, Plenum Press, 1978, vol. 4.

9. Watanabe H, Mishina T, Ohe H: Staging of bladder tumors by transrectal ultrasonotomography and UI Octoson. *Urol Radiol* 5:11–16, 1983.

10. Jewett HJ, Strong GH: Infiltrating carcinoma of the bladder: Relation of depth of penetration of the bladder wall to incidence of local extension and metastases. *J Urol* 55:366–372, 1946.

11. Sukov RJ, Scardino PT, Sample WF, et al: Computed tomography and transabdominal ultrasound in the evaluation of the prostate. *J Comput Assist Tomogr* 1(3):281–289, 1977.

12. Itzchak Y, Singer D, Fischelovitch Y: Ultrasonographic assessment of bladder tumors. I. Tumor detection. *J Urol* 126:31–33, 1981.

13. Singer D, Itzchak Y, Fischelovitch Y: Ultrasonographic assessment of bladder tumors. II. Clinical staging. *J Urol* 126:34–36, 1981.

14. McLaughlin IS, Morely P, Deane RF, et al: Ultrasound in the staging of bladder tumours. *Br J Urol* 47:51–56, 1975.

15. Rifkin MD, Kurtz AB, Pasto ME, Goldberg BB: Unusual presentations of cystitis. *J Ultrasound Med* 2(1):25–28, 1983.

16. Morgan CL, Grossman H, Trought WS, Oddson TA: Ultrasonic diagnosis of obstructed renal duplication and ureterocele. *South Med J* 73(8):1,016–1,019, 1980.

17. Griffin J, Jennings C, MacErlean D: Ultrasonic evaluation of simple and ectopic ureteroceles. *Clin Radiol* 34:55–57, 1983.

18. Mittelstaedt CA, Gosink BB, Leopold GR: Gray scale patterns of pelvic disease in the male. *Radiol* 123:727–732, 1977.

19. Goodman JD, Macchia RJ, Macasaet MA, Schneider M: Endometriosis of the urinary bladder: Sonographic findings. *AJR* 135:625–626, 1980.

20. Albert NE: Leiomyoma of bladder preoperative diagnosis by ultrasound. *Urology* 17(5):486–487, 1981.

21. Torres WE, Sones PJ Jr, Thames FM: Ultrasound appearance of a pelvic arteriovenous malformation. *J Clin Ultrasound* 7:383–385, 1979.

22. Church PA, Kazam E: Computed tomography and ultrasound in diagnosis of pelvic lipomatosis. *Urology* 14(6):631–633, 1979.

23. McLean GK, Edell SL: Determination of bladder volumes by gray scale ultrasonography. *Radiology* 128:181–182, 1978.

24. Harrison NW, Parks C, Sherwood T: Ultrasound assessment of residual urine in children. *Br J Urol* 47:805–814, 1976.

25. Pedersen JF, Bartrum RJ Jr, Grytter C: Residual urine determination by ultrasonic scanning. *AJR* 125(2):474–478, 1975.

26. Rees M, Joseph AEA: Ultrasound-guided suprapubic puncture: A new, simple way of releasing a blocked Foley balloon. *Br J Urol* 53:196, 1981.

27. Wexler JS, McGovern TP: Ultrasonography of female urethral diverticula. *AJR* 134:737–740, 1980.

28. White RD, McQuown D, McCarthy TA, Ostergard DR: Real-time ultrasonography in the evaluation of urinary stress incontinence. *Am J Obstet Gynecol* 138(2):235–237, 1980.

29. Leissner KH, Tisell LE: The weight of the human prostate. *Scan J Urol Nephrol* 13:137–142, 1979.

30. Denkhaus H, Dierkopf W, Grabbe H, Donn F: Comparative study of suprapubic

sonography and computed tomography for staging of prostatic carcinoma. *Urol Radiol* 5:1–9, 1983.

31. Greenberg M, Neiman HL, Brandt TD, et al: Ultrasound of the prostate. *Radiology* 141:757–762, 1981.

32. Greenberg M, Neiman HL, Vogelzang R, Falkowski W: Ultrasonographic features of prostatic carcinoma. *J Clin Ultrasound* 10:307–312, 1982.

33. Henneberry M, Carter MF, Neiman HL: Estimation of prostatic size by suprapubic ultrasonography. *J Urol* 121:615–616, 1979.

34. Aguirre CR, Tallada MB, Mayayo TD, et al: Evaluation comparative du volume prostatique par l'echographie transabdominale, le Profil uretral et la radiologie. *J d'Urologie* 86(8):675–679, 1980.

35. Miller SS, Garvie WHH: The evaluation of prostate size by ultrasonic scanning: A preliminary report. *Br J Urol* 45:187–191, 1973.

36. Bissada NK, Finkbeiner AE, Redman JF: Accuracy of preoperative estimation of resection weight in transurethral prostatectomy. *J Urol* 116:201–202, 1976.

37. Nakamura S, Niijima T: Transurethral real-time scanner. *J Urol* 125:781–783, 1981.

38. Holm HH, Northeved A: A transurethral ultrasonic scanner. *J Urol* 111:238–241, 1974.

39. Gammelgaard J, Holm HH: Transurethral and transrectal ultrasonic scanning in urology. *J Urol* 124:863–868, 1980.

40. Harada K, Tanahashi Y, Igari D, et al: Clinical evaluation of inside echo patterns in gray scale prostatic echography. *J Urol* 124:216–220, 1980.

41. Harada K, Igari D. Tanahashi Y: Gray scale transrectal ultrasonography of the prostate. *J Clin Ultrasound* 7:45–49, 1979.

42. Resnick MI, Willard JW, Boyce WH: Transrectal ultrasonography in the evaluation of patients with prostatic carcinoma. *J Urol* 124:482–484, 1980.

43. Watanabe H, Saitoh M, Mishina T, et al: Mass screening program for prostatic diseases with transrectal ultrasonotomography. *J Urol* 117:746–748, 1977.

44. Sekine H, Oka K, Takehara Y: Transrectal longitudinal ultrasonotomography of the prostate by electronic linear scanning. *J Urol* 127:62–65, 1982.

45. Brooman PJC, Griffiths GJ, Roberts E, et al: Per rectal ultrasound in the investigation of prostatic disease. *Clin Radiol* 32:669–676, 1981.

46. Peeling WB, Griffiths GJ, Evans KT, Roberts EE: Diagnosis and staging of prostatic cancer by transrectal ultrasonography. A preliminary study. *J Urol* 51:565–569, 1979.

47. Rifkin MD, Kurtz AB, Choi, HY, Goldberg BB: Endoscopic ultrasonic evaluation of the prostate utilizing a transrectal probe: Prospective evaluation and acoustic characterization. *Radiology* 149:265–271, 1983.

48. Kohri K, Kaneko S, Akiyama T, et al: Ultrasonic evaluation of prostatic carcinoma. *Urology* 17(2):214–217, 1981.

49. Holm HH, Gammelgaard J: Ultrasonically guided precise needle placement in the prostate and the seminal vesicles. *J Urol* 125:385–387, 1981.

50. Hastak SM, Gammelgaard J, Holm HH: Ultrasonically guided transperineal biopsy in the diagnosis of prostatic carcinoma. *J Urol* 128:69–71, 1982.

51. Rifkin MD, Kurtz AB, Goldberg BB: Technique for ultrasonically guided transperineal prostatic biopsy. *AJR* 139(4):745–747, 1983.

52. Fornage BD, Touche DH, Deglaire M, et al: Real-time ultrasound-guided prostatic biopsy using a new transrectal linear-array probe. *Radiology* 146:547–548, 1983.

53. Rifkin MD, Kurtz AB, Goldberg BB: Prostate biopsy utilizing transrectal ultrasound guidance: Diagnosis of nonpalpable cancers. *J Ultrasound Med* 2:165–167, 1983.

54. Sample WF, Gottesman JE, Skinner DG, Ehrlich RM: Gray scale ultrasound of the scrotum. *Radiology* 127:225–228, 1978.

55. DiGiacinto TM, Patten D, Willscher M, Daly K: Sonography of the scrotum. *Med Ultrasound* 6:95–101, 1982.

56. Richie JP, Birnholz J, Garnick MB: Ultrasonography as a diagnostic adjunct for the evaluation of masses in the scrotum. *Surg Gynecol Obstet* 154:695–698, 1982.

57. Leopold GR, Woo VL, Scheible FW, et al: High-resolution ultrasonography of scrotal pathology. *Radiology* 131:719–722, 1979.

58. Wilson PC, Valvo JR, Gramiak R, Frank IN: Automated water-path ultrasonic examination of scrotum. *Urology* 18(1):94–99, 1981.

59. Glazer HS, Lee JKT, Melson GL, McClennan BL: Sonographic detection of occult testicular neoplasms. *AJR* 138:673–675, 1982.

60. Rifkin MD, Foy PM, Kurtz AB, et al: Varicoceles: The role of diagnostic ultrasound. *J Ultrasound Med* 2(6):271–276, 1983.

61. Rifkin MD, Foy PM, Goldberg BB: Acoustic characterization of the testis and epididymis. *Medical Ultrasound* (in press).

62. Foy PM, Rifkin MD: Hydroceles: Acoustic characterization and diagnosis. *Med Ultrasound* 7(3):91–94, 1983.

63. Subramanyam BR, Balthazar EJ, Raghavendra BN, et al: Sonographic diagnosis of scrotal hernia. *AJR* 139:535–538, 1982.

64. Rifkin MD, Jacobs JA: Simple testicular cyst diagnosed preoperatively by ultrasound. *J Urol* 129:982–983, 1983.

65. Vick WC, Bird KI, Rosenfield AT, et al: Ultrasound of the scrotal contents. *Urol Radiol* 4:147–153, 1982.

66. Becker JM, Ritchie WGM, Goldenberg NJ: Ultrasound of the scrotum and its contents. *Semin Ultrasound* 3(4):348–355, 1982.

67. Orr DP, Skolnick ML: Sonographic examination of the abnormal scrotum. *Clin Radiol* 31:109–113, 1980.

68. Arger PH, Mulhern CB Jr, Coleman BG, et al: Prospective analysis of the value of scrotal ultrasound. *Radiology* 141:763–766, 1981.

69. Blei L, Sihelnik S, Bloom D, et al: Ultrasonographic analysis of chronic intratesticular pathology. *J Ultrasound Med* 2:17–23, 1983.

70. Lupetin AR, King W, Rich P, Lederman RB: Ultrasound diagnosis of testicular leukemia. *Radiology* 146:171–172, 1983.

71. Bird K, Rosenfield AT, Taylor KTW: Ultrasonography in testicular torsion. *Radiology* 147:527–534, 1983.

72. Friedman SG, Rose JG, Winston MA: Ultrasound and nuclear medicine evaluation in acute testicular trauma. *J Urol* 125:748–749, 1981.

73. Albert NE: Testicular ultrasound for trauma. *J Urol* 124:558–559, 1980.

12

Aspiration and Biopsy Techniques

Matthew D. Rifkin
Barry B. Goldberg

INTRODUCTION

Nonsurgical percutaneous aspiration has been a diagnostic and therapeutic procedure for over a century. One of the first cases was reported in 1867 involving drainage of a renal cyst.[1] Extensive evaluation and use of the procedure began in the 1940s,[2,3] with widespread evaluation and refinement occurring since that time.[4-9]

The kidney was the first organ to be studied. The primary goal was to differentiate between cystic and solid lesions.[2-9] Aspiration of cysts, antegrade pyelograms, and aspiration biopsies of the kidneys and other structures were usually performed blindly or localized by palpation. The advent of fluoroscopy allowed more accurate placement of the needle. With the intravenous administration of iodinated contrast, anatomic detail of space-ccupying lesions or dilated collecting systems allowed for accurate procedures.[2-9] Proper needle placement in other organs was still dependent on palpation or mass effect seen on the available imaging modalities including fluoroscopy and angiography.

The development and use of diagnostic ultrasound in the 1970s allowed for visualization of structures that had previously alluded diagnosis. This new imaging modality increased preoperative diagnostic ability. In addition, it made accurate needle placement for aspiration and biopsy of both cystic and solid lesions of many organs possible, often eliminating the need for surgical intervention. Diagnostic studies were soon supplemented with therapeutic procedures, including percutaneous drainage of both obstructed and infected areas.

The refinement in body computed tomography permitted lesions poorly identified by ultrasound to be accurately evaluated. All imaging modalities previously used for guidance are now employed on an individual basis, with the concurrent use of multiple imaging techniques as needed for proper diagnosis and therapy. This chapter deals primarily with ultrasonically guided procedures.

481

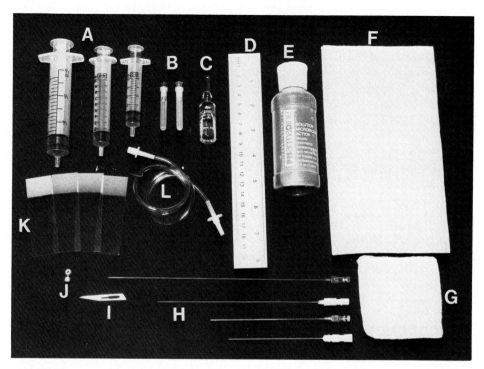

Figure 12-1 Standard aspiration-biopsy material. A = syringes; B = needles; C = local anaesthetic; D = ruler; E = antiseptic solution; F = sterile drapes; G = sterile gauze; H = aspiration-biopsy needles; I = #11 blade; J = needle stop; K = slides; L = extension tubing.

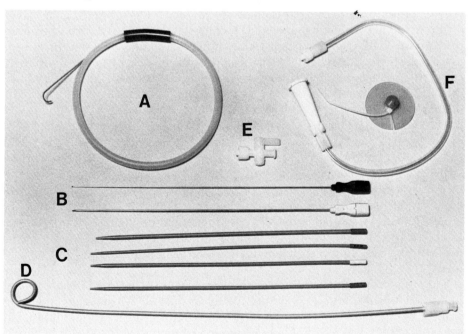

Figure 12-2 Nephrostomy or abscess drainage setup. A = flexible metal guide wire; B = percutaneous aspiration needles; C = soft tissue dilators; D = pigtail catheter; E = stop cock; F = attachments to drainage bag.

Equipment

The techniques for aspiration, biopsy, or drainage of a specific area are similar irregardless of the organ or type of structure being evaluated. In general, the approach (which is discussed in greater detail for each procedure) should follow the least invasive tissue pathway to the area to be treated.

The basic equipment (Fig. 12-1) required for any of these procedures are:

Betadine
Sterile gauze
25-gauge needle for skin anaesthesia
22-gauge needle for deeper anaesthesia
5 to 10 cc syringe for anaesthesia
Local anaesthetic
20 to 50 cc syringe for aspiration
#11 blade
18,20,22-gauge spinal, chiba, and/or cutting needles
Needle stop
Sterile bowls

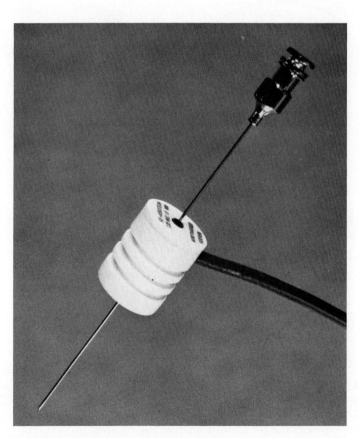

Figure 12-3 A-mode and M-mode biopsy transducer with needle placed through slot.

Sterile gloves

Sterile drapes

Ruler

Extension tubing

There are numerous commercially prepared kits that include most of the above materials. Water soluble, iodinated contrast material is often required for cyst aspirations. Biopsy procedures require glass slides and containers with appropriate fixatives for cytologic studies. Nephrostomy and abscess drainage procedures require aerobic and anaerobic microbacteriologic cultures, sheathed catheters, dilators, and a pigtail catheter (Fig. 12-2).

Unlike other imaging modalities, using ultrasound to guide needle placement allows for constant monitoring of both the site being studied and the needle as it is placed in the lesion. Redirection of the needle can be made immediately if

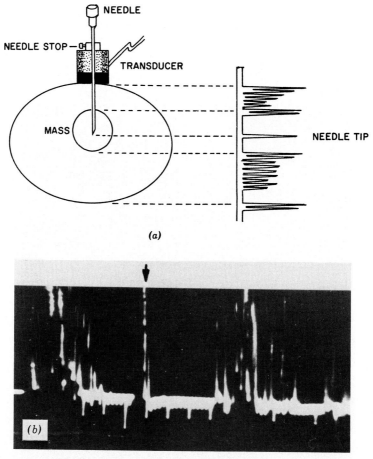

(a)

(b)

Figure 12-4 (*a*) Diagram of A-mode aspiration. Needle with stop placed through transducer into fluid-filled mass. The needle tip is delineated as a bright reflection on A-mode (right) in an anechoic region. (*b*) A-mode study of anechoic area with needle tip (arrow) clearly demarcated in the central portion of mass.

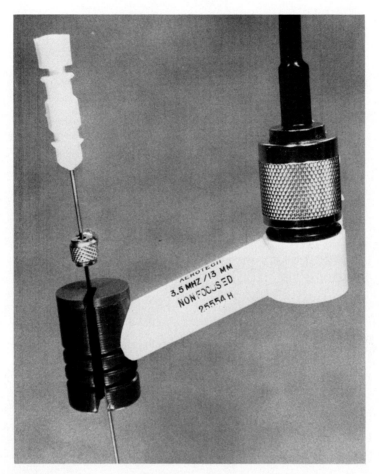

Figure 12-5 B-mode contact scan biopsy transducer for use with an articulated arm. The needle is placed in open slot for easy removal of transducer following appropriate needle placement.

required. The first of the various transducers used was a small, round device, approximately 2 cm in diameter, with a centrally placed slot for the needle (Fig. 12-3).[10,11] It is attached to the microprocessor via a flexible wire and is used with the A-mode, or when available, M-mode capabilities of the ultrasound unit. This transducer is able to differentiate a fluid-filled from a solid mass or area and can readily detect the needle tip located in the central portion of a cystic structure (Fig. 12-4). The ability to visualize the needle is directly proportional to its size. Needles larger than 20-gauge are routinely visualized, while those of a smaller gauge are not. In most cases, only the needle tip is noted with A-mode guidance. When M-mode assistance is used, visualization of the entire needle tract may be seen. The transducer, like most others to be described, can be gas-sterilized for reuse.

Transducers have also been developed for use with gray scale articulated arm B-scan units (Fig. 12-5)[12] and linear array real-time equipment.[13,14] The

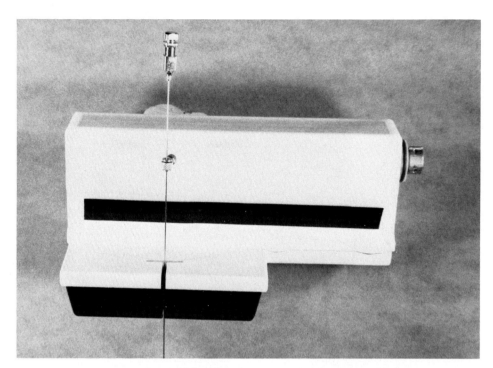

Figure 12-6 Linear array real-time transducer with needle placed in open slot.

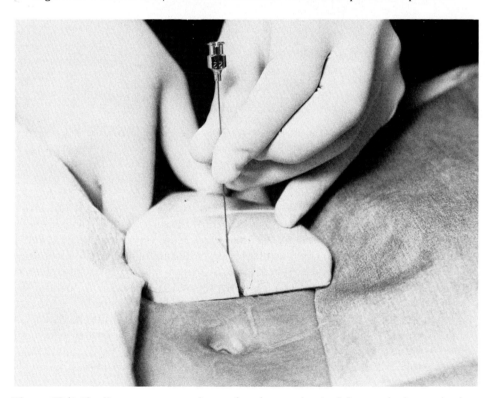

Figure 12-7 Flat linear array transducer placed on patient's abdomen during aspiration biopsy. The needle is placed through the slotted opening.

486

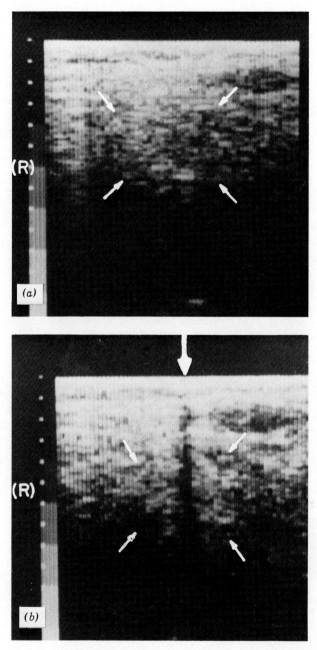

Figure 12-8 (*a*) Linear array ultrasonogram demonstrating mass (arrows). (*b*) Linear array biopsy transducer with defect from needle as it enters the skin interrupting direct contact of the transducer crystals (large arrow). The line defect is the path of the needle when inserted in a perpendicular fashion. The mass is denoted by small arrows.

newer real-time transducers (Fig. 12-6) are relatively compact compared to some of the early devices. Flat, small transducers that permit the use of large-bore needles and intraoperative procedures are widely available (Fig. 12-7). This equipment has been designed to allow the needle to be placed through the transducer without obstructing the scanning ability of the unit. Guides are available that allow the needle to be removed following placement in the desired site, while some transducers fix the needle in the slot. Visualization of the tip or pathway of the needle (Fig. 12-8) is site dependent. The entire needle is usually not seen when the puncture of solid lesions is guided by linear array equipment.

Mechanical sector scanners have also been used for biopsies.[15] Because of the shape and expense to produce a dedicated biopsy transducer, clip-on devices have been developed (Fig. 12-9). These add-on devices are either reusable following gas sterilization or disposable. The benefit of the sector scan devices as compared to most linear array transducers is that the needle path, which is slightly obliqued from the ultrasound beam, is usually visualized in its entirety in both cystic (Fig. 12-10) and solid (Figs. 12-11 and 12-12) lesions. This permits immediate redirection of the needle if needed and accurate placement in the desired location.

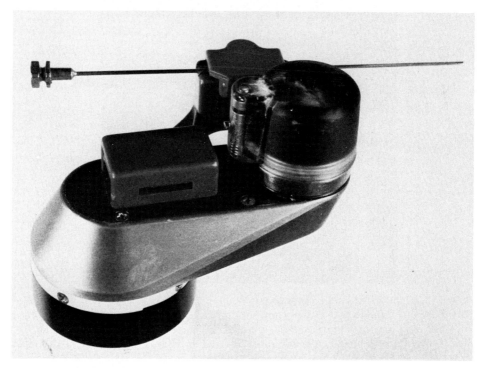

Figure 12-9 Real-time sector scan head with disposable offset biopsy guide attached with needle in place.

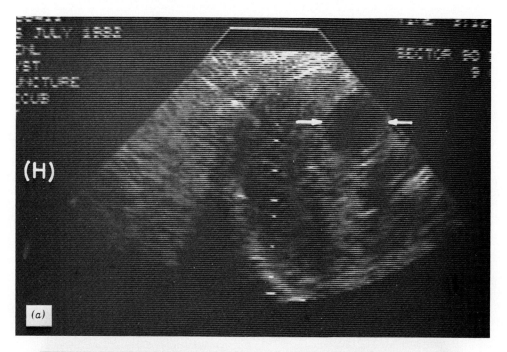

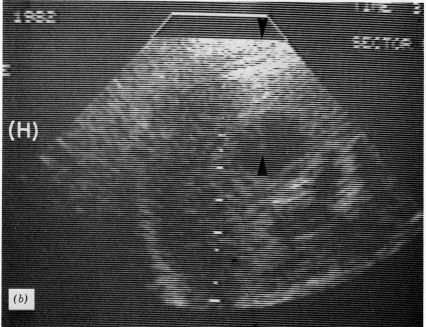

Figure 12-10 Intrahepatic mass. An intrahepatic fluid-filled mass (arrows) is noted before (*a*) and during needle aspiration guided by an offset sector scanner (*b*). The entire needle (arrowheads) is noted entering the lesion from an oblique angle. H = toward patient's head.

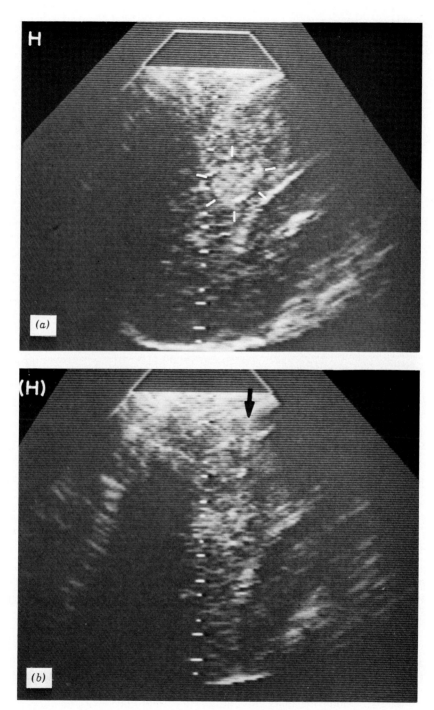

Figure 12-11 Cavernous hemangioma. (*a*) Mechanical sector scan, real-time evaluation of liver demonstrates a well-defined echogenic mass (slashes) within the hepatic tissue. (*b*) Biopsy needle (arrow) is seen as it courses through liver tissue with the tip placed directly into the echogenic mass that proved to be an hemangioma.

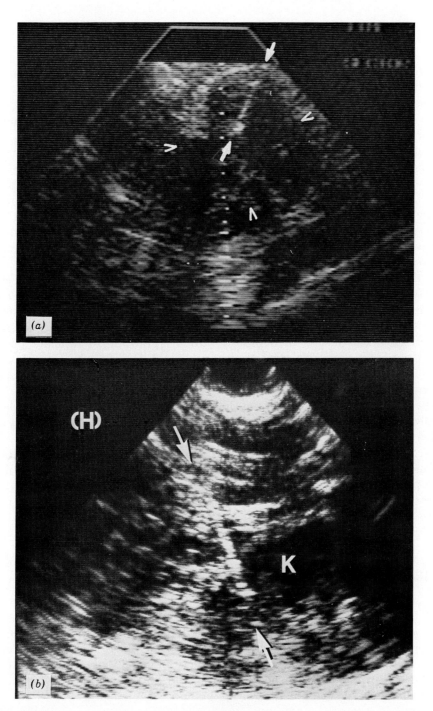

Figure 12-12 (*a*) Carcinoma of the pancreas. Real-time sector scan ultrasonic evaluation of the abdomen during biopsy of mass with the needle visualized in place during biopsy. The needle (arrows) is well defined in the center of the mass (arrowheads), which proved to be an adenocarcinoma. (*b*) Renal biopsy. The biopsy needle (arrows) is clearly defined entering the parenchyma of the kidney (K). (H) = toward patient's head.

491

Technique

Ultrasonically guided aspirations or biopsies permit continual visualization of the entire needle during the actual procedure. Thus, the path and placement as well as areas to be avoided by the needle are rapidly determined. The needle can be repositioned or changed during insertion as required. If the structure to be studied is adequately identified on the sonogram, then ultrasound is usually the imaging modality of choice for guidance. After obtaining the appropriate informed consent and inquiring about possible allergic history to the medication to be used (local anaesthetic, sedative, water soluble iodinated contrast material, etc.), the patient can be placed in the position, that is, supine, prone, decubitus, oblique, etc. that will facilitate the proper place for puncture. A line of site is obtained that is the shortest distance from skin to lesion and traverses the least dangerous course. In general, the puncture of two or more spaces, that is, pleural, peritoneal, retroperitoneal, or multiple organs, should be avoided. Because the needle is visualized during the procedure, a perpendicular position from the skin to the lesion is not required. Angled needle placement can be used as necessary. The appropriate position for needle puncture is marked. The patient is prepared in a sterile manner, and sterile drapes are placed. Skin and deeper subcutaneous anaesthesia is administered. If necessary, the skin is then incised with a #11 blade to facilitate needle placement. This is particularly important to avoid deviation from the desired location when a flexible needle, such as the chiba, is employed or if catheter placement for drainage is anticipated.

The sterile aspiration biopsy transducer is then used to confirm the angle of needle placement and the depth of the lesion. A stop may be placed on the biopsy needle in order to avoid inadvertent placement of the tip through the desired tissue. The needle is placed in the orifice of the biopsy transducer through the skin and is continually monitored as it is positioned into the lesion. Slow positioning with direct visual guidance of the needle can be used. When entering a cyst, a quick jab may be necessary to puncture the capsule. The type of procedure to be performed, which is discussed below, is then completed.

ASPIRATION

Renal Cyst Aspiration

The advent of ultrasound and the improved equipment has led to the development of criteria for diagnosis of renal masses.[16] Differentiating renal cysts from solid lesions is so accurate that it is no longer necessary to aspirate all renal cysts for diagnostic purposes.[17] The major criteria for invasive diagnostic procedures of fluid-filled masses of the kidneys include lesions:

1. That are not distinctly characteristic of simple cysts on the ultrasound examination
2. Where the renal cyst is causing obstruction to the collecting system
3. Where there is pain from the affected kidney

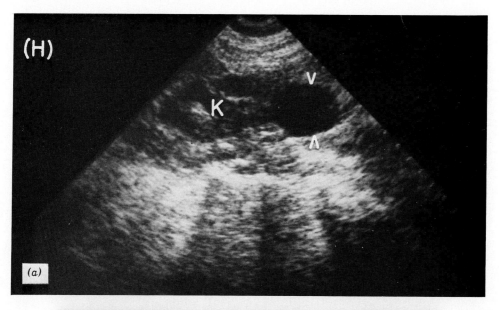

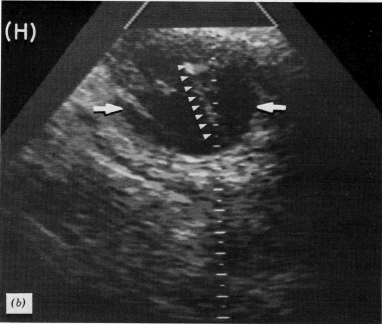

Figure 12-13 Renal cyst. (*a*) Real-time sector scan of the left kidney (K) demonstrates a well-defined fluid-filled mass (arrowheads) distorting the lower pole. This lesion has the ultrasonic characteristics of a simple cyst. (H) = toward patient's head. (*b*) Enlarged image of renal cyst puncture demonstrates the clearly visualized needle (arrowheads) within the partly collapsed cyst (arrows). (H) = toward patient's head. (*c*) Radiograph of a cyst (arrows) following percutaneous aspiration and placement of iodinated contrast and air. The slight irregularity of the walls (arrowheads) is due to inadequate redistension of the benign cyst with air and fluid. Multiple radiographs of the lesion with the patient in various positions will clarify this situation.

493

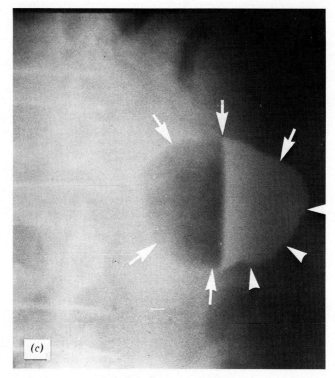

Figure 12-13 (*continued*)

4. Where no definable cause is noted in a patient with sepsis and who has a cyst of the kidney

5. Where two diagnostic imaging modalities result in conflicting and/or indeterminate results

6. Where the patient suffers from renin-dependent hypertension[18,19]

When the lesion being aspirated is located, the patient is positioned for the procedure. A posterior, or posterolateral approach, inferior to the crux of the hemidiaphragm, is preferable in order to avoid involvement of the bowel, other abdominal organs, pleura, or lung parenchyma. The angle is noted and the distance marked. A small (20- or 22-gauge, noncutting) stiff needle is preferable to a flexible needle because there is less chance that the tip will deviate during insertion. Following the previously described puncture technique, a distinct "pop" is often felt as the needle traverses the cyst's capsule. The stylet is then removed from the needle. If the pressure of the cystic fluid is greater than hemispheric pressure, it will flow spontaneously. If the intracystic pressure is less than the atmospheric pressure, aspiration is required. A syringe attached to an extension tube is secured to the needle allowing free movement of the needle during the patient's respiratory excursion.

Fluid is then removed for analysis. Simple cysts are filled with clear, translucent, slightly yellowish fluid. This should be sent for cytologic evaluation.

Chemical evaluation of the fluid has also been employed in the past. It has been reported that fat content and LDH levels are frequently elevated in tumors.[20,21] If cloudy, purulent, or hemorrhagic material is obtained, further tests including aerobic and anaerobic bacteriologic cultures and a hematocrit should be ordered.[22,23] Amylase levels of the fluid can determine if the lesion may be pancreatic in origin.[24] Water-soluble iodinated contrast material can be instilled to evaluate the walls of these cysts.

Ideally, the injection of both contrast and air (in equal amounts to the fluid withdrawn), together with the remaining fluid, produces a triple contrast radiographic examination. The instillation of the materials should be done under fluoroscopic control to avoid possible extravasation.[25] Thus, this procedure may use two imaging modalities, since radiographs of the kidneys are then obtained in multiple projections.

Simple benign cysts classically have smooth, well-defined walls (Figs. 12-13 and 12-14), although septations are not uncommon (Fig. 12-15). Hemorrhagic material within a simple cyst appears as filling defects.[26–29] Necrotic tumors or

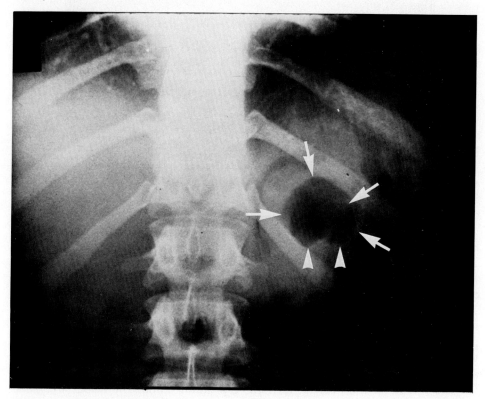

Figure 12-14 Renal cyst. Radiographs of a patient with a severe allergy to iodine. Following percutaneous aspiration of a benign renal cyst, air was instilled as a contrast material. The dependent portion of the mass (arrowheads) is filled with the cyst's fluid causing poor definition, while the air distended the remainder of the wall, which is sharply marginated (arrows). Multiple radiographs to visualize all the walls are necessary for complete evaluation.

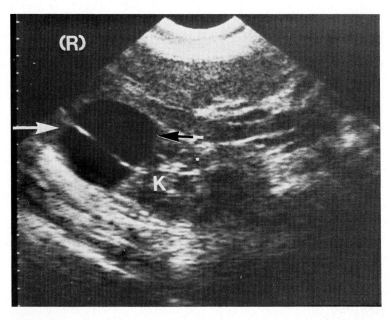

Figure 12-15 Renal cyst with septation. Transverse B-scan of the right kidney (K) demonstrates a fluid-filled mass (arrow) with thick echogenic septation, which was proven on cyst aspiration.

neoplastic degeneration of the wall of the cyst have irregular margins (Figs. 12-16 and 12-17).

The necessity of obtaining all these tests following cyst puncture is unclear. Although it occurs, it is very rare that the fluid of cysts with concurrent neoplasms has a negative cytology.[25,30] Radiographic evaluation of the wall of the cyst is imperative when the fluid obtained is not clearly translucent.

Many agents have been instilled into renal cysts to permanently decrease their size. Quinicrine, talc, and pantopaque were previously thought to offer great benefit, but their long-term success has yet to be medically proven. Leakage of some of the materials are quite irritating in the perirenal space requiring exact placement of the needle if this technique is to be employed.[31–34]

Major complications, including perirenal hemorrhage, pneumothorax, arteriovenous malformation, and urinomas have been reported to occur in approximately 10 percent of cases.[35] These problems were slightly more common when the needle was "fixed" to the transducer or aspiration syringe directly and no extension tubing was used. In these cases, the kidney and the cyst wall may be torn as it moves with normal respiration. Pneumothoraces are more commonly noted when the renal masses involve the left side, particularly the upper poles. Perirenal hemorrhage (less than 5 percent) were more commonly seen with lesions that were situated in the anterior portion of the kidney. No appreciable differences were noted with different sized needles. Minor complications include microscopic (6 percent) and macroscopic (0.5 percent) hematuria and extravasation of contrast material following its administration (1.7 percent). Infection of the cyst following puncture is rare.[36]

Other Cystic Lesions

Aspiration of other fluid-filled lesions in the abdomen has been successfully performed with minimal complication. Hepatic and mesenteric cysts are usually easily studied. While pancreatic pseudocysts can be aspirated for diagnostic purposes, if indicated, leakage of material from uncomplicated pancreatic pseudocysts may be quite damaging to the surrounding structures. Therefore, a small-gauge (22) needle should be employed. Cytologic evaluation and selected chemical studies including amylase, bilirubin, and others, depending on the type of fluid noted, should be obtained.

Ascites

When aspiration of ascitic or pleural fluid is required for therapeutic or diagnostic purposes, it can often be done blindly. However, when there is a

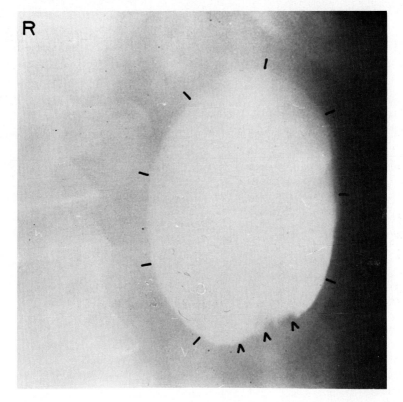

Figure 12-16 Renal adenocarcinoma. Radiograph of the kidney following needle aspiration and contrast administration demonstrates well-defined walls superiorly (slashes) with an area of irregularity of the inferior wall (arrowhead). The fluid aspirated was serosanginous, and the lesion proved to be an adenocarcinoma.

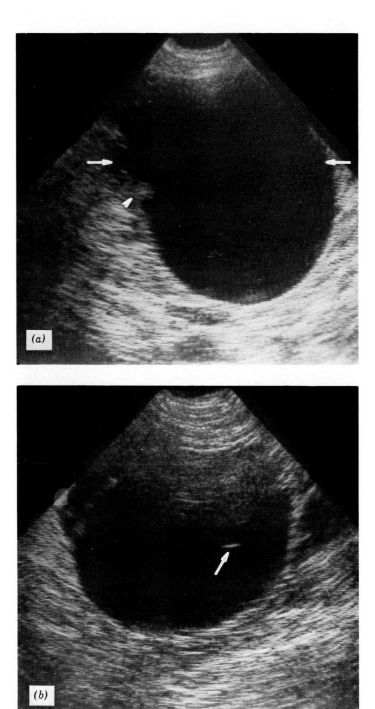

Figure 12-17 Renal cyst with wall thickening. Longitudinal image (*a*) of a large renal cyst (arrows) with smooth walls is replacing the majority of the kidney. There is a small protuberance from the wall noted (arrowhead). The renal cyst aspiration demonstrates (*b* and *c*) the needle tip as it is progressively placed in the lesion (arrow). A biopsy of the wall irregularity (*d*) shows the needle (arrow) at the protuberance (arrowhead), which was adherent hemorrhage.

498

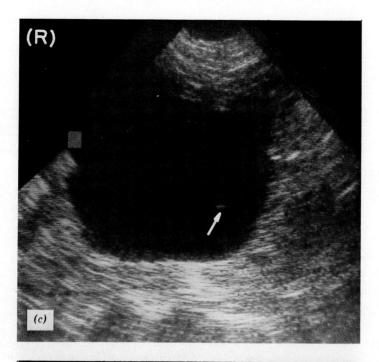

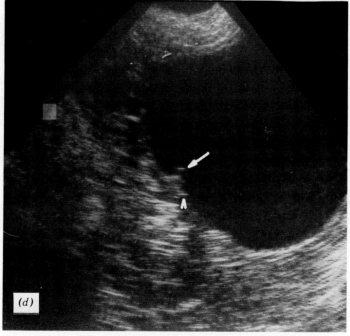

Figure 12-17 *(continued)*

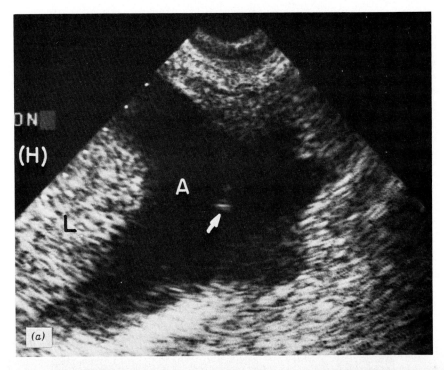

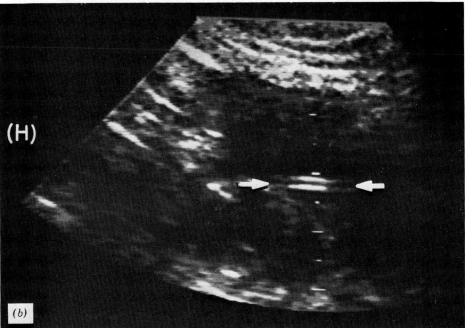

Figure 12-18 Ascites. (*a*) A small amount of loculated ascites (A) is noted inferior to the liver (L). The needle tip (arrow) was placed in this area under sonographic guidance. (*b*) An indwelling catheter denoted by the parallel lines of the tube (arrows) was subsequently placed for continuous drainage. (H) = toward patient's head.

small amount of fluid or it is loculated, ultrasonic guidance is quite beneficial (Fig. 12-18).

Suprapubic Bladder Aspiration

The ability to place a needle through the lower anterior abdominal wall into the urinary bladder is advantageous for diagnostic purposes, including cystourethrography,[37,38] and more importantly, for proper identification of possible bacteriologic organisms in urinary tract infections.[39] This technique is used most often in the neonatal and pediatric age group and in patients who cannot urinate on demand and in whom urethral catheterizations are to be avoided. When performed without visual guidance, the procedure has distinct, although minimal, morbidity.[37,40,41] The use of sonically guided suprapubic punctures has allowed more accurate needle placement with subsequent lower morbidity.[42]

BIOPSIES

Abdomen

Biopsies of solid intraabdominal structures have been performed for years using palpation, endoscopic (ERCP), fluoroscopic, and various cholangiographic guidance. The development of ultrasound and CT permitted accurate visualization and biopsies of small lesions.[43-47] The choice of guidance procedure, either ultrasound or CT, depends on the size, type, and placement of the lesion. Using ultrasound is often faster than CT, and it allows the biopsy needle to be visualized continually during placement. In general, if the mass is adequately demonstrated on ultrasound, the biopsy can be performed using that modality (Figs. 12-11, 12-12 and 12-19). If visualization is limited, CT is usually the modality of choice. The indications for a percutaneous nonsurgical aspiration biopsy include:

1. Patients who are poor surgical candidates and require tissue diagnosis
2. Patients with a known primary lesion and in whom other perhaps metastatic lesions are noted
3. Patients with known malignancy who have been successfully treated and now require evaluation of possible recurrence

There are no absolute contraindications to an aspiration biopsy. Patients who have been anticoagulated or have a bleeding diathesis require treatment of the disorder if possible and careful observation. Highly vascular lesions such as hemangiomas have been biopsied without significant complications (Fig. 12-11). A small-gauge needle, however, should be used.

The technique for aspiration biopsy of a solid mass is similar to cyst aspiration. The pop which is felt when a fluid-filled mass is punctured, is absent in solid lesions. Certain masses, particularly carcinoma, may feel hard or gritty, whereas others, such as lymphoma, may have no distinct sensation. A small 22-gauge needle is usually used to enter the lesion. Its placement is then noted on the sonogram. The stylet is removed and a 20 cc syringe is tightly attached to the needle (thus "fixing" the lesion). Vacuum suction is applied to the syringe continuously while it is gently moved in an in-out fashion with simultaneous clockwise–counterclockwise rotation. Suction is gently decreased while the needle is removed. This allows a small number of cells to be obtained for cytologic diagnosis. Occasionally, a small core of tissue is suctioned for cell block histologic evaluation.

If possible, a cytologist should be present for immediate consultation. A small droplet of material can be placed on a slide and immediately smeared and fixed. The remainder of the aspirate can be suspended in a saline solution for further evaluation.

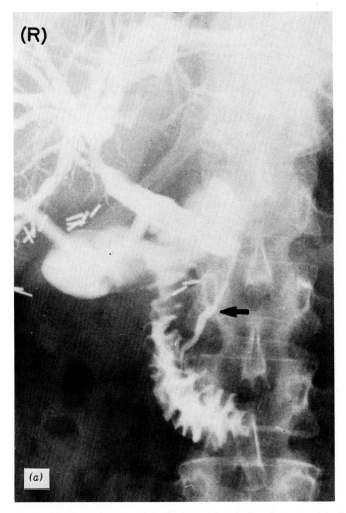

Figure 12-19 Pancreatic carcinoma. A transhepatic cholangiogram (*a*) demonstrates marked thinning and irregularity of the distal common bile duct (black arrows). The longitudinal sonogram (*b*) delineates the mass (white arrows), and the biopsy with ultrasound (*c*) shows the needle tip (arrowhead) in the mass, a pancreatic cancer.

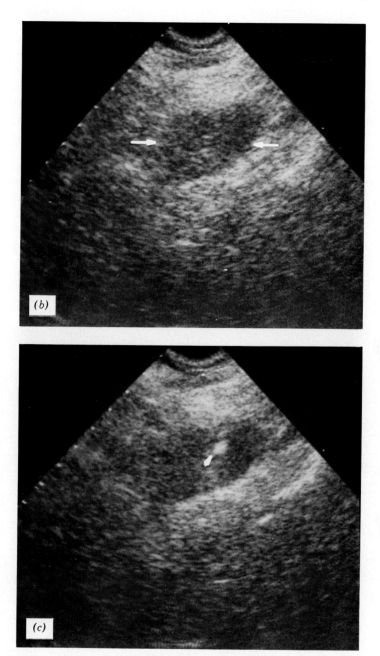

Figure 12-19 (*continued*)

The diagnosis is obtained in 75 percent of the cases with a single pass and increases to 85 to 90 percent when 4 to 5 passes of the needle are made at a single sitting.[43] When a cytologist is present during the procedure, a single aspiration may yield the diagnosis without the need for additional punctures. More punctures would be required only when the cytologist needs more tissue.

Small-gauge cutting needles may yield adequate tissue when the chiba needle aspirations are inconclusive. Slightly greater diagnostic accuracy without increase in complications has been obtained in aspiration of hepatic lesions with an 18-gauge needle instead of a 22-gauge needle.[48]

The complications of the procedure are uncommon.[43,47,49–52] Small hematomas and transient sepsis are uncommon, usually requiring no further therapy.[53] Passage of the needle through the adjacent structures, particularly the bowel, has been shown to be of no clinical significance. Experimentally, perforations of the bowel with a 22-gauge needle in laboratory animals seal immediately, and the actual puncture site cannot be visualized.[54] Extravasation or development of pancreatitis is quite unusual, particularly when a noncutting needle is used.[55] Theoretically, pneumothoraces may occur when lesions in the upper abdomen are biopsied through the pleura, but these are clinically uncommon.

The spread or seeding of malignant cells is theoretically a worrisome complication which has been reported in biopsies using large bore needles.[56–58] It is distinctly rare in cases where small, 22-gauge needles have been employed.[59]

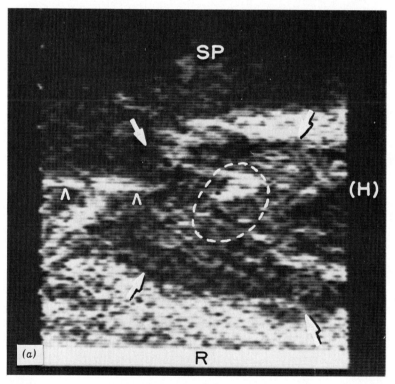

Figure 12-20 Transrectal longitudinal sonogram of the prostate. The ultrasonic probe is placed into the rectum (R). An ultrasonically guided biopsy needle (arrowheads) is placed under sonographic guidance (*a*, *b*, and *c*) into an area of focal echogenicity (circled), which proved to be an adenocarcinoma. SP = symphysis pubis; H = toward patient's head; Arrows = prostatic margins.

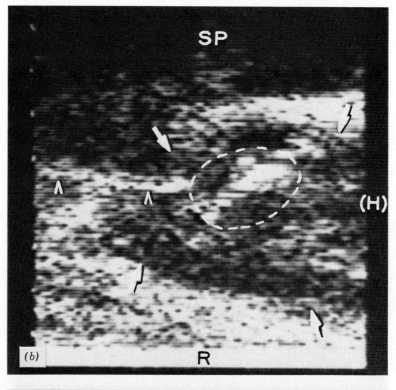

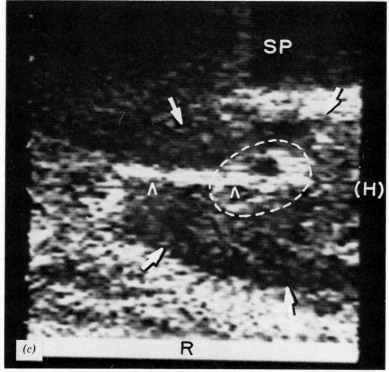

Figure 12-20 (continued)

505

Prostate

Recently, transrectal sonographic evaluation of the prostate gland has demonstrated effective differentiation between normal and abnormal portions of the gland.[60] The ability to differentiate clearly benign and malignant disease is not yet possible. Thus, techniques have been developed for ultrasonically guided percutaneous transperineal biopsy of the prostate with a specially designed ultrasound probe placed in the rectum (Fig. 12-20).[61-62]

DRAINAGE PROCEDURES

Percutaneous Nephrostomy

Percutaneous or antegrade nephrostomy was initially reported as viable diagnostic procedure in the 1950s.[63,64] The technique relied on fluoroscopic or blind guidance and was used to diagnose and alleviate renal obstruction and pyonephrosis.[63-75] Using ultrasound for guidance has made the procedure commonplace and decreased the risk of possible complications.[74-83] The percutaneous approach under sonographic control permits needle placement into renal pelves that are only minimally dilated.

The indications for percutaneous nephrostomy include:

1. The need to evaluate the cause for a patient's renal obstruction
2. Short-term relief of obstruction
3. Diagnosis and treatment of infection of a dilated collecting system

When the patient's clinical condition is severely compromised by chronic disease, metastatic disorders, or generalized illness, and when general anaesthesia is contraindicated, this procedure assumes greater importance.[82,83] Long-term urinary diversion in patients with chronic or terminal disease has been a useful therapeutic procedure effective for up to two years.[73,83]

The technique is similar to renal cyst aspiration. Care must be taken to ensure that anatomic compartments other than the retroperitoneum are not invaded. This is particularly important when an indwelling catheter placement is planned. Both ultrasound and fluoroscopic guidance is usually required. The patient is placed in a slightly obliqued prone position. Ultrasonic guidance is used to mark the appropriate puncture site. A posterolateral approach below the twelfth rib is desirable to allow for patient mobility following catheter placement. A portion of renal parenchyma should be traversed, if possible, to stabilize the catheter. The initial puncture is similar to other percutaneous procedures. If the procedure is purely diagnostic, a 20- or 22-gauge sheathed catheter is inserted into the renal pelvis, urine is removed for bacteriologic, and if required, cytologic evaluation. If needed to prove adequate needle placement, a small amount of water-soluble iodinated contrast material should be injected under fluoroscopic control. Overdistension of the collecting system should be avoided to reduce possible extravasation. Adequate contrast material must be instilled into the collecting system to yield the proper diagnosis. Care must be taken so that the renal pelvis, calyces, and ureter are not overdistended causing rupture or leakage.

Various techniques may be employed for successful drainage-catheter placement. A two-puncture technique involves a diagnostic puncture using a small-gauge needle, which can be removed after withdrawing a small amount of fluid for laboratory studies. A larger bore needle is then placed into the collecting system. The stylet is removed from the large-gauge needle, and a flexible guidewire is advanced into the renal collecting system. The latter steps should be performed under fluoroscopic visualization to avoid aberrant placement of the wire. Sequential dilation of the subcutaneous tissue with standard angiographic dilators is followed by placement of a pigtail catheter with multiple side holes. The wire is then withdrawn (Fig. 12-21).

When an indwelling catheter is planned, the initial puncture may involve a different needle. A trocar type needle is of large caliber. A flexible pigtail catheter can be placed directly over the outer diameter or through the inner lumen depending on the needle. The use of this device eliminates the necessity of a second puncture. It should be attempted only with a moderate to grossly dilated renal pelvis. When adequate placement of this drainage catheter is noted, the likelihood of inadvertent removal can be reduced by suturing it to the skin.

There are no major contraindications except for possible bleeding disorders. The procedure may be technically difficult in individuals in which there is minimal renal pelvic dilatation. It should be avoided when the patient is markedly obese, uncooperative, or incoherent and may unwittingly remove the drainage catheter.

Complications are similar to those described with renal cyst aspiration. They include hemorrhage, pneumothorax, and perirenal hematoma. The risk of developing a urinoma or secondary infection from the indwelling catheter is minimal.[84]

The initial catheter technique for other manipulative procedures of the urinary tract is similar to that used for percutaneous nephrostomy.[75–78] These procedures include ureteral stent placement, ureteral stricture dilatation, calculus and foreign body extraction, and nephroscopy and are beyond the scope of this text.

Percutaneous Abscess Drainage

Percutaneous aspiration of abdominal abscess collections for diagnostic purposes has long been an accepted modality. Initially, once an abscess was located and diagnosed, medical and surgical therapy was initiated.[85] The development of acceptable catheter drainage techniques of the urinary system has resulted in similar successful, nonsurgical therapy of intraabdominal abscess collections.[86–98] The procedure has been proven to aid the surgeon in preoperative[94,97] and postoperative[98] patient care. It has also negated the need for surgical intervention in up to 90 percent of patients.[89–92,95]

Percutaneous abscess drainage should be limited to those lesions that are unilocular (Fig. 12-22), well defined (Fig. 12-23), and demonstrate an acceptable and safe route of entry (Fig. 12-24). The majority of spontaneous and other abdominal abscesses are amenable to percutaneous drainage.[90] Both transperitoneal and extraperitoneal approaches can be used without further dissemination of sepsis.[91]

The technique is essentially identical to placement of an indwelling percu-

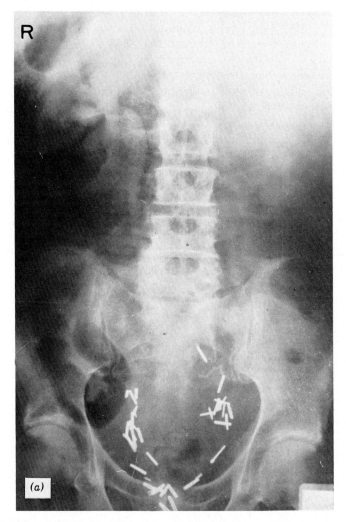

Figure 12-21 Percutaneous nephrostomy. (*a*) Intravenous urogram in patient with urinary bladder carcinoma (surgical clips are noted from partial cystectomy) demonstrates bilaterally poor renal function and moderate pelvocalyceal dilatation. R = patient's right. (*b*) Longitudinal gray scale ultrasonogram notes the collecting system of the right kidney is slightly dilated (arrows). L = liver; H = toward patient's head. (*c*) Transverse sonogram demonstrates the dilated calyces and renal pelvis (arrows). R = patient's right; S = spine; L = liver. (*d*) Radiograph with pigtail catheter coiled into the renal collecting system, which is filled with radiopaque water-soluble, iodinated contrast material. R = patient's right.

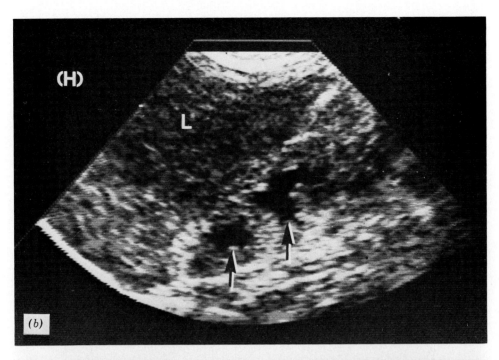

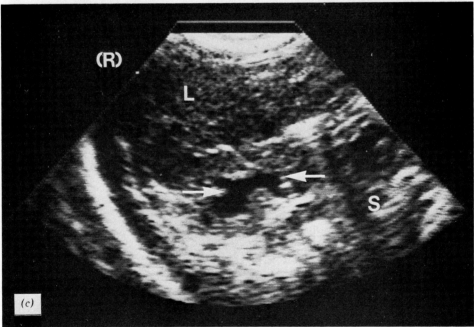

Figure 12-21 (*continued*)

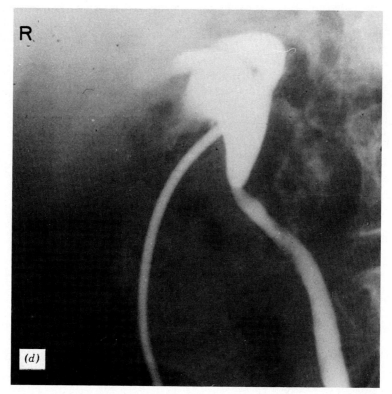

Figure 12-21 (*continued*)

taneous nephrostomy catheter. Either the pigtail or trocar type of catheter can be used. The size, 8 to 14 French, depends on the type of material obtained and the adequacy of drainage. Antibiotics should be administered systemically before puncture and often intracavitary immediately following placement.[90] The catheter position should be chosen so it assumes a dependent position that facilitates drainage. Dependent drainage or attachment to suction has been used,[89,91] but intermittent flushing of the drainage catheter with sterile saline has also been employed with successful results.[91]

When the abscess cavity has cleared and the patient is clinically improved (Fig. 23), the catheter can be withdrawn slowly over a period of days in a similar fashion to a surgically placed drain or by rapid removal. The drainage is usually complete within 7 to 21 days of catheter placement.[89–92,98]

Aspirations and biopsies via a percutaneous approach are safe, accurate, and often clinically necessary. When applicable, the approach using ultrasonic guidance appears to have the greatest degree of flexibility as compared to other imaging modalities. The basic technique can be expanded to include a large variety of procedures.

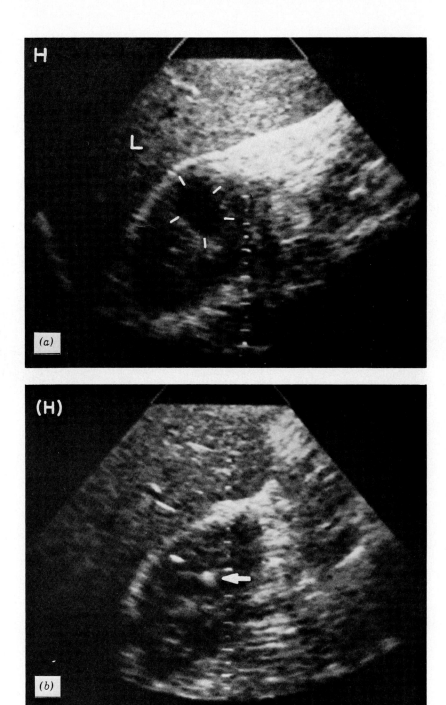

Figure 12-22 Infected renal cyst. (*a*) Gray scale longitudinal sonogram of right kidney from an anterior approach demonstrates an anechoic collection without enhanced sound through transmission (slashes). L = liver; H = toward patient's head. (*b*) Following drainage of pus from an infected renal cyst, the fluid-filled mass has been decreased in size. The catheter placement is noted by echogenic focus (arrow). H = toward patient's head.

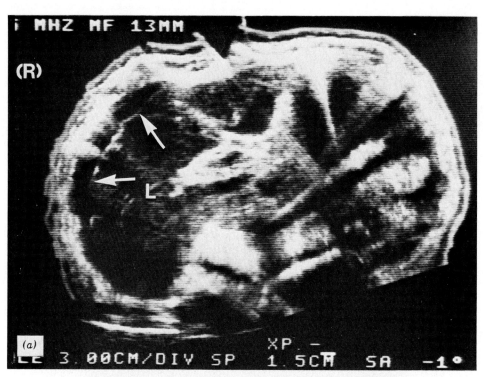

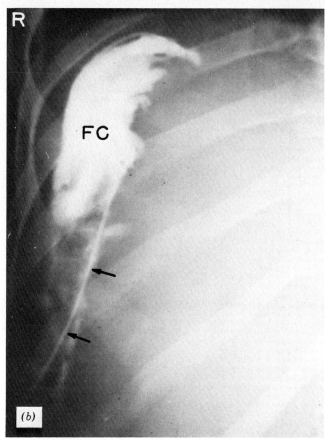

Figure 12-23 Subdiaphragmatic collection. (*a*) Transverse ultrasonogram demonstrates a unilocular subdiaphragmatic fluid collection (arrows), between the right flank and the liver (L). R = patient's right. (*b*) Radiograph of drainage catheter (arrows) in place in fluid collection (FC), which proved to be a subdiaphragmatic infected hematoma. R = patient's right side.

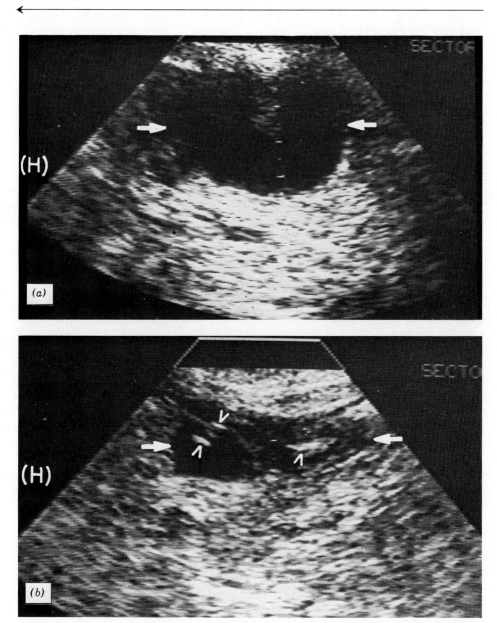

Figure 12-24 Abscess. (*a*) Sector scan of abdomen demonstrates an anteriorly placed, unilocular, fluid-filled collection (arrows). (*b*) The abscess has decreased in size (arrows) after drainage. The catheter is placed into the collection and is defined by bright acoustic reflectors (arrowheads) from the pigtail catheter, which is coiled in the abscess.

513

REFERENCES

1. Thompson H: Enormous sac connected with the kidney, recognized as such during life, and repeatedly emptied by tapping. *Trans Pathol Soc*, 13:128, 1867.

2. Lindblom K: Diagnostic kidney puncture in cysts and tumors. *AJR* 68:209, 1952.

3. Ainsworth WL, Vert JA: The differential diagnosis between renal tumor and cyst. *J Urol* 66:740, 1951.

4. Pearman RO: Percutaneous needle puncture and aspiration of renal cysts: A diagnostic and therapeutic procedure. *J Urol* 96:139, 1966.

5. Devine CJ Jr, Buttarazzi PJ, Devine PC, et al: Aspiration or exploration to confirm diagnosis of renal masses. *JAMA* 204:100, 1968.

6. Thornbury JR: Needle aspiration of avascular renal lesions. *Radiology* 105:299, 1972.

7. Jeans WD, Penry JB, Roylance J: Renal puncture. *Clin Radiol* 23:298, 1972.

8. Vestby GW: Percutaneous needle puncture of renal cysts. *Invest Radiol* 2:449, 1967.

9. Clarke BG, Goade WJ Jr, Rudy HL, Rockwood L: Differential diagnosis between cancer and solitary serous cyst of the kidney. *J Urol* 75:922, 1956.

10. Goldberg BB, Pollack HM: Ultrasonic aspiration-biopsy transducer. *Radiology* 108:667, 1973.

11. Goldberg BB, Pollack HM: Ultrasonic aspiration transducer. *Radiology* 102:187, 1972.

12. Becker JA, Schneider M, Staiano S, Cromb E: Needle aspiration and B-mode scanning. *Invest Radiol* 10:173, 1975.

13. Goldberg BB, Cole-Beuglet C, Kurtz AB, Rubin CS: Real-time aspiration-biopsy transducer. *J Clin Ultrasound* 8:107, 1980.

14. Otto R, Deyhle P: Guided puncture under real-time sonographic control. *Radiology* 134:784, 1980.

15. Lindgren PG: Ultrasonically guided punctures. *Radiology* 137:235, 1980.

16. Pollack HM, Goldberg BB, Bogash M: Changing concepts in the diagnosis and management of renal cysts. *J Urol* 111:326, 1974.

17. Pollack HM, Banner MP: Comparison of computed tomography and ultrasound in the diagnosis of renal masses. *Clin Diagn Ultrasound*. 2:25, 1979.

18. Hoard TD, O'Brian DP: Simple renal cyst and high renin hypertension cured by cyst decompression. *J Urol* 115:326, 1976.

19. Rockson SG, Stone RA, Gunnells JC Jr: Solitary renal cyst with segmental ischemia and hypertension. *J Urol* 112:550, 1974.

20. Lang EK: The differential diagnosis of renal cysts and tumors. *Radiology* 87:883, 1966.

21. Viamonte M Jr, Roen S, Raskin MM, et al: Why every renal mass is not always a surgical lesion: The need for an orderly, logical, diagnostic approach. *J Urol* 114:190, 1975.

22. Stables DP, Jackson RS: Management of an infected simple renal cyst by percutaneous aspiration. *Br J Radiol* 47:290, 1974.

23. Limjoc UR, Strauch AE: Infected solitary cyst of the kidney: Report of a case and review of the literature. *J Urol* 96:625, 1966.

24. Nosher JL: Aspiration with amylase determination in differentiating pancreatic from renal cysts. *J Urol* 123:94, 1980.

25. Raskin MM, Roen SA, Serafini AN: Renal cyst puncture: Combined fluoroscopic and ultrasonic technique. *Radiology* 113:425, 1974.

26. Jackman RJ, Stevens GM: Benign hemorrhagic renal cyst. *Radiology* 110:7, 1974.

27. Harris RD, Goergen TG, Talner LB: The bloody renal cyst aspirate: A diagnostic dilemma. *J Urol* 114:832, 1975.

28. Ambrose SS, Lewis EL, O'Brien DP, et al: Unsuspected renal tumors associated with renal cysts. *J Urol* 117:704, 1977.

29. Sinclair DJ, Ritchie GW: Renal carcinoma diagnosed by cyst puncture: A case of mistaken identify. *Br J of Radiol* 44:885, 1971.

30. Buttarazzi PJ, Poutasse EF, Devine CJ, et al: Aspiration of renal cyst. *J Urol* 100:591, 1968.

31. Raskin MM, Poole DO, Roen SA, Viamonte M Jr: Percutaneous management of renal cysts: Results of a four-year study. *Radiology* 115:551, 1975.

32. Mindell HJ: On the use of pantopaque in renal cysts. *Radiology* 119:747, 1976.

33. Raskin MM, Roen SA, Viamonte M: Effect of intracystic pantopaque on renal cysts. *J Urol* 114:678, 1975.

34. Wahlquist L, Grumstedt B: Therapeutic effect of percutaneous puncture of simple renal cysts. *Acta Chir Scand* 132:340, 1966.

35. Lang EK: Renal cyst puncture and aspiration: A survey of complications. *AJR* 128:723, 1977.

36. Lockhart JL, Wacksman J, White RD, et al: Renal cyst puncture and abscess formation. *Urology* 10:98: 1977.

37. Simon G, Berdon WE: Suprapubic bladder puncture for voiding cystourethrography. *J Pediatr* 81:555, 1972.

38. Fletcher E, Forbes W, Gough M: Suprapubic micturating cystourethrography in infants. *Clin Radiol* 29:309, 1978.

39. Monzon OT, Ory EM, Dobson HL, et al: A comparison of bacterial counts of the urine obtained by needle aspiration of the bladder catheterization and midstream: Voided methods. *N Engl J Med* 259:764, 1958.

40. Weathers WT, Wenzl JE: Suprapubic aspiration of the bladder. *Am J Dis Child* 117:590, 1969.

41. Mandell J, Stevens PS: Supravesical hematoma following suprapubic urine aspiration. *J Urol* 119:286, 1978.

42. Goldberg BB, Meyer H: Ultrasonically guided suprapubic urinary bladder aspiration. *Pediatrics* 51:70, 1973.

43. Ferrucci JT, Wittenberg J, Mueller PR, et al: Abdominal malignancy by radiologic fine-needle aspiration biopsy. *AJR* 134:323, 1980.

44. Hancke S, Holm HH, Koch F: Ultrasonically guided percutaneous fine-needle biopsy of the pancreas. *Surg Gynecol Obstet* 140:361, 1975.

45. Zornoza J, Wallace S, Ordonez N, Lukeman J: Fine-needle biopsy of the liver *AJR* 134:331, 1980.

46. Izumi S, Tamaki S, Natori H, Kira S: Ultrasonically guided aspiration needle biopsy in disease of the chest. *Am Rev Respir* 125:460, 1982.

47. Nosher JL, Plafker J: Fine needle aspiration of the liver with ultrasound guidance. *Radiology* 136:177, 1980.

48. Pagani JJ: Biopsy of focal hepatic lesions. *Radiology* 147:673–675, 1983.

49. Isler RJ, Ferrucci JT Jr, Wittenberg J, et al: Tissue core biopsy of abdominal tumors with a 22-gauge cutting needle. *AJR* 136:725, 1981.

50. Yeh H: Percutaneous fine needle aspiration biopsy of intra-abdominal lesions with ultrasound guidance. *Am J Gastroenterol* 75:148, 1981.

51. Staab EV, Jaques PJ, Partain CL: Percutaneous biopsy in the management of solid intra-abdominal masses of unknown etiology. *Radiol Clin North Am* 17:435, 1979.

52. Kidd R, Freeny PC, Bartha M: Single pass fine-needle aspiration biopsy. *AJR* 133:333, 1979.

53. Holm HH, Als O, Gammelgaard J: *Clin Diagn Ultrasound* 1:137, 1978.

54. Goldstein HM, Zornoza J, Wallace S, et al: Percutaneous fine needle aspiration biopsy of pancreatic and other abdominal masses. *Radiology* 123:319, 1977.

55. Evans WK, Ho CS, McLoughlin MJ, Tao L-C: Fatal necrotizing pancreatitis following fine-needle aspiration biopsy of the pancreas. *Radiology* 141:61, 1981.

56. Gibbons RP, Bush WH Jr, Burnett LL: Needle tract seeding following aspiration of renal cell carcinoma. *J Urol* 118:856, 1977.

57. von Schreeb T, Arner O, Skousted G, Wikstad N: Renal adenocarcinoma. *Scand J Urol Nephrol* 1:270, 1967.

58. Wolinsky H, Lischner MW: Needle tract implantation of tumor after percutaneous needle biopsy. *Ann Intern Med* 71:359, 1969.

59. Ferrucci JT, Wittenberg J, Margolies MN, Carey RW: Malignant seeding of the tract after thin-needle aspiration biopsy. *Radiology* 130:345, 1979.

60. Brooman PJC, Griffiths GJ, Roberts E, et al: Per rectal ultrasound in the investigation of prostatic disease. *Clin Radiol* 32:669, 1981.

61. Holm HH, Gammelgaard J: Ultrasonically guided precise needle placement in the prostate and seminal vesicals. *J Urol* 125:885, 1981.

62. Rifkin MD, Kurtz AB, Goldberg BB: Technique for ultrasonically guided transperineal prostate biopsy: Preliminary experience with a longitudinal linear array transducer. *AJR* 139(4):745–747, 1983.

63. Casey WC, Goodwin WE: Percutaneous antegrade pyelography and hydronephrosis. *J Urol* 74:164, 1955.

64. Goodwin WE, Casey WC, Woolf W: Percutaneous trocar (needle) nephrostomy in hydronephrosis. *JAMA* 187:891, 1955.

65. Lundin E, Wadstrom LB: Translumar pyelography. *Acta Chir Scand* 130:267, 1965.

66. Link D, Leff RG, Hildel J, Drago JR: The use of percutaneous nephrostomy in 42 patients. *J Urol* 122:9, 1979.

67. Saxton HM, Ogg CS, Cameron JS: Needle nephrostomy. *Br Med Bull* 28:210, 1972.

68. Ogg CS, Saxton HM, Cameron JS: Percutaneous needle nephrostomy. *Br Med J* 4:657:1969.

69. Burnett LL, Correa RJ Jr, Bush WH Jr: A new method for percutaneous nephrostomy. *Radiology* 120:557, 1976.

70. Barbaric ZL, Davis RS, Frank IN, et al: Percutaneous nephropyelostomy in the management of acute pyohydronephrosis. *Radiology* 118:567, 1976.

71. Walsh PC, Kaufman JJ, Smith RB, Goodwin WE: Percutaneous antegrade pyelography in hydronephrosis. *Urology* 1:537, 1973.

72. Sherwood T, Stevenson JJ: Antegrade pyelography: A further look at an old technique. *Br J Radiol* 45:812, 1972.

73. Stables DP, Holt SA, Sheridan HM, Donohue RE: Permanent nephrostomy via percutaneous puncture. *J Urol* 114:684, 1975.

74. Newhouse JH, Pfister RC: Percutaneous catheterization of the kidney and perinephric space trocar technique. *Urol Radiol* 2:157, 1981.

75. Bigongiari LR: The Seldinger approach to percutaneous nephrostomy and ureteral stent placement. *Urol Radiol* 2:141, 1981.

76. Pollack HM, Banner MP: Percutaneous nephrostomy and related pyeloureteral manipulative techniques. *Urol Radiol* 2:147, 1981.

77. Castaneda-Ziniga WR, Clayman R, Smith A, et al: Nephrostolithotomy: Technique for urinary calculus removal. *AJR* 139:721, 1982.

78. Newhouse JH, Pfister RC: Therapy for renal calculi via percutaneous nephrostomy: Dissolution and extraction. *Urol Radiol* 2:165, 1980.

79. Babcock JR Jr, Skolnick A, Cook WA: Ultrasound-guided percutaneous nephrostomy in the pediatric patient. *J Urol* 121:327, 1979.

80. Pederson JF: Percutaneous nephrostomy guided by ultrasound. *J Urol* 112:157, 1974.

81. Pederson JF, Cowan DF, Kristensen JK, et al: Ultrasonically-guided percutaneous nephrostomy. *Radiology* 119:429, 1976.

82. Saxton H: Percutaneous nephrostomy technique. *Urol Radiol* 2:131, 1981.

83. Perinetti E, Catalona WJ, Manley CB, et al: Percutaneous nephrostomy: Indications, complications and clinical usefulness. *J Urol* 120:156, 1980.

84. Portela LA, Patel SK, Callahan DH: Pararenal pseudocyst (urinoma) as complication of percutaneous nephrostomy. *Urology* 13:570, 1979.

85. Altemeier WA, Culberston WR, Fullen WD, Shook CD: Intraabdominal abscesses. *Am J Surg* 125:70, 1973.

86. Caldemone AA, Frank IN: Percutaneous aspiration in the treatment of renal abscess. *J Urol* 123:92, 1980.

87. Hietala S, Beachley MC, Girevendulis A, Wheeler WE: Combined radiographic and ultrasonographic approach in diagnosis of renal inflammatory lesions. *Urology* 10:486, 1977.

88. Gerzof SG: Percutaneous drainage of renal and perinephric abscess. *Urol Radiol* 2:171, 1981.

89. vanSonnenberg E, Ferrucci JT, Mueller PR, et al: Percutaneous drainage of abscesses and fluid collections: Technique, results, and applications. *Radiology* 142:1, 1982.

90. VanSonnenberg E, Ferrucci JT, Mueller PR, et al: Percutaneous radiographically guided catheter drainage of abdominal abscesses. *JAMA* 247:190, 1982.

91. Gerzof SG, Robbins AH, Johnson WC, et al: Percutaneous catheter drainage of abdominal abscesses. *N Engl J Med* 305:653, 1981.

92. Johnson WC, Gerzof SG, Robbins AH, Nabseth DC: Treatment of abdominal abscesses. *Ann Surg* 194:510, 1981.

93. MacErlean DP, Owens AP, Hourihane JB: Ultrasound guided percutaneous abdominal abscess drainage. *Br J Radiol* 54:394, 1981.

94. Snyder SK, Hahn HH: Diagnosis and treatment of intra-abdominal abscess in critically ill patients. *Surg Clin North Am* 62:229, 1982.

95. Gerzof SG, Robbins AH, Birkett DH, et al: Drainage of abdominal abscesses guided by ultrasound and computed tomography. *AJR* 133:1, 1979.

96. Conrad MR, Sanders RC, Mascardo AD: Perinephric abscess aspiration using ultrasound guidance. *AJR* 128:457, 1977.

97. Yaremchuke MJ, Kane R, Cady B: Ultrasound-guided catheter localization of intrahepatic abscesses: An aid in open surgical drainage. *Surgery* 91:482, 1982.

98. Martin EC, Karlson KB, Fankuchen EI, et al: Percutaneous drainage of postoperative intra-abdominal abscesses. *AJR* 138:13, 1982.

Index